HUMOR AND HEALTH PROMOTION

HEALTH PSYCHOLOGY RESEARCH FOCUS

Additional books in this series can be found on Nova's website
under the Series tab.

Additional E-books in this series can be found on Nova's website
under the E-book tab.

PERSPECTIVES ON COGNITIVE PSYCHOLOGY

Additional books in this series can be found on Nova's website
under the Series tab.

Additional E-books in this series can be found on Nova's website
under the E-book tab.

HUMOR AND HEALTH PROMOTION

PAOLA GREMIGNI
EDITOR

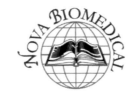

Nova Science Publishers, Inc.
New York

LIBRARY OF CONGRESS CATALOGING-IN-PUBLICATION DATA

Humor and health promotion / editor, Paola Gremigni.
    p. cm.
 Includes index.
 ISBN 978-1-61942-657-3 (hardcover)
 1. Wit and humor--Therapeutic use. I. Gremigni, Paola.
 BF575.L3.H866 2011
 152.4'3--dc23
                2011050985

Published by Nova Science Publishers, Inc. † New York

This book is dedicated to the memory of my Mother Norina (1914-2010).

CONTENTS

PREFACE

Humor is a human activity that occurs in all type of social interaction and serves a number of important social, cognitive, and emotional functions. That laughter is the best medicine is a common claim and there is a continually expanding research on this subject. Interest in humor has grown in recent years, especially in relation to its clinical applications. However, there seems to be little systematic knowledge of it among psychologists and other health professionals. Two of the main reasons are the difficulty of defining humor univocally and unambiguously, and the difficulty of measuring the health benefits of laughter. A number of scientific studies done in clinical settings seem to support the benefits of humor therapy, although other studies found contradictory results or null findings.

This book aims to identify the different components of humor (cognitive, emotional, expressive, and social), to provide and integrative review of theory and research results in most areas of psychology of humor and examine the role of humor in the therapeutic and healing process and in healthcare contexts. I believe that only an integrated approach may support a positive influence of humor on the individuals and communities well-being.

The book is designed to be used as a research handbook for those interested in conducting their own research on humor. It is also intended for practitioners in healthcare, counseling, psychotherapy, education, and social work who are interested in effective application of humor. Finally, I believe that this book will be of interest to the general public. In fact, we are attempting to reach a broad audience by providing enough information to make all chapters accessible for those readers who are not familiar with psychological theories and methods.

In treating a subject that is still relatively new, we have chosen to dedicate a part of the book to introduce the research on humor as a field of rigorous studies and scientific foundations. In this way we hope to enable understanding of the mechanisms and psychological and social functions of humor. The central part of the book is dedicated to the influence of humor on the individual health and its application in various areas of clinical intervention. Humor therapy is used in mainstream, alternative medicine, and in psychotherapy. It can take many forms and it is especially important with children and the elderly. Nevertheless, not everyone will appreciate humor therapy; therefore, it is important to know when humor will be therapeutic and when it will be inappropriate. Measuring humor skills is also an important issue, thus a review of psychometric instruments to assess humor skills completes the book. This book is unique in its focus on both a theoretical approach to humor and a discussion on clinical applications.

I would like to acknowledge and warmly thank all the contributors. My task as the editor was greatly facilitated by the enthusiasm and the full involvement of Alberto Dionigi. We are particularly honored of the positive response to our initial inquiry by Prof. Willibald Ruch.

In: Humor and Health Promotion
Editor: Paola Gremigni

ISBN: 978-1-61942-657-3
© 2012 Nova Science Publishers, Inc.

Chapter 1

THE PSYCHOLOGY OF HUMOR

Alberto Dionigi[1] and Paola Gremigni[2]
[1]Department of Education, University of Macerata, Italy
[2]Department of Psychology, University of Bologna, Italy

ABSTRACT

Lay definitions and interpretations that ordinary (non-academic) people give to the word "humor" do not capture the complexity of this concept. In this chapter, we try to shed light on the concepts of humor and sense of humor, highlighting the differences and difficulties in finding clear definitions of them. After a brief history of the term "humor", we focus on the psychology of humor, identifying different areas of research, and giving some idea of the work that has been conducted so far. Current research suggests that a multidimensional conceptualization of the sense of humor may include a cognitive ability, an aesthetic response, a habitual behavior pattern, an emotion-related temperament trait, an attitude, and a coping strategy or defense mechanism. Besides these aspects, a considerable relevance has been recently given to humor styles that are related to personality differences among individuals and have been recognized as critical functions in which humor may be used.

INTRODUCTION

Interest in humor has grown in recent years, particularly in relation to its clinical applications. The reason is that it seems to have beneficial effects on physical and mental health of people. If we think about the role of humor in everyday life, we realize that it is a vital role. For example, humor and laughter help us manage our daily mood, as well as the disposition of other influential people in our life. However, humor is not as easy to define as it seems. Explaining the relationship between humor and health is even more complex than trying to define humor.

Humor is everywhere: in literature, art, media, history, philosophy, family, workplace, school, interpersonal relationship, and even health. There are virtually unlimited ways in which humor can come: irony, satire, caricature, nonsense, wit, paradox, jokes to name just a few. When people talk about humor, refers to a positive quality represented by the ability to make funny comments, to tell jokes, to amuse people and appreciate the incongruities of life. These qualities may capture the essence of what is named a "lay definition", but humor is much more than making people laugh or be able to laugh at funny things. Most people assume that something is humorous when evokes laughter. This may be right for stand-up comedians who use laughter as a measure of their success, but the concept of humor, as it stands today, is complex and difficult to define in clear, unambiguous and concerted terms.

Humor is a daily experience for centuries. However, over time, this phenomenon has been treated indifferent ways. Various disciplines have dealt with humor based on different perspectives and approaches. This has allowed each discipline to establish a theoretical framework to guide the research on humor. Therefore, it is difficult today to agree on a single, coherent approach to the study of humor.

In this chapter, we try to answer, although not exhaustively, the first question posed in this book: what is humor? Other authors will answer this and other questions about how humor works, and how it might be used for therapeutic purposes.

A BRIEF HISTORY OF THE WORD "HUMOR"

First of all, we need to answer the questions: where does the word *humor* come from and what does it mean? Usually, people try to find an answer in dictionaries. A possible definition of humor refers to a "construct based on a sympathetic heart, not in a superior spirit (like wit), moral sense or even haughtiness (like mock/ridicule), or vitality/high spirits (like fun)" [1]. This is a pretty benevolent definition, which fails to include the aggressive aspects of humor [2].

The term "humor", as we refer to it nowadays, entered the field only in the late 16th century [3]. At the beginning, the word humor (better *umor*) had the meaning of fluid in Latin and was connected to human health. The Greek physician Hippocrates, known as the Father of Medicine, proposed that the body contains four different fluids (i.e. blood, phlegm, yellow bile, and black bile), and that these four *humors* are present in balanced proportions, in a man. Any imbalance of humors makes people becoming ill.

Humors also identified differences in the personality of the individuals. If a person had an over-plus of blood, then he was classified as optimistic or "sanguine" (Latin *sanguis* = blood). A generous amount of phlegm, on the other hand, made people "phlegmatic". Too much yellow bile identified individuals who apt to be "choleric" and short tempered (the word "bile" is *choler* in Latin). The black bile, in a too large amount, made people "melancholic". For many centuries, this concept was held as the basis of medicine and became much elaborated when Galen introduced a new aspect. The four basic temperaments were then associated with the four basic elements that were thought of as representing states of matter as well as basic substances (i.e., fire, water, air, and earth). Over time, any character abnormality or eccentricity was referred to as a *humour*.

With advances in medical science, the concept of "humoral" pathology was abandoned and in the 16th century arose the idea that humor was responsible for labile behavior or character in general, so humor referred to a more or less dominant mood feature either positive (good humor) or negative (bad humor). During this century, the meaning of humor was extended to include behaviors deviating from the established social norms, expressed though odd and eccentric behaviors that eventually became objects of derision. For example, in 1598, Ben Johnson wrote a play entitled *Every Man in His Humour,* the story of a young man with an eye for a girl, who had trouble with a phlegmatic father. Jonson embodied in four of the main characters the four humors of the medieval medicine. Because of people laughed at humors, humor became synonymous with "funny".

A subsequent significant step in redefining humor was represented by Humanism, which extended the idea that people should not be derided for the peculiarities of their temperament, because they are not responsible for them. With Humanism people began to smile kindly at the imperfections of the human nature. In this period, humor began to be seen as a talent, which involved the ability to make others laugh. The frequent association of "good" and "humor" eventually made the neutral term *humour* into a positive term. In the latter half of the 18th century, the word *humourist* started to identify the person who continually creates and produces humor to entertain others [4].

The medical theory of humors was definitively abandoned in the 19th century, when Rudolf Virchow delivered his lectures on cellular pathology at the Pathological Institute of Berlin. The concept of pathology established a more solid foundation in physiological and pathological histology. In this period, the definition of humor was influenced by the philosophy that contributed to the definitive distinction between "wit" and "humor". Samuel Taylor Coleridge claimed that humor arises "whenever the finite is contemplated in reference to the infinite" [3: 141]. With this meaning, in the 19th century, humor became one of the English cardinal virtues and a person who lacked a sense of humor was considered incomplete. The political predominance of the British Empire made humor as a lifestyle model spread around the world.

Nowadays, although much research has been conducted, the experts have not yet reached an agreement on the humor terminology. According to Ruch [5], there are different and conflicting terminological systems. Here, we want to mention two of them. The first one, defined as "historical nomenclature", originates from the field of aesthetics, where the *comic* (or the *funny*) is distinguished from other aesthetic qualities (e.g., beauty, harmony, and tragic). In this frame, humor is *one* aspect of the comic (other elements are wit, fun, nonsense, sarcasm, etc.). It represents a smiling attitude towards life and its imperfections.

The other terminological system (widely used by researchers) conceives humor as the umbrella-term for *all* phenomena in this field. In this frame, humor is treated as a neutral term, which is no longer limited to a positive sense.

Hence, it is obvious that humor is a complex term. Therefore, we can refer to humor as to "anything people say or do that is perceived to be funny or evokes mirth and laughter in others" [6: 20], with the knowledge that this is one of the multiple meanings of humor.

THE PSYCHOLOGY OF HUMOR

Talking about the psychology of humor, we could take into account two areas, psychology and humor, but we want to consider this area as a gestalt, where the whole is much more that the sum of the parts. Psychology is the scientific study of behavior and cognitive processes at both individual and group level. Its constant aims are to explore basic principles, looking at general laws, and understand individual differences. Humor is an extremely complex phenomenon that involves basic principles and mechanisms, as well as individual differences and subjective perceptions. For example, the adjectives "funny", "humorous", and "amusing" connote primarily subjective responses to things and events rather than objective characteristics. Therefore, it is difficult to determine what exactly makes an act or a statement humorous. As such, humor has become over time an intriguing object of study of psychologists. Martin [6: 2] says that "humor touches on all branches of academic psychology: … cognitive, social, biological, clinical, health, educational, and industrial-organizational psychology". In combining psychology with humor, we can say in Willibald Ruch's words: "the psychology of humor refers to the study of humor and people, not humor of humorous material only" [5: 1-2].

Psychology of humor is organized into four main areas depending on its goals [5]. The first goal is to *describe* behaviors and phenomena involved in humor (e.g., cognitive processes involved in the creation and appreciation of jokes). A second aim is to *explain* humor behavior, seek in general laws that can be applied to many different people. A third aim is to *predict* how people will behave in certain situations, depending on individual humor characteristics. The fourth aim is to *control* humor behavior. It means helping people learn to self-control undesirable humor behaviors and deal with situations and relationships related to humor. Researchers focus on different areas of interest as humor has various aspects and effects. For example, cognitive psychologists are more interested in the cognitive processes involved in the perception, comprehension, appreciation, and production of humor. Social psychologists focus on analyzing the role of humor within groups of people. Developmental psychologists study how humor develops trough the lifespan and within the relationship between parents and children. Clinical psychologists and psychotherapists are more interested in research that involves the role of humor in mental and physical health [6].

Although studying humor empirically may seem strange to ordinary people, the research in this field has a long history. Towards the end of the 19th century, the psychology began to be accepted as a legitimate field of study, and since then it has offered a valuable contribution to the research on humor [5]. The first empirical studies of the "comic" by psychologists were conducted at the end of the 19th century. The first survey on tickling and laughter was conducted more than 100 years ago by Hall and Allin, [7] who collected responses from about 3000 people on nearly 4000 items on a questionnaire they sent out requesting a description of all situations which individuals considered being humorous. Other empirical studies were conducted by Kraepelin, Heymans, Lipps, Martin, and Hollingworth. A sense of humor is one of the traits Hollingworth [8] termed "admirable".

Later, at the beginning of the 20th century, Sigmund Freud's work gained worldwide attention to the psychology of humor and his book *Jokes and Their Relation to the Unconscious* [9] had a significant impact on modern thought and research in this field. According to Freud's humor theory the joking situation is a "safety valve" for expressing forbidden thoughts and feelings that are normally inhibited. The energy of repression is released in the form of laughter. Subsequent psychological theorists emphasized the positive role of a style of humor that is non-hostile and self-deprecating, while remaining self-accepting, as characteristic of a healthy personality. We can mention, about this approach, Maslow [10], Allport [11], and Vaillant [12]. Outside of these major contributions, the psychology of humor has received little recognition in the scientific scene until the third decade of the 20th century. In the seventies, the research on humor had a strong experimental and cognitive focus related to the development of the emerging cognitive psychology. This gave impetus to the study of mental processes involved in humor. In the eighties, research on humor was more directed towards the study of personality, as well as to applications such as health and treatment. This change was facilitated by the resonance of the story of Norman Cousins. In "Anatomy of an Illness" [13], he recounts his recovery from ankylosing spondylitis following a self-prescribed treatment regimen involving daily laughter and massive doses of vitamin C. The popularity of alternative approaches to medicine in that time favored the acceptance of humor and laughter as ways of healing by ordinary people. The scientific community also began to take into account the role of emotions and humor in the healing process.

From that time, several studies have been conducted endeavoring to confirm the idea that people with a greater sense of humor are less likely to developing symptoms such as distress, anxiety and depression and are better able to face stressful events. Research began to emphasize the role of humor as a helpful resource that promotes psychological adjustment. It was parallel to the growth of interest in positive emotions that took place in the nineties. Emblematic, the *American Psychologist* devoted its millennial issue to the emerging science of positive psychology, which was defined as the study of positive emotion, character, and institutions [14].

Coming to the current situation, according to Martin [6], from a psychological perspective, the humor process can be divided into four basic components: a social context, a cognitive-perceptual process, an emotional response, and the vocal behavioral expression of laughter.

Regarding the social context humor is a social phenomenon. People tend to laugh and kid more often when they are with other people than when they are alone [15,16]. Obviously, people laugh even when they are alone, such as reading comic books, or watching a comedy show on television, or remembering a comical experience. However, these situations can be seen as "pseudo-social" because one is still responding to the authors of the book, or to the characters on TV, or remembering events, which involved other people [6].

The cognitive-perceptual process of humor regards the cognitions that are used in the production, understanding and appreciation of humor. To produce humor the person should handle data that come from the environment or memory, play with ideas, words or actions, and, eventually, produce a humorous, verbal utterance or a nonverbal action which will be perceived as funny.

In the reception of humor, we gather information (usually by eyes and ears), process the meaning of this information and evaluate it as humorous or nonsense.

With regard to the emotional aspects of humor, we must remember that the perception of humor evokes an emotional response. Research shows that exposure to humorous stimuli produces an increase positive affect and mood [17]. A recent brain imagining research showed that exposure to funny cartoons activates the reward network in the limbic system of the brain. Some researchers consider humor an emotion that is elicited by specific cognitive processes [2003].

The mirthful enjoyment of humor has an emotional component characterized by laughter and smile. Laughter is a way of expressing or communicating to others the fact that one is experiencing the feeling of mirth, although humor, laughter and smile are not always related.

All subfields of psychology seem to contribute to the understanding of humor and laughter. However, the study of humor it is not relegated to psychological domain, but it is also a subject of study of other disciplines, such as biology, linguistics, philosophy, neuroscience, sociology, literature, and religious studies. For this reason, it has been set up the *International Society for Humor Studies* (ISHS), a multidisciplinary scholarly and professional organization dedicated to the advancement of humor research. Many of the Society's members are university and college professors in the Arts and Humanities, Biological and Social Sciences, and Education. The Society also includes professionals in the fields of counseling, management, nursing, journalism, and theater. The ISHS publishes a quarterly journal entitled *Humor: International Journal of Humor Research* and holds annual international conferences.

Another significant association is represented by the Association for Applied and Therapeutic Humor (AATH). Members who join the AATH are from the medical, education and public speaking communities, including professionals who comprise humor and laughter into their lives and work, people committed to humor and laughter, scholars and researchers who study humor and laughter, and all who think they would benefit from this organization.

THE SENSE OF HUMOR

Sense of humor is a universal human trait [19]; in fact, anthropologists did not find a society or group that lacks it [20].

Nowadays, nothing seems to be as valued as having a sense of humor; we seek it out in others and are proud to claim it in ourselves. We often assume that people who have a strong sense of humor are also brilliant, happy, socially confident, and healthy. However, as humor is a complex phenomenon, involving cognitive, emotional, behavioral, physiological, and social aspects, the conceptualization of a sense of humor is a difficult task, because it refers both to a number of relatively stable humor-related personality traits and to individual difference variables [1]. Furthermore, as Ruch [21] pointed out, there is a collection of expressions related to the same thing (e.g., *sense of humor, humorous temperament humor styles, creation of humor, wit* etc.) and often the same expression is used for quite distinct aspects of humor. Indeed, no single element can adequately capture the concept of sense of humor.

People tend to refer to the term "sense of humor" as to a positive ability, which led to tell jokes and funny stories in order to divert others, to appreciate humorous incongruities and be amused by them, to be cheerful, have a humorous perspective in coping with stress, and so on [2]. Martin [22: 17] gives a definition of a sense of humor as the "habitual individual differences in all sorts of behaviors, experiences, affects, attitudes, and abilities relating to amusement, laughter, jocularity, and so on."

Recently, there has been an increasing interest in the personality construct of sense of humor. Humor researchers and ordinary people agree that there is a wide variability across individuals in the extent to which they possess a sense of humor. Having or lacking a sense of humor are common evidence to explain why people behave the way they do [6].

When humor researchers investigate sense of humor and personality, they come into dichotomous questions. Is it better distinguishing among many but close components, or considering a few broad traits or even a unidimensional concept? And again, are components of the sense of humor referring to a typical behavior/temperament, or to an ability? These questions are given different answers, so does not exist univocal means to conceptualize and measure sense of humor.

Research indicates how the sense of humor is a multifaceted construct, which must be seen as a group of loosely related traits [5,6]. Martin [23] gives a theoretical and multidimensional conceptualization of the sense of humor as:

1. *A cognitive ability* (e.g., ability to create, understand, reproduce, and remember jokes;
2. *An aesthetic response* (e.g., humor appreciation, enjoyment of humorous material);
3. *A habitual behavior pattern* (e.g., tendency to laugh frequently, to tell jokes and amuse others, to laugh at others jokes);
4. *An emotion-related temperament trait* (e.g., habitual cheerfulness) ;
5. *An attitude* (e.g., bemused outlook on the world, positive attitude toward humor);
6. *A coping strategy or defense mechanism* (e.g., tendency to maintain a humorous perspective in the face of adversity)

These different components of sense of humor are not necessarily highly inter-correlated and are often necessary different measurement approaches to evaluate each of them [23]. This means that if we want to use "sense of humor" as an umbrella-term for humor as a personality trait, we have to exempt this expression from its benevolent definition [21]. We should also take into account that sense of humor refers to a personality trait that should be descriptive of all forms of humor behavior, including the negative ones.

Several measurement approaches have been developed to evaluate the sense of humor reflecting the many different ways of conceptualizing it. Interestingly, since ten years ago, self-report humor measures did not distinguish between potentially adaptive and harmful functions of uses of humor in relation to the well-being [23,24].

Sense of Humor as a Cognitive Ability

Referring to humor as a cognitive ability means taking into account the ability to create, understand, reproduce, and remember jokes and funny remarks. From this view point, sense of humor represents a cognitive ability strictly related to the capacity to recognize and be amused by incongruities of life.

The first reference to humor as a cognitive ability can be attribute to Koestler's early cognitive, scientific approach to humor in *The Act of Creation* [25]. Starting from that point, cognitive psychologists began to explore the cognitive mechanisms of humor interpretation, and several studies have been conducted to investigate the role of cognitive processes in developing and improve sense of humor.

Most people, when asked to answer the question "what do you mean with a sense of humor?" usually respond that it is the capacity to produce humor by creating witty remarks about the circumstances in which people are. Respondents tend to say "create" and not "recreate", linking this ability to intelligence, creativity and so on. This relationship has been empirically studied by Feingold and Mazzella [26,27] who found that humor cognition is a rational variable related to intelligence and creativity, whereas motivation and communication aspects of humor are related to social and temperamental variables.

There is a substantial difference between producing and reproducing humor. Some people love to entertain folks reproducing jokes and stories listen before, but this does not mean that they possess a great sense of humor; they are just brilliant tellers. One of the first studies that made a distinction between humor production and reproduction [28] showed that these two dimensions are uncorrelated in individuals.

One of the most used ways to measure empirically the capacity to produce verbal humor is represented by requiring people to write funny captions for cartoons. Participants may be asked to list as many funny captions as they could do in 10 minutes. Later, some judges may rate the funniness of cartoons using a Likert scale. This open-ended humor production has been tested as a reasonably valid measure of spontaneous humor ability [26,27].

Sense of humor as a cognitive ability does not consist only in the production ability. Most of us bear in mind a scene when someone telling a joke, in front of a non-appreciation of it, accuses the listener of not having a sense of humor. Here, the reference is about understanding firstly and appreciation then. Also, appreciation of humor involves ability. It is well known that jokes differ in complexity, and some are hard to get. However, recent studies [29,30] suggested that appreciation of humor is related to competence rather than intelligence.

Humor comprehension is a fascinating subject. In the elderly, humor comprehension functions in a different fashion than in younger adults. In a recent research [31], a sample of older adults were tested in their ability to complete jokes, as well as their cognitive capabilities in areas of intellectual reasoning, short term memory, and cognitive flexibility. The results showed that older adults tend to have lower performance on both test of cognitive ability and humor comprehension than younger adults.

Finally, the relationship between humor and memory is a controversial subject. Research has shown that people who are presented with a series of hilarious sentences or cartoons tend to remember the amusing information, forgiving the non-humorous information [32-34].

Sense of Humor as an Aesthetic Response

When we talk about aesthetic response we are fully in the realm of affects. An aesthetic response refers to the reaction a person has to an object based on his or her perception of the object [35]. The response is based on the qualities of the object. Although there is not any accepted definition of aesthetic response, there seem to be some consensus that the concept involves the registering of affect or pleasure due to the conscious or unconscious influences of characteristics of an object [36].

What does it mean that sense of humor is an aesthetic response and which is its relationship with individual personality?

First of all, we should define humor appreciation. From theoretical studies investigating humor appreciation and humor comprehension, we can define humor appreciation as the experience of finding something amusing. It can be inferred by the intensity and duration of smiling and laughing, or by individual funniness ratings given in response to humorous stimuli [25,27,30,37]. Having a sense of humor led to the difference demonstrated in the enjoyment of humorous material. When talking about sense of humor we employ the term "sense" that in its etymological definition means "sensible knowledge". Now, we can find a connection between aesthetic behavior and sense of humor through the action of senses. In order to enjoy humor, it is necessary to understand it without conscious reflection and thought. Nothing like humor may represent the aesthetic response, which is non-conceptual but emotional and cannot be expressed by words and, in a certain way, even understood [38].

Humor as a Habitual Behavior Pattern

Everybody knows people who are defined as terribly funny: these people tend to laugh frequently, to tell jokes and amuse others, to laugh at others jokes, and everybody wants to stay with them. These people do not have to work hard to produce humor, laughter, and cheerfulness in folks.

Humor researchers are particularly interested in the influence of family on development of a sense of humor in children and how children use humor in regard to others. In particular, two theories arose about how the relationships with parents affect individual differences of humor: *modeling/reinforcement* and *stress/coping* [39].

According to the first model, children learn a sense of humor by observing their parents: a mother and a father who joke and laugh constantly maintain a high probability to transmit such behavior to their children. Parents also affect the humor experience: a child who lives every day in a playful and fun atmosphere will spend more time in the pleased way he has been taught [2]. The following model refers to humor as a coping strategy: family environment characterized by stressful experience makes children using humor to overcome difficult situations and show hostile feelings in a socially acceptable way.

McGhee [39] found that the absence of mothers' cure is associated with an increased sense of humor in children. This is more pronounced in females who tend to face difficult situations with humor and clowning. These children develop a sense of humor more focused to deal with conflict situations in order to attract others attention and seek care.

Two key signals in behavior pattern are smiling and laughter. They represent not only natural reactions to humor, but also behavioral reactions that convey positive emotions and funniness felt by people. Laughter, much more than smile, represents the first signal of humor. While smile can be displayed with different purposes (most of them are pro-social), laughter represents the critical component of happiness. The differences between them will be thoroughly discussed in subsequent chapters.

Humor as an Emotional-Related Temperament Trait

Having a sense of humor is strictly related to have habitual cheerfulness and optimism. Some people tend to be more cheerful, optimistic and humorous than others. These qualities may help people making life happy while facing difficulties, having a higher sense of perspective and seeing life philosophically. Life of course has its light and dark sides. Optimists tend to take more the light sides than the dark ones. Optimism is a dispositional psychological attribute that refers to positive expectations and future objectives, related with dimensions like perseverance, achievement, physical health, and well-being [40].

Research on cheerfulness as a temperamental trait has a long tradition in personality psychology. At the beginning of the 20[th]century, Meumann [41] identified cheerfulness as one of 12 basic temperaments, which are based on the structure of affective and volitional dispositions.

Interest in state and trait cheerfulness arose in the context of experimental studies on smiling and laughing. A graduated sequence was identified: loudly laughter, moderate laughter, broad smile, gentle smile, and the expression of mere cheerfulness. Nowadays a large number of studies have been conducted in this field; to see the state of the art of this topic, see Ruch and Hofman's chapter in this book.

Humor as an Attitude

Think of humor as an attitude is to take it as the ability to have a positive outlook of life and the world and a positive attitude toward humor itself. These terms are strictly related to positive thinking. Humor is an attitude because it represents a way of thinking, an approach, an outlook. As we become aware of this attitude, then we may ask ourselves about the character of our thinking. If it is too negative, we can work on it trying to learn more effective ways of thinking.

Humor is also a form of enjoyment. Paul McGhee [42] describes humor as an attitude that can help enjoying experiences that cannot match one's mental patterns. Thus, humor may give people an opportunity to be at odds with the rules of the society.

As an attitude, humor may help people facing adverse conditions making them laughing at themselves, reducing tension, building confidence, and bringing joy to others.

Humor may be seen as the ability to "connect the dots". Humor makes possible to establish relationships that normally people do not see immediately.

Finally, people usually think they cannot change, because their personality is already structured. Humor may help them to change, and this attitude can be cultivated, as some programs aimed (see Dionigi's chapters in this book).

Humor as a Coping Strategy

See humor as a way of coping with stress represents a critical element in defining individual sense of humor. It recalls the notion of humor as a healthy defense mechanism. In this view, humor may help alleviate the negative consequences of adversity by maintaining a humorous perspective. This approach involves putting ideas, concepts, or situations together that are usually separate in surprising or unexpected ways [43].

Using humor as a coping mechanism is related to the idea that humor contributes to emotional health and resistance to stress. People with a greater sense of humor are also thought to be more socially competent than unhumorous people [6].

Lefcourt and colleagues [44] proposed two forms of humor coping: the first one is an emotion-focused coping strategy, which reduces negative emotional outcomes by finding humor in stressful situations. The second one is a problem-focused coping strategy used to modify the stressful situation itself. In the case of the first form of humor coping, the positive effects of humor may be explained through its role in the cognitive appraisal of threatening and stressful situations. Humor, in fact, has been described as producing a cognitive-affective shift or a restructuring of the situation, so that it appears less threatening. This led to a concomitant release of emotion associated with the perceived threat and reduces the physiological arousal [6].

HUMOR STYLES

Humor is of vital importance in people lives. In order to understand humor's dynamic nature, we have seen that it is necessary to implement a multidimensional conceptualization taking a global view of it, considering also the negative uses such as sarcasm and ridicule.

To develop their model, Martin and colleagues [23] adopted both a rational and an empirical method to find out potentially adaptive and maladaptive styles of humor.

Examining the previous theoretical studies for uses of humor found that it is a double-edged sword. It can build stronger relationships and help people to cope with life (adaptive), or it can be corrosive, eating away at self-esteem and antagonizing others (maladaptive). These researchers proposed four humor styles that were able to explain these differences. The four distinct humor styles are in turn divided in two positive and two negative.

Affiliative humor involves funny, non-hostile jokes, and natural witty used to divert others in a respectful way. It is aimed at others and used, in an adaptive manner, to facilitate relationships and reduce interpersonal conflict [45]. People who use affiliative humor are perceived as pleasant and non-threatening and, as a result, they attract people to them, thereby bringing people together.

These individuals may make fun of themselves, while maintaining their positive self-image, with the purpose of making other feel better. The goal of this form of humor is to strengthen interpersonal bonds and help with the creation of new relationships. This styles associated with "extraversion, cheerfulness, self-esteem, intimacy, relationship satisfaction, and predominantly positive moods and emotions" [6: 53].

Self-enhancing humor is often used as an adaptive coping mechanism, allowing the individual to choose a humorous outlook on life and maintain a realistic approach in stressful situations. Self-enhancing humor makes stressful situations tolerable.

This style is most in line with previous theories on coping humor. A person who makes use of this style has a hilarious outlook on the situations that faces and does not take things too seriously. People high in this style are not necessarily extroverted, but prefer to keep a humorous and positive outlook on life. However, self-enhancing humor, while not directly oriented towards the other individual in an interaction, can contribute to a more productive and light-hearted social interchange.

Aggressive humor represents the tendency to use humor for the end of belittle others and includes the use of sarcasm, ridicule, derision, and so on. This negative humor style can be useful to the self, but only by ridiculing, teasing, demeaning, or mocking others in an attempt to make one feel better.

Although this style can be beneficial in the immediate, it can be harmful when used over repeatedly over time because it use could offend people and undermine interpersonal bonds.

Self-defeating humor is also a negative style. It involves the use of self-disparaging humor, in order to entertain people by doing or saying funny things at one's own expense. In contrast to self-enhancing humor, which is an effective coping strategy, this style is postulated to be a conflict avoidant process [46].

People who use self-defeating humor are trying to raise their status by endearing themselves to others. They tend to be emotionally needy, and this acting-out behavior is assumed to be related to global low-self-esteem and an inability to confront others [23].

With reference to the relationships between the four scales, average correlations are typically found between self-enhancing and affiliative humor and aggressive and self-defeating humor, indicating that the two positive and the two negative styles.

CONCLUSION

Many books on humor have been written. Everyone who approaches this fascinating subject try to answer some questions: what is humor? What is amusing? What is a sense of humor? Why people laugh and what they laugh at? How does the personality modulate humor appreciation and production? And so on.

Our purpose in this chapter was to answer, although not exhaustively, some of these questions taking into account what humor experts said and what results of recent studies showed. Trying to do so, we realized that is almost impossible to lock up humor in a confined area or get an unambiguous definition.

Finally, we particularly focused on the field of psychology of humor not only because we are psychologists, but mostly because today psychology is one of the disciplines that most fundamentally and importantly influence humor research, although it is not the only one.

REFERENCES

[1]   Ruch, W. (2001). The perception of humor. In A.W. Kaszniak (Ed.), *Emotion, Qualia, and Consciousness*. (pp. 410-425). Tokyo: Word Scientific Publisher.

[2]   Ruch, W. (1998). Foreword and overview. Sense of humor: A new look at an old concept. In W. Ruch (Ed.), *The Sense of Humor: Explorations of a Personality Characteristic*, (pp.109-142). Berlin: Mouton de Gruyter.

[3]   Schmit-Hidding, W. (1963). Europaische Schliusselworter. Band I. *Humor and Witz*. Munchen: Huber.

[4]   Wickberg, D. (1998). *The Sense of Humor: Self and Laughter in Modern America*. Ithaca, NY: Cornell University Press.

[5]   Ruch, W. (2008). Psychology of Humor. In V. Raskin (Ed.), *The Primer of Humor Research. New York*, NY: Mouton de Gruyter.

[6]   Martin, R. A. (2007). *The Psychology of Humor. An Integrative Approach*. New York: Academic Press.

[7]   Hall, G., Allin, A. (1897). The psychology of tickling, laughing, and the comic. *American Journal of Psychology, 9*, 1-41.

[8]   Hollingworth, H.L. (1911). Experimental studies in judgment: Judgment of the comic. *Psychological Review, 18*, 132-156.

[9]   Freud, S. (1960 [1905]). *Jokes and their Relation to the Unconscious*. New York: Norton.

[10] Maslow, A. H. (1954). *Motivation and Personality*. New York: Harper.

[11] Allport, G. W. (1961). *Pattern and Growth in Personality*. New York: Holt, Rinehart and Winston.

[12] Vaillant, G. E. (1993). The wisdom of the ego. Cambridge, MA: Harvard University Press.

[13] Cousins, N. (1979). *Anatomy of an Illness as Perceived by the Patient: Reflections on Healing and Regeneration*. New York: W. W. Norton.

[14] Seligman, M. E. P., Csikszentmihalyi, M. (2000). Positive psychology: An introduction. *American Psychologist, 55,* 5-14.

[15] Martin R. A, Kuiper, N. A. (1999). Daily occurrence of laughter: Relationships with age, gender, and Type A personality. *Humor: International Journal of Humour Research, 12*(4), 355-384.

[16] Provine, R. R., Fischer, K. R. (1989). Laughing, smiling, and talking: Relation to sleeping and social context in humans. *Ethology, 89(2),* 115-124.

[17] Szabo, A. (2003). The acute effects of humor and exercise on mood and anxiety. *Journal of Leisure Research, 35(2),* 152-162.

[18] Mobbs, D., Greicius, M. D., Abdel-Azim, E., Menon, V., and Reiss, A. L. (2003). Humor modulates the mesolimbic reward centers. *Neuron, 40,* 1041–1048.

[19] Hinde, R. A.(1974) *Biological Bases of Human Social Behaviour*. New York: McGraw-Hill.

[20] Apte, M. L. (1985). *Humor and laughter: An anthropological approach*. Ithaca, NY: Cornell University Press

[21] Ruch, W. (2007). *The Sense of Humor: Explorations of a Personality Characteristic* (Mouton Select). Berlin and New York: Mouton de Gruyter.

[22] Martin, R. A. (1998). Approaches to the sense of humor: A historical review. In W. Ruch (Ed.), *The Sense of Humor: Explorations of a Personality Characteristic* (pp. 15-60). Berlin, Germany: Walter de Gruyter.

[23] Martin, R. A., Puhlik-Doris, P., Larsen, G., Gray, J., Weir, K. (2003). Individual differences in uses of humor and their relation to psychological well-being: Development of the humor styles questionnaire. *Journal of Research in Personality, 37*: 48-75.

[24] Kuiper, N. A., Martin, R. A. (1998). Is sense of humor a positive personality characteristic? In W. Ruch (Ed.), The *Sense of Humor: Explorations of a Personality Characteristic*, (pp. 159-178). New York: Mouton de Gruyter.

[25] Koestler, A. (1964). *The Act of Creation*. London: Hutchinson.

[26] Feingold, A., Mazzella, R. (1991). Psychometric intelligence and verbal humor ability. *Personality and Individual Differences, 12,* 427-435.

[27] Feingold, A., Mazzella, R. (1993). Preliminary validation of a multidimensional model of wittiness. *Journal of Personality* 61, 439-456.

[28] Babad, E. Y. (1974) A multi-method approach to the assessment of humor: A critical look at humor tests. *Journal of Personality*, 42, 618-631.

[29] Derks, P. Staley, R. E, Haselton, M. G. (2007). "Sense" of humor: Perception, intelligence, or expertise? In W. Ruch (Ed.), *The Sense of Humor: Explorations of a Personality Characteristic*, (pp. 143-158) New York: Mouton de Gruyter.

[30] Cunningham, W. A., Derks, P. (2005). Humor appreciation and latency of comprehension. *Humor, International Journal of Humour Research, 18,* 389–403.

[31] Mak, W., Carpenter, B. D. (2007). Humor comprehension in older adults. *Journal of the International Neuropsychological Society, 13,* 606-614.

[32] Schmidt, S. R. (1994). Effects of humor on sentence memory. *Journal of Experrimental Psychology, Learning, Memory, and Cognition, 20*, 953– 967.

[33] Schmidt, S. R. (2002). The humour effect: Differential processing and privileged retrieval. *Memory, 10*, 127–138.

[34] Schmidt, S. R., Williams, A. R. (2001). Memory for humorous cartoons. *Memory and Cognition, 29*, 305–311.

[35] Berlyne, D. E. (1974), *Studies in the New Experimental Aesthetics*, New York: John Wiley and Sons.

[36] Bamossy, G., Scammon, D. L., Johnston M. (1983). A Preliminary Investigation of the Reliability and Validity of an Aesthetic Judgment Test. In R. P. Bagozzi, A. M. Tybout, and A. Arbor, (Eds.) *Advances in Consumer Research. Association for Consumer Research*, (volume 10, pp. 685-690). Ann Arbor, Mich.: Association for Consumer Research.

[37] Vaid, J., Hull, R., Heredia, R., Gerkens, D., Martinez, F. (2003). Getting a joke: The time course of meaning activation in verbal humor. *Journal of Pragmatics, 35,* 1431–1449.

[38] Nunez-Ramos R., Lorenzo, G. (1997). On the aesthetic dimension of humor. *Humor: International Journal of Humor Research, 10,* 105–116.

[39] McGhee, P. E. (1979). *Humor, its Origin and Development.* San Francisco: W. H. Freeman.

[40] Peterson, C., Bossio, L. M. (1991). *Health and Optimism.* New York: Oxford University Press.

[41] Henman, L. D. (2001). Humor as a coping mechanism. *Humor: International Journal of Humor Research, 14,* 83–94.

[42] McGhee, P. E. (2010). *Humor: The lighter path to resilience and health.* Bloomington: Author House.

[43] Martin, R. A. (2001). Humor, laughter, and physical health: Methodological issues and research findings. *Psychological Bulletin, 127,* 504–519.

[44] Lefcourt, H. M., Davidson, K., Prkachin, K. M., Mills, D. E. (1997). Humor as a stress moderator in the prediction of blood pressure obtained during five stressful tasks. *Journal of Research in Personality, 31*, 523-542.

[45] Lefcourt, H. M. (2001). *Humor: The Psychology of Living Buoyantly.* New York: Kluwer Academic.

[46] Kuiper, N. A., McHale, N. (2009). Humor styles as mediators between self-evaluative standards and psychological well-being. *Journal of Psychology: Interdisciplinary and Applied, 143(4),* 359-376.

In: Humor and Health Promotion   ISBN: 978-1-61942-657-3
Editor: Paola Gremigni   © 2012 Nova Science Publishers, Inc.

Chapter 2

HUMOR THEORIES

Alberto Dionigi

Department of Education, University of Macerata, Italy

ABSTRACT

In this chapter the focus is on the major theories which are referred to when it comes to humor. The aim is to answer questions like: What is humor? What makes us laugh? What are the necessary elements to make something funny? Why is humor so enjoyable and why are we motivated to look for it?

These questions have interested many thinkers over the centuries and several theories have been proposed since the earliest times in an attempt to give an answer.

There are several theories which try to explain this fascinating construct, but none of them, if taken individually, may be said to be exhaustive. This chapter introduces those of greatest interest and still important for research, in order to give a theoretical and scientific explanation. I consider it important to emphasize how some of them, although much in vogue in the past, today have lost plausibility and credibility because of inconsistent scientific evidence.

In fact, even if the term "theory", in several cases, is used more for tradition than for strict relevance, often it is only unsystematic observations or individual propositions that identify one or more features (sometimes as presumed essence).

The basic distinction that I suggest is between theoretical propositions (for example those developed by philosophers such as Aristotle, Plato and Kant), proper theories (with general and systematic characteristics, besides agreeing or not with what they say), such as those of Freud or even Bergson, (although pre-scientific, because they do not fully meet the criteria of verifiability and falsifiability) and scientific models, which in turn distinguish themselves in macro-models, such as the Semantic Script Theory of Humor and General Theory of Verbal Humor, and models that frame an important aspect in a specific disciplinary perspective (perception of incongruity with or without resolution).

INTRODUCTION

Humor is an enigma. There is no aspect of our lives that is not open to humor: at home, at work, in relationships with friends and in all areas of our lives we find this fascinating phenomenon. But what is humor? What happens at a psychological level to make us feel and live a situation as fun? What is the function of humor and why do we appreciate it so much?

Many illustrious thinkers have previously approached this complex concept: personalities such as Plato, Aristotle, Descartes, Hobbes, Kant, Schopenhauer, Darwin, Freud and Bergson have tried to answer these questions, and since humor has become ground for scientific research, scholars have increasingly brought their contribution to the definition and explanation of this fascinating phenomenon.

In fact, thanks to growing interest in humor, a large number of theories were born: a recent review lists more than one hundred [1]. Despite the large number of theories, the authors note that many of them don't differ much from each other. For this reason, several experts on the subject have tried, little by little, to systematically categorize them.

Most of the humor theories proposed are based on concepts which are vague and not clearly defined, being unable to set the minimum requirements for humor to exist and being not falsifiable [2]. Each of these theories explores few aspects of humor without giving a complete picture. Some thinkers present themselves as discoverers of the necessary and sufficient conditions, which involves providing a full explanation of the phenomenon. Severe criticism, however, has systematically debunked these claims, even if it still acknowledged that sometimes the model proposed has a descriptive, explanatory and predictive value. A recent attempt of radical and total explanation from an evolutionary perspective was submitted by Hurley, Dennett and Adams [3].

There are several options for classifying humor theories and there is an agreement among the authors on the fact that none of these theories, taken individually, is able to explain each and every aspect of it, showing no weaknesses. Given the topic of this volume, I find it appropriate to dwell more specifically on psychological humor theories. The purpose of this chapter, in fact, is not to provide a comprehensive analysis of the humor theories that have been submitted over the years, but to present a review of the theoretical and empirical work done so far, in order to describe and explain individual differences in senses of humor. For this reason I will focus on the three theories that have proved to be of major interest in psychology and which having greatly influenced the investigation of individual differences and the production of research material: psychoanalytic theories, superiority theories, and incongruity theories [4]. These theories differ in many ways, but particularly in the relative emphasis placed on the structure of humor content versus the centrality of social context in the elicitation of amusement. Incongruity theories emphasize the irony and surprise of humor content [5-8], while psychoanalytic and superiority theories emphasize, among other aspects, antagonistic social relationships between humorists and targeted individuals, groups or objects in a given context [6,9]. It must be remembered that "classification" of theories means forcefully simplification, as by focusing more on certain aspects, they leave out other relevant ones.

This chapter also addresses the *Semantic Script Theory of Humor* [7] and its extension, the *General Theory of Verbal Humor* [10], a theoretical model that had an enormous impact on the last twenty years of humor research. Despite its matrix starting from linguistics, it has the value of an interdisciplinary model or, better, over-disciplinary as comprehensive of multiple approaches. Some of the *Knowledge Resources* mentioned in the GTVH, such as, for example, the Target (TA) and Logical Mechanisms (LM), in fact, bring references to social psychology, for the first and cognitive psychology for the latter.

PSYCHOANALTIC THEORY

One of the most important theories of humor is the psychoanalytic theory. It is inscribed within a broader framework of theories, often referred to as "relief" theory. This theory is based on the idea that humor engenders some kind of release when it is experienced.

The Relief Theory appears around the eighteenth century, as by focusing on the phenomenon of laughter, especially in relation to the nervous system: the medical world of that time, in fact, was already aware of the connection between brain, sense organs and muscles through the nerves.

Nerves were thought to carry not lector-chemical impulses, but liquids and gases called "animal spirits" which included both blood and air. In his first version of the Relief Theory, the nervous system was represented as a network of tubes inside which the animal spirits build up pressure that calls for release [11]. Over the next two centuries, thinkers such as Herbert Spencer and Sigmund Freud added new elements to this earlier theory.

Spencer's thought, expressed in the text *On the Physiology of Laughter* states that in our body, emotions take the form of nervous energy. So, for example, when we are angry with someone, we produce precise movements, such as approaching the person and tightening our fists. If the energy reaches a certain level, we even come to attack the other person [12].

Laughter, according to Spencer, has a similar explanation. The movements arising in this case are not aimed to to attack anyone, but only work as a release of a burst of energy, which is why Spencer says that the movements of laughter "have no object".

Within the Relief Theory, a particular position is the one of Sigmund Freud who, in his famous book Jokes *and Their Relation to the Unconscious* of 1905, brings an important contribution that will give life to the Psychoanalytic Theory of Humor. This contribution will be later taken up and deepened in some aspects with a short article entitled "Humour" [13].

Freud, whose theory has significantly influenced research until the first half of the XX century and was initially influenced by the writer and philosopher Herbert Spencer, believes that laughter has the function of discharging a burst of repressed and instinctual energy, due to sexual and aggressive impulses. When the energy channeled into the nervous system is no longer needed, it is released through laughter.

Freud distinguishes three different types or categories of phenomena related to laughter: *Jokes* (German Witz, sometimes translated as "*wit*", even if the two terms do not coincide), the *comic* and *humor*. Each one dissipates the psychic energy, saved and conserved in the form of laughter, in a different way.

Freud describes these three different kinds of sources of mirthful pleasure as follows:

"Pleasure in the joke seemed to come from savings in expenditure on inhibition [esp. repression], comic pleasure from savings in the imagining of ideas (when charged with energy), and humorous pleasure from savings in expenditure on feeling. In all three methods…the pleasure comes from a saving; all three [involve] methods for regaining from the activity of the psyche a pleasure which in fact was lost only with the development of that activity. For the euphoria that we try to reach along these routes is nothing other than the temper of a time in our life when we were wont to defray the work of our psyche with the slightest of expenditures: the temper of our childhood – when we…had no need of humour to feel happy in our life." [9: 226]

Jokes

The first category to which Freud refers is that of the wit or jokes. He divides jokes into two categories: *tendentious* and *non–tendentious*.

Freud believes that the release of libidinal energy (aggressive and sexual) is the cause of *tendentious jokes*, while the cognitive "joke-works" are called *non-tendentious* jokes.

The pleasure produced by jokes is based primarily on the formal aspect, which Freud calls "joke-work" techniques, and consists of linguistic and conceptual manipulations of various kinds, including displacement, condensation, unification, indirect representation. These techniques act as "distracting" factors of the superego, allowing unconscious sexual and aggressive impulses, which would normally be suppressed, to emerge into consciousness to be quickly unloaded.

In the first category, the *tendentious jokes*, the person is allowing for the release of an economy of sexual and/or aggressive desires or thoughts. Through jokes, people can express their prohibited ideas in a socially acceptable manner, allowing for temporary relief. Such inhibition is due to their individual experience as a result of their society and culture.

In *non-tendentious* wit, pleasure is taken in the individual's ability to regress to a more childlike state of mind. At these times the individual ceases to think in terms of morality, rationality and logic and embraces a more playful mode of thought. The change in cognitive functioning is the source of the amusement one feels from such an experience.

All this does not cause guilt in the human, both because censorship is momentarily distracted by the cognitive complexity (wit) included in the joke, and because the individual is not always aware of the intensity degree of the aggressive or sexual impulses contained in the joke.

Freud [9] catalogued jokes by form, by technique, and by purpose. He also compared them to dreams: he argued that both dreams and jokes provide an understanding of the unconscious mind and the importance of the non-rational, non-linear thought processes of condensation, displacement, and indirect representation.

Here are some examples drawn from Freud's work on the techniques used in the jokes [9]. To the extent to reveal the unconscious influence, there are some mechanisms which produce a comic effect, very similar to the work that the mind accomplishes through dreams. Here I will focus on three main techniques: condensation, displacement and representability.

- The first technique consists of condensing two words or two fragments of words, creating a neologism that can appear absurd. It is such neologism which has a comic effect on those to whom the joke is told.

One example cited by Freud is the one built around the word "*alcoholidays*": an invented word told by a 'sport', about the Christmas season. In this example the comic effect comes from the new word pronounced, which comes from the abbreviation and combination of two other words: *alcohol* and *holidays*. Here, the condensation expresses the idea that holidays are conducive to alcoholic indulgence [9: 16].

- The second technique consists of using a single word twice. An example given by Freud was the following:

Two Jews meet near a bathing establishment. "Have you taken a bath?" asked one. "How is that?" replies the other. "Is one missing?" [9: 93].

The technique lies in the double meaning of the word *take*. In the first case the word is used in a colorless idiomatic sense, while in the second it is the verb in its full meaning. The joke, therefore, lies in the expression "take a bath".

- The third technique is that of the double meaning or multiple use of the same word. Freud reports this technique in several jokes. Here below there is an example:

A doctor, as he came away from a lady's bedside, said to her husband with a shake of his head: "I don't like the look of her". "I've not liked her looks for a long time." The husband hastened to agree. The doctor was of course referring to the lady's condition: but he expressed his anxiety about the patient in words which the husband could interpret as a confirmation of his own marital aversion [9:37].

In conclusion, for a joke to be effective, two important functions must be fulfilled: it must involve cognitive activity and must help the expression of repressed sexual or aggressive drives. Although Freud hypothesized that most of the jokes involve the release of sexual and aggressive drives, he proposed the existence of non-aggressive and non-sexual jokes, where the fun is due just to the cognitive process involved (joke-work), which allows regressing, for a short time, to a less logical and more childlike way of reasoning [2].

Some authors [14], however, have noted how Freud was unable to carry examples of innocent jokes; these authors have thus reached the conclusion that they do not exist: so all the jokes are biased but on a different degree.

Comic

It is a category of phenomena related to laughter and based on non-verbal sources of joy, such as *slapstick comedy* and circus clown.

Freud [9]explains that in the comic laughter comes from a comparison between two representations: the one that would be expected in a normal situation and the one which actually comes from the comical object. The psyche uses a certain representative energy to acknowledge situations from the outside world, such energy is always ready when you pay attention to external objects; but if they behave inconsistently towards the expectation, the amount of energy waiting to be used becomes superfluous and is released through the pleasure of laughter.

All this happens with no relation to the unconscious, in fact in comic the investment and the energy release take place in the preconscious and are immediately willing to come to the surface.

The key element is the inadequacy of the mental energy expenditure when comparing what is normal for the subject to the actual mental energy expenditure of the comical object. For this reason the clowns may look funny with their excessive movements.

Freud gives the example of a person who is waiting to catch a ball that was thrown. The person submits his/her body to tensions that will make him/her able to with stand the impact of the ball; and, if it appeared that the ball grabbed were too light, unnecessary and clumsy movements would make the scene comical in the eyes of the spectators. In this way, the person would have allowed the expectation to encourage for an excessive expenditure of movement [9].

Freud believes that the economy of comic, working only in the preconscious and referring to a spending and saving of representative energy, is not directly linked to desire (as is the case for jokes).

Humor

The last category proposed by Freud is that of *humor*. In this theme, expounded in his famous work *Humour* in 1928, Freud emphasizes the role of humor in fostering not only the triumph of ego, but also the principle of pleasure [13].

Freud theorized that humor has the capacity to reduce stress, anxiety, or other negative responses and individual feels towards a given situation. In fact, Freud held humor in very high regard, stating that it is the greatest of all the defense mechanisms a person can utilize [13].

According to Freud, humor occurs in stressful or negative situations in which people normally tend to experience unpleasant emotions such as fear, sadness, anger, etc.

The pleasure of humor comes from the release of energy, which is associated with negative emotions, and is now excessive: this type of humor is found mostly in the ability to laugh at our fears, weaknesses and mistakes.

Freud recognized the impact humor could have on the psychological state of the individual through what he called the "saving in feeling". The "saving" occurs when a person is faced with a situation which would otherwise result in some strong negative emotion. Instead of the negative outcome, the individual is able to use humor to reduce the perceived seriousness of the situation. By way of this purposeful reduction of the threat, the person can cope better with the situation.

According to Freud [13] though the comic and jokes may be experienced by everyone, humor is a rare and precious gift that is owned by only a few lucky people; in this perspective, it acts as a parental superego attempting to comfort the anxious ego. In humor a special condition takes place, where the super-ego acquires the characteristics of tolerance and benevolence towards the ego, becoming reassuring, and where the feared problems of the world end up looking like a childish game about which one can joke and have fun. This point of view, as opposed to the classical psychoanalytic theory, shows the benign side of the superego.

To Know More

It must be said that Freud is not the only psychoanalyst who has dealt with humor: Lacan [15] viewed humor as an important aspect of the individual's developing capacity to address the limitations imposed by society, mortality, and the unspeakable terror of the real. He compared the relationship between action and desire within the psychosocial structures of tragedy and comedy [15]. Given the importance of this theory in the early part of last century, Freud's assumptions have been extensively investigated in several psychological studies.

Freud states that the creation of jokes and witty comments is an unconscious process through which one can bring out to consciousness repressed contents. Morreall [11] argues that this definition is weak, because a large part of the jokes are written by comedians and professional authors who approach this task through conscious strategies to generate set-ups and punch lines. The mechanical explanation of how the nervous energy is released during the jokes, also seems to be problematic.

Freud states that we use psychic energy to repress hostile and sexual thoughts and feelings. Trough jokes, we "elude the censor" and allow this thoughts and feelings to arise from it. The energy released would be used to suppress hostile feelings and thoughts. This is difficult to verify by experimentation. According to the Freudian theory, people who appreciate more sexual and aggressive humor are supposed to suppress more aggression and sexual impulse.

Eysenck's experiments [16] instead, gave opposite results: people who give free rein to their sexual and aggressive feelings are those who appreciate the most this type of humor, while little feedback has been received by the hypothesis that individuals who usually tend to repress their sexual and aggressive instincts show greater appreciation of jokes containing such issues. Some research however, shows that people find aggressive jokes less funny when this feature gets pointed out [16]. The vision of the comic also has theoretical and practical deficiencies. In comic it is assumed that the energy saved would be otherwise used to think.

Freud says, for example, that we use a large amount of energy to explain how clowns manage to accomplish their task, while a small amount of energy is spent thinking about how we would do the same thing. Since the large amount of energy has been used, this is compared with the small amount, and the difference is unnecessary and available to be dissipated through laughter.

But if this energy is used to think about the two movements, and in fact we do think about the two movements, one wonders where the surplus of energy is. Both packets get utilized and nothing is left over [11].

Freud's ideas here, about the "mimetic representation" of motion, are idiosyncratic and have strange implications. If, for example, we thought of climbing the stairs, we would use more energy than if we thought of lifting a foot. If Freud were talking about real energy that burns up calories, exhausting weight-loss diets would not be necessary, one would only need to think of running around town [11]. On the other hand, from a Lacanian perspective, jokes are examples of unconscious formations that combine metaphor and metonymy, condensation, and displacement [17].

Given the scientific inconsistency and the idea that an "hydraulic model" of psychic energy built on Freud's theory - which sees the humor as dissipation of excessive stress - would not be consistent with the modern one of the nervous system, Freud's theory was dropped from the empirical research in the early eighties, although some other contributions are found in the psychoanalytic literature.

The Relief Theory and psychoanalytic theory in particular, have the advantage of putting the focus on some important issues emerging in every theory about humor: the predominance of aggressive and sexual themes in most jokes, the feelings of emotional pleasure and appreciation that are generated by the humor and a strong motivation to generate them.

These aspects still are of great interest to researchers and theorists today, yet one of the major limitations consists of focusing mostly on the intra-psychic dynamics, and less on the relational context and social function.

SUPERIORITY AND DISPARAGEMENT THEORIES

As we have seen, the psychoanalytic theory of humor is based on the assumption that laughter is a manifestation of censored or suppressed aggressive and sexual drives. Indeed, there is evidence that humor is based largely on aggression and hostility.

In particular, finding a note of aggression in humor is something quite common, and some authors postulate that all humor is aggressive [14]. Many examples are brought daily to our attention: consider, for example, how many times during the day we make fun of other people, or think of the satirical broadcasts where sarcasm and derision reign supreme. It is believed that laughter is a reaction generated by a sense of superiority felt by the listener towards the protagonist of the story.

There are several theories of humor that lead back to the expression of aggression. One of the earliest theories postulated, which finds its roots in Greek philosophy, focuses on the feeling of increased self-esteem, control, confidence that accompanies humor, and the experience of superiority over the object of ridicule.

Plato (428-248 BC) was the first to address this matter: in his text "Philebus" he proposed that at the base of comicality is a close association between pain and pleasure: pleasure because one enjoys the ignorance or faults or ills of others (by which one feels superior to others); pain because the individual who laughs for these reasons shows bad spirited feelings. According to this view, the derision of the enemy can be considered a legitimate source of pleasure, while laughing at one's friends is a sign of perversion [11].

Aristotle, associated the ridiculous to the ugly and deformed, just like the comic mask; he claimed that this attitude did not involve any pain or damage. It also introduced the concept of surprise, regarded as the fundamental cause of the laughter, which occurs when a discussion takes an unexpected turn. Aristotle viewed comedy as an imitation of the behavior of individuals who are worse than average and considered it a "species of the ugly"[11]. People who make excessive use of humor are considered vulgar because they are trying to be funny at all costs and their goal is to provoke a laugh, no matter who might be the ridiculed object and without worrying if causing discomfort or discontent. Comedy, especially the unregulated, embodies the negative but, as opposed to Plato, Aristotle considers benign and non-destructive forms of comedy to be tolerable.

Although these philosophers can be regarded as precursors, it was Hobbes in the seventeenth century to first define and ensure that it be adopted, the "Superiority Theory."

He states in his treatise on *Human Nature*:

> "Men laugh at mischance and indecencies, wherein there lies not wit or jest at all… Also men laugh at the infirmities of others… I may therefore conclude that passion of laughter is nothing else but sudden glory arising from sudden conception of some eminence in ourselves, by comparison with the infirmity of others, or with our own formerly…"[18]

He further explains this simple point in the Levithan:

> "Sudden glory is the passion which makes those Grimaces called laughter, and is caused either by some sudden act of their own, that pleased them; or by the apprehension of some deformed thing in another, by comparison where they suddenly applaud themselves."

Humor is supposed to arise from a sense of superiority (hence the name "Superiority Theory"), from the denigration of another person or our major past mistakes or our foolishness.

Hobbe's idea of the sudden glory which humor confers as another is ridiculed has been built on by Ludovici [19] and Rapp [20]. Ludovici claims that the motivation for superiority humor is a form of "superior adaptation", the realization and feeling of pleasure at having adapted better to societal norms than the person being ridiculed. Rapp states that superiority humor ties back to the human's primitive self, a form of "trashing laughter" or joy taken in defeating an adversary, a modern adaptation of "the roar of triumph in an ancient jungle duel" [20: 21].

Items related to the theory of Hobbes were proposed in 1900 also by Bergson who gave a major contribution in the history of theories about humor, writing the essay "Le Rire" [21] in which he condensed his vision of the nature of comicality.

According to Bergson [21], laughter comes only when we become insensitive and indifferent, because we cannot laugh at a person who causes feelings of affection or pity. Another key point of his theory is that comicality does not exist outside of what is properly human. He also discusses the mechanization of the living as laughter occurs in those situations where there is rigidity or mechanical nature of the character, of the spirit or body. The mechanization of the living contrasts the *élan vital*, understood as a principle of nature in the evolution and development of organisms, and laughter is a social gesture that helps to correct this behavior, in fact, by being considered as a form of derision, it can be used as a means to force adherence to the norms of the community. Another important point of his thought is to assess laughter as social (in fact we would not enjoy comedy if we felt isolated), as it loses its meaning and vanishes outside the context of the social group in which it is formed.

Laughter, therefore, is a spontaneous impulse which allows us to overcome, in ever new and original forms, the obstacles we are faced with; in this sense, laughter corrects those behaviors that would endanger the survival of the species.

The most important theorist contemporary to the superiority theory is Charles Gruner, an expert on language and communication, and a professor at the University of Georgia. He sees humor as playful aggression and speaks of "the game of humor". This is not a real aggression as there is no real physical attack resulting in injury, but rather it resembles the playful fight of children or animals. Gruner emphasizes the idea that humor is a game where there is competition, challenge and winners and losers. The fun caused by humor is thus similar to joy or to the feeling of victory after a grueling competition[14].

Gruner's theory of humor contains a three-part thesis: the first and most important element is that every humorous situation has a winner and a loser. Second, a salient aspect is represented by incongruity. Finally, humor always has an element of surprise. In Gruner's theory, all these three elements are present in a humoristic topic.

Gruner, to elaborate his formulation, bases it on evolutionary theory: it is thanks to aggression, competition, curiosity and ability to use resources that humans have managed to climb to the top of the food chain and become masters of the earth.

In accordance with what was postulated by Hobbes, to Gruner laughter also originates from a "roar of triumph" after a hard fought battle, also present in primates. Darwin [22] had already become aware of a particular form of laughter emitted by young chimpanzees. Chimpanzees and other apes, in fact, produce a sound similar to laughter when they play among themselves or when they get tickled. In support of this theory, Van Hoff and Preuschoft [23] found that although laughter is an innate characteristic peculiar to man, it also appears in a prototypal form in primates.

Provine [24] has shown that the laughter of humans is the evolution of the characteristic sound that chimpanzees emit after performing physical activities and during play (the so-called *pant pant* laugh), which, during evolution and through ritualization, has assumed the characteristic sound "ah ah".

Gruner affirms that during evolution, humans have had to spend two million years in an endless struggle for survival, during which they have experienced the tensions that accompany competition, and that they suddenly become loose, resulting in a laugh. During physical struggle with another person, in fact, a great deal of emotional and physical energy is created, caused by the secretion of adrenaline; at the end of the battle, the winner needs to release this excess tension, and this occurs through laughter. Laughter therefore functions to restore balance in the body and to manifest the victory deriding the enemy.

With the evolution of language, people have become able to "defeat" the enemy by turning it into a game, making fun with words rather than physical aggression. Men realized that were able to also try entertainment by building comments that ridiculed others, inventing stories that debase groups, people or ideas. Nowadays, this type of humor is evident in slapstick comedy, in verbal errors, and in the laughter resulting from ridicule of people from other ethnic groups.

According to this theory, to understand any humorous material it is necessary to identify only those who are ridiculed, how and why, since the necessary condition for a stimulus to be humorous is that there is any form of aggression.

Gruner bases the first criteria, that all humor has a winner and a loser, on basic human nature. Based on Darwin's Theory of Evolution, he explains that humans have always had a competitive nature imbedded in their psyche. Over the course of thousands of years, individuals have started to "compete" through humor, instead of brutal physical combat. The "winner," in this sense, is the one who successfully makes fun of the "loser".

The second point of Gruner's theory is that of incongruity. He states that in order to be humorous the act has to in some way deviate from the norm. Most aspects of everyday life are not funny, simply because they have become commonplace in our lives. This is why we find sitcoms so amusing, they place fairly normal characters in shameful situations, situations most people never face.

The third criterion of Gruner's theory which must be present is surprise: if a joke is too predictable, we are not surprised, and we do not laugh. Therefore, a stimulus must be unexpected in order to be humorous.

There are some possible critical points to this superiority theory that have been exposed by humor researchers during the years. The first is that not every situation containing a winner and loser, incongruity, and surprise is necessarily humorous. For these reasons he points out that only certain events are actually humorous. For example, sporting events are held every day with winners and losers, but typically don't make us laugh. Moreover, car accidents meet both the incongruity and surprise criteria, but just aren't funny.

Second, the surprise tenant of Gruner's model has some obvious exceptions. People who have seen their favorite movies many times and still laugh, demonstrate that they can find them humorous even if they are not surprised by the jokes. On the other hand, most people will stop laughing at even the funniest jokes after hearing them several hundred times.

Another criticism of this theory is that some forms of innocent humor, such as simple puzzles or word games, do not appear to adhere to the theory of superiority. These categories appear, in fact, devoid of aggressiveness. Riddles and word games would be nothing more than a "duel of wit", in which individuals try to show their intellectual superiority by exhibiting a mastery of language and cognition. This is also the reason why people tend to react to the play of words with the murmurs that are seen as an admission of inferiority. Research reported, after analyzing a large number of different types of jokes, the presence, in each of them, of an expression of playful aggression [14].

Another criticism of this theory is self-deprecating humor. How can laughing at yourself be explained in terms of the theory of superiority? Along with Hobbes, Gruner also says that it is possible to laugh at our own stupidity or past failures feeling superior compared with the person who we were in the past, and, if the event is reported in the present, it is a part of ourselves which laughs at the other. All of us, in fact, put on different roles, try on different moods and possess personal characteristics which often conflict with each other: the sense of humor is what keeps all these aspects in balance. People who have no sense of humor are rigid, and unable to see their own funny side.

This aspect of superiority theory can be seen by examining the Woody Allen joke: "I wouldn't join any club that would have me as a member." The joke is simultaneously using both the control and resistance aspects of superior humor. Allen is controlling another's laughter by allowing others to laugh at him for not being superior (while in effect he can achieve high status through making fun of himself). Conversely the superiority motivation of humor can provide an interpretation of the joke as Allen's response to anti-Semitic clubs with exclusion laws. This explanation of Allen's humor, using superiority humor to appear weak or create a sense of strength, highlights the complexity of humor in that, even using only one theory, the joke still does not provide a simple classification scheme [25].

To Know More

If Gruner can be defined as one of the current leading theorists of the superiority theory, over the years a large number of scholars have made their contributions to this theory. In this regard, Ford and Ferguson [26] have proposed an interesting and updated review with reference to disparagement humor, bringing psychoanalytic review, superiority, and social identity theories.

The superiority theory introduced by Hobbes was extended by Wolf et al. [27] who introduced the concept of affiliation. They state that "affiliated objects are those objects towards which a subject adopts the same attitude as he does towards himself " [27: 344]. In their opinion, affiliated objects must be seen as psychological extensions of the self. In this vision, a person should experience self-esteem enhancement upon perceiving disparagement of people or groups with whom they are not affiliated. In accord with Wolf et al. [27], people should be more amused upon witnessing disparagement of unaffiliated targets (i.e., members of a social out-group) than affiliated targets (i.e., members of an in-group). The researchers found partial support for their and also Middleton [28] also provided partial support for superiority theory.

La Fave and colleagues introduced the concept of identification class to predict amusement with disparagement humor [29,30]. Identification Class is defined in terms of both affiliation (group membership) and attitude toward a class or category of persons. Identification Class may be a positive attitude if the person identifies himself with the class of persons, or negative attitude, if the person does not. This theory is also known as vicarious superiority theory and suggests that people are sometimes amused by humor that disparages their in-group because of the fact that the recipient does not identify with the in-group.

In contrast to vicarious superiority theory Zillmann and Cantor proposed a "dispositional model of humor" in which they suggest that indiscriminate aggression is not humorous and stated that one or more of the following is present humor is enhanced: the object of the aggression is not seriously injured; there are social/environmental cues for laughter; the object is a hated instead of a loved object; there is an equal level of aggressive retaliation; the object is a member of a different class than the aggressor and/or the audience.

These aspects are clear in Ruch and Hehl's works [32]. The researchers found that this model works well in predicting the behavior of groups which believe they are traditionally 'superior'. A classic example is that men appreciate jokes more in which women are disparaged.

Bryant [33] found that a moderate amount of hostility expressed in put-down humor was higher appreciated than either mild or intended hostility. For this reason, has been suggested a curvilinear (inverted-U) rather than a linear relationship between hostility and funniness.

The superiority/disparagement theory of humor seems to highlight humor as a rather negative human activity, associated with aggression, hostility, and derision. It is important to remember that several theoretical approaches to humor, derived from this theory, have taken a more positive perspective. According with this point of view, humor enhances self-esteem and feelings of competence. In this way, humor emphasizes positive feelings of well-being [2]. In this regard Holland pointed out "we can state the disproportion the other way around, calling the purpose of laughter not so much a glorifying of the self as a minimizing of the distresses menacing the self" [34: 45] and Kallen stated: "I laugh at that which has endangered or degraded or has fought to suppress, enslave, or destroy what I cherish and has failed. My laughter signalizes its failure and my own liberation" [35: 59].

Knox defined humor as playful as a species of liberation [36].

The research presented seems to support that aggression is likely to be present to perceive funniness. Willibald Ruch and colleagues investigated which factors are involved in humor appreciation, using factor analyses of jokes and cartoons [37-39]. These researchers consistently found three stable factors: one related to content factor (sexual humor) and two related to structural aspects of the humor (labeled incongruity-resolution and nonsense). Interestingly, Ruch's investigations did not reveal aggressive topics as content factor. Ruch and colleagues included a large number of jokes and cartoons containing hostile and aggressive themes in their studies, but instead of forming a separate factor, they loaded on one or other of the two structural factors suggesting that hostility is not a very salient dimension in people's responses to humor.

INCONGRUITY THEORIES

Many different theories have something to say about the cognitive and perceptual aspects of humor. Incongruity theories of humor focus more specifically on the cognitive aspects and less on the social and emotional aspects of humor. It is believed that the perception of incongruity is the crucial factor in determining whether or not something is funny: to be funny things to be inconsistent, surprising, unique, unusual or different from what we normally would expect in general and generic terms. There should be a "technical" and defined use of the term "incongruity" [40].

Many researchers on humor have refused to accept the idea that hostility, aggression, and superiority are the exclusive basis to appreciate humorous stimuli. These researchers firstly point out that incongruity is quite distinct from degradation, and focus on incongruity, and not degradation, as the central feature of all humor [41].

The idea that the incongruity is the basis of humor has been proposed by various authors over the past two hundred-and-fifty years, the first of which was the Scottish philosopher Frances Hutcheson in 1750 who further developed what has come to be known as the incongruity theory.

In his "Reflections upon Laughter", Hutcheson stated that people do not laugh at the "inferior" beings, such as in asylums, nor do they laugh at animals except when they resemble human beings. Even when someone slips on a banana peel, observers laugh not because they feel superior but because of the incongruity between expectations and reality.

The eighteenth-century writer Beattie claimed that laughter arises from an unusual mixture of attraction and aversion. He stated that "laughter arises from the view of two or more inconsistent, unsuitable, or incongruous parts of circumstances, considered as united in one complex object or assemblage, or acquiring a sort of mutual relation from the peculiar manner in which the mind takes notice of them" [42: 48].

Even Kant echoes this view of incongruity and claims that laughter comes from an expectation which suddenly turns into nothing. Kant noted that "in everything that is to excite a lively convulsive laugh" there must be "something absurd" [43: 223]. Kant's understanding of laughter by way of incongruity resulted from the frustration of understanding. Laughter derives from "a sudden transformation of a strained expectation into nothing."

Schopenhauer (1788-1860) augments Kant's development of the incongruity principle by noting that "a mismatch between conceptual understanding and perception" results in laughter [44]. Schopenhauer believed that laughter is the result of the unexpected. For this reason incongruity plays a fundamental role in provoking laughter.

In his statement, Schopenhauer, seems to take into account only the intellectual element in humor: humor depends on the pleasure of finding unexpected connections between ideas. In his idea, humor is different from serious intellectual effort because the connection cannot be taken seriously [41]. Moreover, the laughter from incongruity that Schopenhauer and Kant identified seems to depend on what emotion arises out of the unexpected situation [45]. Incongruity can be an element which augments the effect of other types of laughter, such as superiority.

Spencer states that all humor can be explained as "descending incongruity." With the adjective "descending" he implies a judgment of value. Even if it can be related to some aspect of superiority theory, he thinks that it is the incongruity, and not the descent or "degradation," that is the important feature [41]. In his thought laughter is an overflow of nervous energy that must escape.

It was Koestler [46] who provided the most interesting contribution to cognitive psychology with the work, The Act of Creation. The author argues the existence of a close link between three creative activities, namely the field of humor that of scientific research and art, embodied respectively in the clown, the wise and the artist. For Koestler, the boundaries between these art forms are fluid and their common characteristic is "the perception of a situation or an idea from two angles consistent with each other, but usually incompatible" [46: 35], i.e. the perception of incongruity.

Koestler argues that the essence of creativity lies in: "the perceiving of a situation or idea in two self-consistent but habitually incompatible frames of reference." He coins the expression "bisociation" to characterize this act and uses the term "matrices of thought" to describe "any pattern of activity governed by a set of rules."

The "bisociative shock" has the effect of making explicit what was implicit or taken for granted and may be followed by cognitive processing that leads to the birth of a new idea.

"Laughter is a luxury reflex which could arise only in a creature whose reason has gained a degree of autonomy from the urges of emotion, and enables him to perceive his own emotions as redundant to realize that he has been fooled." [46: 96].

As an example consider the following joke cited by Koestler:

"Chamfort tells a story of a Marquis at the court of Lousis XIV who, on entering his wife's boudoir and finding her in the arms of a Bishop, walked calmly to the window and went through the motions of blessing the people in the street. 'What are you doing?' cried the anguished wife. 'Monsignor is performing my functions,' replied the Marquis, 'so I am performing his.'" [46: 96].

He argues that in this anecdote the context of adultery is suddenly bisociated with that of "the division of labor, the quid pro quo". In terms of creativity, "the crucial point about the Marquis' behavior is that it is both unexpected and perfectly logical - but of a logic of usually applied to this type of situation."

Koestler, in agreement with what is postulated in the superiority theory, affirms that a stimulus, to be humorous, in addition to containing an incongruity, it must be accompanied by an aggressive component. Over the years, proponents of the theory of incongruity have abandoned this vision of "hybrid", focusing purely on the incoherent aspects of humorous situations.

Humor, according to incongruity theories, may be said to consist in the finding of "the inappropriate within the appropriate" [41].

Incongruity Theory has been the dominant theory of humor for the past two decades. Although there has been tinkering with the theory on some minor issues [47- 49] it has been widely accepted that humor recognition requires the perception of an incongruity.

The term "incongruity" is often used as a unifying element, to which other vocabulary used in humor can be traced, such as "conflict, ambiguity, dissonance, disagreement" [40]. Although these terms have specific connotations distinguishable from each other, they belong to a single semantic field. Among these, the incongruity refers to the cognitive context, but it can also be used in other areas. In modern research the term incongruity appears to be used in two major ways. In the first case, it is used in a broad (potential) sense and incongruity is a possible aspect or type of humor. In the second case, incongruity is used in a narrow (actual) sense and it represents a characteristic which, though important and common, may, however, not be present [40].

A representative definition of this position is furnished by McGhee [50] who states that "The notions of congruity and incongruity refer to the relationship between components of an object, event, idea, social expectation, and so forth. When the arrangement of the constituent elements of an event is incompatible with the normal or expected pattern, the event is perceived as incongruous" [50: 6-7]. On this point of view, humor seemed to be essentially a cognitive or intellectual experience, and that incongruity was a necessary (although not sufficient) prerequisite [50].

In the early seventies, debate developed in reference to the role of incongruity in humor that is still relevant today. There are two main positions under consideration: one describes the humor as a two-stage process, called resolution of incongruity in which after incongruity has been perceived, it is necessary to find a cognitive rule that "resolves" it, the other, called perception of incongruity, considers only the incongruous stimulus as a necessary requirement for us to talk about humorous experience [40].

THE INCONGRUITY-RESOLUTION MODEL

Although the psychology of humor and the cognitive processes underlying the recognition of incongruity have long been accepted as the best explanation of humor [50,41], it seems that simply noting the incongruous as the cause does little more than explain humor with something that needs further explanation.

Not just any incongruity qualifies as humor: some incongruities are simply confusing or threatening. Morreall [11] proposed an example to illustrate the insufficiency of incongruity as a definition of humor. He suggests that if one opens the bathroom door to find a tiger in the bathtub, this will certainly be incongruous with one's expectations, but it will probably lead to fear rather than amusement.

The main positions are closed in what is known as Incongruity- Resolution Theory, whose main advocates are Suls [51-53] and Schultz [54]. The usual statement of the incongruity-resolution (IR) model postulates that humor is created by a multistage process in which an initial incongruity is created, and then some further information causes that incongruity to be resolved [55].

Shultz [51] when proposing the Incongruity- Resolution (I-R) theory, hypothesized that the punch line creates an incongruity, introducing information that is not compatible with our initial mental set for understanding the joke. This approach allows the subject to mentally trace back what he has heard (or read), in search of the ambiguity that can be interpreted in different ways and allows the punch line to make sense. The ambivalent element that "solves" the joke may take different forms: phonological, lexical, superficial, profound or not linguistic. To explain Shultz's concept, I report one of his example, cited in Ritchie [55]:

Why did the cookie cry? Because its mother had been a wafer so long.

Shultz says that the answer is initially seen as incongruous, with wafer interpreted as "a type of cookie", but then resolution occurs with the realization that there is an alternative interpretation, "away for", that is the ambiguous term.

Another example, is the one proposed by Rothbart and Pien, cited in Ritchie [55]:

> Why did the elephant sit on the marshmallow? Because he didn't want to fall into the hot chocolate.

Here, the authors say that in the question presents an incongruous situation, and the answer both explains (resolves) it and adds a new incongruity.

Ritchie [55] reports the evolution of two theories arising from this debate: The Surprise Disambiguation theory and the two-stage model. According to the first, the initial part of the comic experience (*set up*) has two different interpretations, one very obvious to the listener, the other implicit. The significance of the punch clashes conflicts with the obvious, although compatible, interpretation, and tends to conjure up another hidden meaning, provoking entertainment.

In the example below:

> Why do birds fly south in winter? It's too far to walk.

There is a hidden ambiguity regarding the focus of the initial question. This is disambiguated in a surprising way by the answer.

In the two-stage model, the *punch line* creates incongruity and, subsequently, it's necessary to find a cognitive rule to allow the content to be in line with what is present in the set-up.

This model was proposed by Suls for humor comprehension. He describes the steps that the subject performs, from receiving the stimulus to the humorous response. The two main stages of the process are described as follows:

"In the first stage, the perceiver finds his expectations about the text disconfirmed by the ending of the joke or, in the case of a cartoon, his expectations about the picture disconfirmed by the caption. In other words, the recipient encounters an incongruity — the punch line. In the second stage, the perceiver engages in a form of problem solving to find a cognitive rule which makes the punch line follow from the main part of the joke and reconciles the incongruous parts. A cognitive rule is defined as a logical proposition, a definition, or a fact of experience."[51: 82]

According to this author, understanding a joke is a task of problem solving; processing of a joke is in fact in two basic steps: first the subject finds a conclusion that is incongruous with respect to the premises; second, a problem solving task is undertaken, trying again to resolve the incongruity, that is, finding something that gives meaning to the conclusion and that reconciles it with the premises. When the cognitive rule is found, the inconsistency is removed and the joke is perceived as funny. If the cognitive rule is not found, the incongruity remains and the joke produces puzzlement instead of amusement. From this point of view, humor lies in the removal or resolution of an incongruity, rather than in the continuous presence of it. The element of incongruity-resolution is defined as "cognitive rule", which may take various forms.

One of the examples put forward by Suls [52: 111] is as follows:

> Fat Ethel sat down at the lunch counter and ordered a whole fruit cake. "Shall I cut it into four or eight pieces?" asked the waitress. "Four," said Ethel, "I'm on a diet."

The conclusion "I'm on a diet" is incongruous with the premises, as eating a whole cake divided into either four or eight slices does not make any difference. You can, however, create a rule that would give cognitive meaning to the conclusion in some way: it could be argued that an increase in the number of shares corresponds to an increase in quantity (eight being twice four, if cut into eight parts, Ethel would eat twice as much cake). If the rule is not found, the inconsistency remains, and the joke is not understood, causing confusion.

Here I report an example by famous comedian Emo Philips cited and explained in Earlywine [56: 28]:

> "My grandfather died peacefully in his sleep, but the kids on his bus were screaming."

We can use the two stage model to illustrate the above joke. Suls points out that the *set-up* of any comedic material leads a person to generate a prediction (about the likely outcome). When the *punch line* does not conform to the prediction, the reader (or the listener) is surprised and looks for a cognitive rule that will make the punch line follow for the material in the set up.

When we read the sentence "My grandfather died peacefully in his sleep", we easily imagine an old person lying peacefully in bed. Suls, also emphasizes that the *punch line* of the joke has to differ from our prediction or we won't find it funny. In this way the *punch line* has to violate one of our assumptions about what's going on and lead to a surprise. So, reading the second part "but the kids on his bus were screaming" we shift from the previous imagine into another, after having found the cognitive rule (all the people were in a bus, and only the old guy was sleeping) and we can find a "solution".

Suls does not explore the possibility that the nature of the resolution (i.e. the content of the cognitive rule) may contribute to the humor, although he suggests that the complexity of the reasoning needed may be a factor. His claim is that it is both necessary and sufficient for humor if there is an incongruous *punch line* which can make sense using a suitable cognitive rule.

Furthermore, the above examples show how the resolution is only partial, and how, ultimately, the illogic remains. What characterizes the process of humor is the persistence, at the end, of an element of incongruity (because it is not entirely resolved) and at the same time its elimination (as it has a perception of congruence). The cognitive rule gives the joke a sense, but its nonsensical base remains.

Although advocates of the "incongruity-resolution" theory see the resolution as a key feature for a joke to be perceived as a humorous, it is recognized that the incongruity is never completely resolved.

Forabosco [40], with regard to this, spoke of "pseudo-resolution", which makes sense only within the fantasy world of the joke. If the joke made complete sense and the incongruity was totally resolved, it would be an unfunny enigma, rather than a joke. In addition, Attardo [57] speaks of pseudo-resolution, arguing that the resolution of the incongruent element does not occur completely, but in fact tends to introduce even more incongruity, but, presenting some distorted real similarity to reality is accepted as a lighthearted resolution. Similarly, McGhee [58] speaks of "assimilation of fantasy" which distinguishes jokes and differentiates them from "assimilation of reality" of non-humorous cognitive processes.

Rothbart and Pien [59] suggested distinguishing between possible and impossible incongruities and between complete and incomplete resolutions. They argue that only possible incongruities can be resolved completely while for an impossible incongruity only a partial resolution is possible and a residue of incongruity is left [60].

Oring uses the term "appropriate incongruity" [61]. He argues that all humor is created by appropriate incongruity, and he gives as examples such as this:

A man goes to see a psychiatrist. The doctor asks him: "What seems to be the problem?" The patient says: "Doc, no one believes anything I say." The doctor replies: "You're kidding!"

His model is non-sequential, in the sense that there is no need for the incongruity to be perceived prior to the resolution [62]. It is not meaningful to ask where the incongruity is located within the processing; the incongruity, in the terminology here, is part of the conveyed scenario. Oring's notion of "appropriate" is a form of partial resolution, allowing (in fact demanding) that the incongruity not be eliminated.

To Know More

Shultz [51], in the demonstration of the theory of two stages, emphasizes what is already supported by McGhee [58] on children, which is that the appreciation of humor is often confined to the first stage (the perception of incongruity). This is due to the fact that children below the age of eight have not yet developed concrete operational thought, so are not in able to appreciate the resolution of incongruity.

Likewise, Nerhardt [63], in a pioneering and fundamental study, ascertained that in order to trigger humor it is not necessary to have the resolution of an incongruity, but merely its presence. He was dissatisfied with the studies of comics and jokes because they referred to various linguistic elements not easily controllable and measurable.

To avoid such problems, Nerhardt devised a methodology called the *weight judgment paradigm*, which consists of manipulating incongruity, which he defined as a difference from expectation. Within this paradigm, the research participants were asked to compare the weight of a series of apparently identical objects with a reference object. Initially dumbbells of a similar weight were evaluated (averaging 500 grams +/- 50 grams), while in the end they were presented with other weights much heavier or lighter than the standard (50 grams or 3000 grams). Curiously, when participants raised these weights, it was usual for them to smile or even laugh out loud and Nerhardt pointed out that the people felt much more amused the more the difference between the object that was lifted and the reference object. This result led to the hypothesis that the amplitude incongruity (the discrepancy in weight) was directly linked to the joy and amusement expressed (from a minimum value, evaluated with a smile, the maximum value of resounding laughter). Deckers used this paradigm in a large number of studies, varying the parameters from time to time, in order to evaluate the effects on the response of joy [64]. Deckers found that a minimum number of initial comparisons is needed to build an expectation about the weight, before a large discrepancy evokes a response of entertainment. The researchers concluded that incongruity without resolution is capable of provoking humor, contradicting the theory of incongruity resolution [63, 64]. At the same time they asserted that, to evoke a response of humor (the emotional climate and the mental set of the perceiver) conditions are necessary other than incongruity. Supporters of the incongruity-resolution model argue that the weight judgment paradigm actually does have a resolution. They assert that participants lift the last weight, recognize the incongruity, and resolve it with the idea that this last weight is some sort of joke. This explanation seems to go a bit beyond the way the model was initially proposed [56]. According to Forabosco [40] there are three key-points to take into account in relation to Incongruity-Resolution Theory:

1. Pseudo-resolution leaves a residual incongruity and that the resolution may not completely reconcile the incongruous parts, just as it has been observed that the resolution of the incongruity may introduce new incongruities [59].
2. If by "resolution" an explicit problem-solving activity is meant in which a "cognitive rule is identified that reconciles the incongruous parts," then it can be said that incongruity alone, without resolution, may be the necessary condition for a humor experience. In this regard McGhee [50] talks about cognitive mastery. Without this, incongruity cannot be accepted and used in the humor context.
3. The relationship between incongruity and congruence can also be seen in terms of incongruity as divergence from the cognitive model of reference. "There is incongruity because the stimulus differs from the model; there is congruence because, thanks to the congruence criterion, the stimulus conforms with a specific model that evisions humor stimuli as stimuli in which there are acceptance and use of the incongruity. Considered in this light, cognitive mastery corresponds to the possibility and ability to refer to this specific cognitive model" [40: 61].

FROM THE SEMANTIC SCRIPT THEORY OF HUMOR TO THE GENERAL THEORY OF VERBAL HUMOR

One particular field of humor is represented by linguistics which includes a large number of subfields, (e.g. phonology, syntax, semantics and pragmatics) [2]. Starting from a linguistic point of view, using Raskin's words "a linguistic theory of humor is supposed to account for the fact that some texts are funny while some others are not and to do it in terms of certain linguistic properties of the text. Ideally, a linguistic theory of humor should determine and formulate the necessary and sufficient linguistic conditions for the text to be funny" [7: 47]. We also must keep in mind that "getting a joke" or perceiving a situation as funny involves mental processes and, whit this, we are in full domain of cognitive psychology. On this regard, Attardo points out how the linguistic humor research of the last years is characterized by a strong cognitive orientation, and he states that "linguists who study humor may well be pleased to find out that they were doing cognitive stylistics all along" [65: 231]. In this chapter, I will focus on two theories that have been proposed and that are of certain scientific interest. They are the Raskin's Semantic Script Theory of Humor (SSTH) and its more developed version, the General Theory of Verbal Humor (GTVH) [10,66,67]. These two theories can be defined as cognitive linguistic in the sense that they explore the interface between language and cognition in highly creative language use. Since a considerable amount of work has been done and written about them, I will explain the basis of the two theories and I will briefly focus on the last development.

The Semantic Script Theory of Humor (SSTH)

The Semantic Script Theory of Humor (SSTH) [7] posits that "a text can be characterized as a single-joke-carrying text if both of the [following] conditions are satisfied:

(i) The text is compatible, fully or in part, with two different scripts.
(ii) The two scripts with which the text is compatible are opposite" [7: 99].

The SSTH carefully develops a formal-theoretical basis for the core concept of script, and it provides a methodology for script identification and analysis. A script is "a cognitive structure internalized by the native speaker and it represents the native speaker's knowledge of a small part of the world" [7: 81]. Every speaker has internalized repertoire of scripts of "common sense" [7]. Beyond script of "common sense" every native speaker may have individual scripts determined by his/her individual background and subjective experience and restricted scripts which the speaker shares with a certain group, such as family, neighbors, colleagues. Thus to understand the meaning that rests behind a joke, sufficient scripts or back ground knowledge of a certain joke are indeed needed [7].

Scripts are evoked by lexical items [66] and are organized in a network made of nodes, namely meanings, semantically linked to each other so that every node can be considered more or less close to another: "The script is a large chunk of semantic information surrounding the word or evoked by it. Formally or technically, every script is a graph with lexical nodes and semantic links between the nodes." [66: 199].

The SSHT assumes that a joke is always related with two different scripts that are *opposed to each other in a special way*. The theory explains that the text of a joke is unambiguous up to the point of the *punch line*. The *punch line* triggers a switch from one script to another and makes the hearer realize that more interpretations of the text are possible from the beginning.

The punch line of the joke turns out to be incompatible with the profiled first script interpretation (*incongruity*), but there is a lexical cue in the text (script-switch trigger) that enables the switch or shift from the first interpretation to the second, back grounded script.

As Raskin points out, the overlap between the two scripts may be partial or total. If the overlap is total, the text in its entirety is compatible with both scripts. On the contrary, if the overlap is partial, some parts of the text, or some details, will not be compatible with one or the other script.

Here I will explain Raskin's general perspective by referring to the following famous joke [7: 100]:

"Is the doctor at home?" The patient asked in his bronchial whisper.
"No", the doctor's young and pretty wife whispered in reply. "Come right in."

In the joke above, the words "doctor", "patient", and "bronchial whisper" all evoke the script for "DOCTOR" while the doctor's wife's reply (script-switch trigger) in the punch line forces the reader to backtrack and reinterpret the text in a different script, in this case the script "LOVER".

As Raskin points out, to recognize as humorous a text, two out of the set of scripts activated must overlap (partially or fully) with the text and be in opposition.

Here the hearer faces a problem. When the answer of the young lady does not respond to the script "DOCTOR" he can hardly fail to notice that a whole different situation has been created: the description of the physical appeal of the doctor's wife and the way she replies appear odd. As soon as the script for "LOVER" is evoked, all the contradictions (The "no" in response to whether the doctor is in, in conjunction with an unexplained invitation to come in; the woman's unexplained whisper, the woman's youth and good looks) are resolved and what initially appeared as incongruent elements, immediately become appropriate and congruent with the text.

However, the overlapping of two scripts is not necessarily a cause of humor per se. Many ambiguous texts present overlapping scripts but they are not funny. This is because there is a second condition in the SSTH to fulfill the joke: the central idea is that in verbal humor, the text must be compatible with two different semantic scripts which must be «opposed». The two overlapping scripts are perceived as opposite in a certain sense, and it is this oppositeness which create the joke [7].

Raskin states that in order to comprehend a humor, the hearer of the jokes must endures several stages. First, he/she must distinguish all the non-self-sufficient elements of the sentence, words that refers to something out the sentence. Second, the hearer needs to relate the sentence to the previous sentence in the joke, which has already been interpreted. Finally, the hearer needs to relate the sentences to the pertinent information not contained in the previous discourse. It is important to note that all the information will include various elements of the hearer's experience and knowledge of the world.

SSHT postulates three levels of abstraction of script opposition with at the highest level of abstraction the opposition between *real* and *unreal*. At a lower level of abstraction these oppositions can take three forms, namely *actual vs. non-actual*, *normal vs. abnormal*, *possible vs. impossible*. At the lowest level these oppositions can be manifested as oppositions like *good vs. bad*, *live vs. death*, *sex vs. non-sex*, etc.

Thus, Raskin defines three types of opposition which might hold between scripts:

1.   a direct negation or antonymy;
2.   a negation or antonymy revealed by a process of paraphrasing;
3.   a local antonymy, namely an opposition valid only within the context and discourse of a specific text.

In Raskin's perspective every local antonymy can be reduced to a general antonymy by means of abstraction. The same holds for the two other types of antonyms. Every humorous text plays in fact on the real/unreal dichotomy, which in turn can be specified in three sub-types of dichotomies: "Each of the jokes describes a certain "real" situation and evokes another "unreal" situation which does not take place and which is fully or partially incompatible with the former (...) [7: 111-112].

Even though they sometimes have to be extracted from more concrete scripts, they remain strictly related to the situation described in the text. For example, in the doctor joke the more concrete script opposition is "PATIENT" vs. "LOVER", which can be reduced to the non-sex related vs. sex related dichotomy. This latter dichotomy can be further reduced to the actual vs. non-actual dichotomy, and to the real vs. non-real. Raskin also states that because the boundaries between the three superordinate dichotomies are not clear-cut, the risk is to be excessively interpretative when referring to these more abstract steps [7].

In this context, Wyer and Collins [68], have developed a theory of humor based on an understanding -processing, which suggests that humor involves the simultaneous activation of two different schemes to understand the same situation / event. The more time passes to find and apply a second scheme, the greater the perceived humor. If finding the second scheme becomes too difficult or too easy, the joke will be less fun, because the perception of fun depends on cognitive elaboration required in reference to the event and its implications. This processing concerns the degree to which each scheme is activated causes the "jumping back and forth" in the understanding of the other script, generating a greater number of possible interpretations and of mental images. The greater the cognitive processing of humor produced by the event, the greater the perception of the event as fun. It should also be pointed out that the possible combinations proposed by SSTH are stored and incorporated with other successful combinations until all the elements in the text have been processed. If these is, at least, one coherent interpretation, that is licensed as «the meaning» of the text, and the semantic theory will classify the sentence/text as «well formed».

The General Theory of Verbal Humor (GTVH)

Although SSTH is a good and testable theory, it shows some limitations. The first lies in the fact that it is known to work only for jokes [66]. Since jokes are not the only source of humor, this theory is expected to fall short when applied to other types of humorous text. A second shortcoming of the theory is that it focuses almost exclusively on the semantics of the joke and no other linguistic subfields [66]. A high degree of social interaction, in fact, involves humorous utterances, either intentional or unintentional, which rely on linguistic formulae.

The SSTH was later broadened by Attardo and Raskin [10] and was renamed General Theory of Verbal Humor or GTVH. The GTVH presented in great detail the knowledge structures that are necessary for generating and processing a joke, broadening its scope, in order to be able to account for any kind of (extensive) humorous texts.

Whether Raskin's theory has been considered a semantic theory, the new theory takes into account such as textual linguistics, the theory of narrativity and a broader conception of pragmatics. This broadening consists of the introduction of five more Knowledge Resources (KR) that must be considered as well as the script opposition from the SSTH when generating a joke.

Attardo and Raskin's [10] revision of the SSTH encompassed six knowledge resources (KRs) ordered hierarchically: script opposition (SO), logical mechanism (LM), situation (SI), target (TA), narrative strategy (NS), and language (LA). The hierarchy of KRs was verified empirically through the application to joke similarity [69], although the LM did not fare entirely as predicted.

Here, I report a brief description of the six KRs given by Ruch, Attardo and Raskin [69]:

Language (LA): the LA is the actual verbalization of the joke, resulting in its text. and it includes all the linguistic components of the text (e.g. word choice, placement of functional elements.).

Narrative strategy (NS): the NS accounts for the fact that any joke has to be cast in some form of narrative organization, that is either as a simple (framed) narrative, as a dialogue (question and answer), as a (pseudo-)riddle, as an aside in a conversation, etc.

Target (TA): the TA selects the butt of the joke. Jokes that are not aggressive have an empty value for the TA.

Situation (SI): any joke must introduce some event or situation such as changing a light bulb, crossing the road, playing golf, etc. The situation of a joke is represented by the objects, participants, instruments, activities, etc.

Logical mechanism (LM): the logical mechanism accounts for the way in which the two senses (scripts) in the joke are brought together. LMs can range from straightforward juxtapositions, as in the tee-shirt slogan reading:

> Gobi Desert Canoe Club

to more complex errors in reasoning, such as false analogies, garden path phenomena, as in:

> Madonna does not have one, the Pope has one but doesn't use it, Bush has a short one, and Gorbachev has a long one. What is it? Answer: a last name.

or figure-ground reversals, as in:

> How many Poles does it take to screw in a light bulb? Five. One to hold the light bulb and four to turn the table he's Standing on. (light bulb: figure; body: ground).

Script Opposition (SO): this KR deals with the script opposition/overlap requirement presented in the SSTH. It should be noted that the SO is the most abstract of all the KRs, which accounts for the fact that the SSTH could collapse all six KRs onto this one (basically ignoring the other five, with some exceptions, such as TA and LA). Script Opposition is seen as the incongruity of the SSTH [57]. This is the one parameter that every joke will contain [66].

As we have seen, one of the most important KR of GTVH is Script Opposition. In this theory, the notion of script is grounded in the work of Schank and Abelson [70]. According to these authors, a script is a schematic structure that impose a sequential, causal ordering on a narrative and which reflect a single top-down interpretation of events based on an abstracted distillation of relevant episodic memories.

Scripts may be activated in three ways: lexically (by association with a single word, called the lexical handle of the script), sententially (by a pattern of words and lexical scripts), and inferentially, as a by-product of common-sense reasoning (e.g., as when one intuits that a joke is racist and activates a Racism script). Not all elements are salient in the same ways, and the more salient are marked to distinguish them from less salient background elements.

GTVH can be applied to longer texts quite easily since he sees longer texts merely as being made of shorter texts combined in different ways. He has, however, felt the need to account for the narrative aspect of longer texts and finds the tools proposed as fulfilling this gap [66].

Recent Findings

SSHT and GVTH have greatly influenced the research on humor in the last 25 years. Several authors have contributed, through their studies, to have their say on these theories, and since GTVH was born, much research has addressed the issue of KR's.

For the sake of brevity, I will just focus on some of the issues which have emerged, and I suggest that the interested readers deepen the specific subjects.

With reference to the LM, recently, has been pointed out that logical mechanisms cannot be studied in isolation from the psychological world of the recipient because of meanings within texts derive from external social contexts and personal cognitive processing [71]. It must be pointed out that LM is not logical, but pseudo-logical, paralogical, or otherwise spurious [10,61]. In order to solve this problem some authors compiled lists of possible LMs [72], but the lists are far from complete and the mechanisms are not well defined [61].

The Script Opposition/Logical Mechanism part of the GTVH corresponds to the incongruity resolution model in a simplified and idealized form. The reality of actual texts is much more complicated because humorous texts often have more than one incongruity [72]. To address this issue has been proposed a distinguishing between *focal* incongruities and *background* incongruities in the text of a joke. Focal incongruities are those that are the object of the punch line and of the resolution, whereas the background incongruities have to do with neither [72].

One of the bigger problem with SSTH that was fully adopted by GTVH is the notion of "opposition" [73]. For this reason, that the main hypothesis of the SSTH about SO encompasses both script overlap (SOv) and script oppositeness (SOp) as the necessary and sufficient requirement for a text to be a joke [74]. Some researchers, moreover, decided to focus on perception of contrariety, giving evidence that the cognitive process involved in the recognition of the incongruity involved in a humorous stimulus is guided by the same basic rules for the recognition of contrariety between perceptual stimuli[75].

According to Oring, despite their brevity, jokes can be incredibly complex affairs. They require close scrutiny and careful analysis. Their parts are not as distinct and identifiable as the parts of a simple machine. Abstract models of jokes are not in-and-of-themselves the problem. They must, however, prove faithful to how a joke works to produce humor [73].

In the end, I would mention the work in progress, to elaborate the evolution of the SSHT and GTVH: the Ontological Semantic Theory of Humor (OSHT) [76]. Differently from the Semantic Script-based Theory of Humor, which claimed that the list of script oppositions was an extra piece of knowledge that it had to use along with regular semantic analysis, in the OSHT the list actually folds onto it, so this disappears as an obstacle to the strict-application status of the Ontological Semantic Theory of Humor. Moreover, the authors claim that the OSHT offers a procedure for discovering the main script opposition in a joke, and to be helpful in shed light onto the controversial theme of LM's. One of the principle aim of this theory is to give a better understanding by the non-linguists and a-theoretical linguists in the humor research community as well as by any scholar interested in humor.

From what emerges, it is clear that the debate and research on SSHT and GTVH are still ongoing and that positions are dynamically open. Finally, I would like to talk about, as cross-disciplinary collaboration between linguistics and psychology and as a trial concerning the GTVH, a couple of works of great interest. First of all, I want to report the work that was conducted to evaluated the hypothesis that subjects' perceptions of similarities between pair of jokes will decrease in a linear fashion as the jokes differ from each other at successively higher levels of the KR hierarchy [77]. The results conformed to predictions, with greater similarities being found between jokes that differed at lower levels of the hierarchy. However, some inconsistencies emerged in the exact ordering of the KRs, particularly in the case of LM.

Another interesting couple of experiment was conducted to exanimate the effects of seriality on joke appreciation [78]. In particular, the aim of the studies was to test if when presented with a series of jokes, people find particular jokes to be less funny if they are similar to ones that they have already seen. Using the GTVH framework, the degree of similarity between jokes was manipulated by varying the number of knowledge resources that they shared. As predicted, the more similar group of jokes were, the more they exhibited a seriality effect, such that those presented later in the series were rated as being less funny than those presented earlier.

CONCLUSION

The purpose of this chapter was not to provide a comprehensive review of the various theories of humor that have been proposed. In fact, even though a large number of different theories of humor have been devised, most of them can be placed into a few general categories.

In this chapter I have discussed the theories that have been most influential in the investigation of individual differences and which have proved of greater interest for research and for the definition of humorous experiences. Each of the theories presented tends to emphasize certain aspects of humor. By combining elements from different theories it is possible to obtain a more complete understanding of this multifactorial phenomenon. Each of the theories reported, on the other hand, substantially contributes to the knowledge of the mechanisms and elements of humor.

The Psychoanalytic theory draws attention to sexuality and aggression issues, the feelings of pleasure and fun which are experienced in the face of humor. Although, at present, they are less interesting for research, they specifically focus on humor related issues that continuously draw the attention of the experts. In particular they try to understand why much humor seems to be based on aggression and sexuality, where does the pleasure caused by humor come from, why are we so fascinated by these themes, and what is the function of humor as a coping strategy. Superiority / disparagement theories focus more on social and emotional aspects, mostly centering on aggression and superiority issues. These theories, in fact, provide some theoretical basis to explain humor as an element of affirmation both on others and on ourselves, laughing at our past weaknesses, and bringing with it a sense of liberation from the constraints of life.

Incongruity theories shed light on the perceptual and cognitive mechanisms involved in the understanding and appreciation of a humorous experience, given by the simultaneous perception of two stimuli which appear incongruous. The cognitive dimension of the sense of humor can be understood as relating to individual differences in the ability to perceive, create and understand humor. The sensitivity to inconsistencies and the possibility of a change of perspective are other important aspects relating to this dimension.

Finally, the last part of the chapter was devoted to the field of linguistics (SSHT and GVTH), two theoretical models that have had an enormous impact on the last twenty five years of humor research and that, even though they begin with a linguistic matrix, represent a supra-disciplinary model, as they include multiple approaches.

In summary, in the current state of the field, there is no unifying theory that can explain humor in a clear and definite manner. Researchers would prefer to focus from time to time on specific aspects and the large amount of emerging research shows how humor is a complex and multifactorial phenomenon.

REFERENCES

[1]   Foot, H. and McCreaddie, M. (2006). *The Handbook of Communication Skills.* London: Routledge.
[2]   Martin, R. A. (2007). *The psychology of humor. An integrative approach.* New York: Academic Press.
[3]   Hurley, M. M., Dennett, D. C., and Adams, R. B. (2011). *Inside Jokes: Using Humor to Reverse-Engineer the Mind.* Massachusetts: Massachusetts Institute of Technology.
[4]   Martin, R. A. (1998). Approaches to the sense of humor: A historical review. In W. Ruch (Ed.), *The Sense of Humor: Explorations of a Personality Characteristic* (pp. 15-60). Berlin, Germany: Walter de Gruyter.
[5]   Attardo S. (1994). *Linguistic Theories of Humor.* Mouton de Gruyter, Berlin: New York.
[6]   Berger, A. A. (1987). Humor: An Introduction. *American Behavioural Scientist, 30*(5), 399-408.
[7]   Raskin, V. (1985). *Semantic Mechanisms of Humor.* Dordrecht: D. Reidel Publishing Company.
[8]   Suls, J. M. (1972). A Two-Stage Model for the Appreciation of Jokes and Cartoons: An Information-Processing Analysis. In J. H. Goldstein and P. E. McGhee (Eds.), *The Psychology of Humor: Theoretical Perspectives and Empirical Issues* (pp. 81-100). New York: Academic Press.
[9]   Freud, S. (1960 [1905]). *Jokes and their Relation to the Unconscious.* New York: Norton.
[10]   Attardo, S., and Raskin, V. (1991) Script theory revis(it)ed: joke similarity and joke representational model. *Humor: International Journal of Humor Research, 4*(3), 293-347.
[11]   Morreall, J. (2009). *Comic Relief: A Comprehensive Philosophy of Humor.* Malden, MA: Wiley-Blackwell.
[12]   Spencer, H. (1860). The physiology of laughter. *Macmillan's Magazine, 1*, 395-402.

[13] Freud, S. (1928). Humour. *International Journal of Psychoanalysis*, *9*, 1-6.

[14] Gruner, C. R. (1997). *The Game of Humor: A Comprehensive Theory of Why We Laugh*. NewBrunswick, NJ: Transaction Publishers.

[15] Lacan, J. (1997), *The Ethics of Psychoanalysis. The Seminar of Jacques Lacan Book VII*. NewYork: Norton.

[16] Eysenck, H. J. (1942). The appreciation of humor: an experimental and theoretical study. *British Journal of Psychology, 32*,191-214.

[17] Dor, J. (1998), *Introduction to the Reading of Lacan: The Unconscious Structured Like a Language*. New York: Other Press.

[18] Hobbes, T. (1650), *Human Nature*, London.

[19] Ludovici, A. M. (1933). *The Secret of Laughter*. New York: Viking Press.

[20] Rapp, A. (1951). *The Origins of Wit and Humor*. Oxford, England: Dutton.

[21] Bergson, H. (1911). *Laughter: An essay on the Meaning of the Comic*. Oxford: Macmillan.

[22] Darwin, C. (1872). *The Expression of the Emotions in Man and Animals*. London: Murray.

[23] Van Hooff, J., A., Preuschoft, S. (2003). Laughter and Smiling: The Intertwining of nature and culture. In F. B. M. de Waal, P. L. Tyack (Eds.), *Animal Social Complexity: Intelligence, Culture, and Individualized Societies* (pp. 260-287). Cambridge, MA: Harvard University Press,

[24] Provine, R. R. (2000). *Laughter: A Scientific Investigation*. New York, NY: Viking.

[25] Lynch, O. H. (2002). Humorous Communication: Finding a Place for Humor in Communication Research. *Communication Theory, 12*(4), 423- 445.

[26] Ferguson, M. A., and Ford, T. E. (2008). Disparagement humor: A theoretical and empirical review of psychoanalytic, superiority, and social identity theories. *Humor: International Journal of Humor Research, 21(3)*, 283–312.

[27] Wolff, H. A., Smith, C. E., and Murray, H. A. (1934). The psychology of humor. *Journal of Abnormal and Social Psychology, 28*, 341-365.

[28] Middleton, R. (1959). Negro and white reactions to racial humor. *Sociometry, 22*, 175-183.

[29] La Fave, L. (1972). Humor Judgments as a function of reference groups and identification classes. In J. H. Goldstein and P. E. McGhee (Eds.), *The Psychology of Humor: Theoretical Perspectives and Empirical Issues* (pp.195-210). New York: Academic Press.

[30] La Fave, L., Haddad, J., and Maesen, W. A. (1996). Superiority, Enhanced Self-Esteem, and Perceived Incongruity Humor Theory. In A. J. Chapman, and H. C. Foot (Eds.). *Humor and Laughter: Theory, Research, and Applications* (pp. 63-91). New Brunswick, NJ: Transaction.

[31] Zillmann, D., and Cantor, J. R. (1972). Directionality of transitory dominance as a communication variable affecting humor appreciation. *Journal of Personality and Social Psychology 24*, 191–198.

[32] Ruch, W. and Hehl, F. J. (1998). A two-mode model of humor appreciation: Its relation to aesthetic appreciation and simplicity-complexity of personality. In W. Ruch (Ed.), *The Sense of Humor*, (pp.109-142). Berlin: Mouton de Gruyter.

[33] Bryant, J. (1977). Degree of hostility in squelches as a factor in humour appreciation. In A. J. Chapman and H. C. Foot (Eds.), *It's a Funny Thing, Humour* (pp. 321-327). Oxford: Pergamon Press

[34] Holland, N. N. (1982). *Laughing: A Psychology of Humor.* Ithaca, NY: Cornell University Press.

[35] Kallen, H. M. (1968). *Liberty, Laughter and Tears: Reflection on the Relations of Comedy and Tragedy to Human freedom.* Dekalb, IL: Northern Illinois University Press.

[36] Knox, I. (1951). Towards a philosophy of humor. *Journal of Philosophy,48,* 541-548.

[37] Ruch, W. (1992). Assessment of appreciation of humor: Studies with the 3 WD humor test. In N. Butcher andC.D. Spielberger, (Eds.), *Advances in Personality Assessment* (pp. 27-75). Hillsdale, NJ: Erlbaum.

[38] Ruch, W. and Hehl, F. J. (1998). A two-mode model of humor appreciation: Its relation to aesthetic appreciation and simplicity-complexity of personality. In W. Ruch (Ed.), *The Sense of Humor*, (pp. 109-142). Berlin: Mouton de Gruyter.

[39] Ruch, W. and Köhler, G. (1998). A temperament approach to humor. In W. Ruch (Ed.), *The Sense of Humor*, (pp. 203-230). Berlin: Mouton de Gruyter.

[40] Forabosco, G. (1992). Cognitive aspects of the humor process: the concept of incongruity. *Humor. International Journal of Humor Research, 5*(1), 45-68.

[41] Monro, D. H. (1988). Theories of Humor. In L. Behrens and L. J. Rosen, (Eds.), *Writing and Reading Across the Curriculum*, (pp. 349-355). Glenview, IL: Scott, Foresman and Company.

[42] Ritchie, G. (2004), *The Linguistic Analysis of Jokes.* London: Routledge.

[43] Kant, I. (1951). *Critique of Judgment.* New York: Hafner.

[44] Morreall, J. (1983). *Taking Laughter Seriously.* Albany, NY: State University of New York Press.

[45] Billig, M. (2005). *Laughter and Ridicule: Towards a Social Critique of Humor.* London: Sage.

[46] Koestler, A. (1964). *The Act of Creation.* London: Hutchinson.

[47] Brône, G., and Feyaerts, K. (2004). Assessing the SSTH and GTVH: A View from Cognitive Linguistics. *Humor: International Journal of Humor Research, 17* (4), 361-372.

[48] Clark, M. (1987). Humor and Incongruity. In J. Morreall (Ed.), *The Philosophy of Laughter and Humor.* (pp.139-155). Albany, NY: SUNY.

[49] Perlmutter, D. D. (2002). On Incongruities and Logical Inconsistencies in Humor: The Delicate Balance. *Humor: International Journal of Humor Research, 15,* 155-168.

[50] McGhee, P. E. (1979), *Humor, Its Origin and Development.* San Francisco: Freeman and Co.

[51] Suls, J. M. (1972). A two-stage model for the appreciation of jokes and cartoons: An information-processing analysis. In J. H. Goldstein and P. E. McGhee, (Eds.), *The Psychology of Humor*, (pp. 81-100). New York: Academic Press.

[52] Suls, J. M. (1976). Cognitive and Disparagement Theories of Humor: A Theoretical and Empirical Synthesis. In A. J. Champman, and H. C. Foot (Eds.), *It's a Funny Thing, Humour* (pp. 41-45). Oxford: Pergamon Press.

[53] Suls, J. M. (1983). Cognitive Processes in Humor Appreciation. In P. E. McGhee, and J. H. Goldstein (Eds.), *Handbook of Humor Research. Basic Issues* (1, pp. 39-57). New York: Springer.

[54] Schultz, T. R. (1976). A cognitive-developmental analysis of humour. In: A. J Chapman and H. C. Foot (Eds.), *Humour and Laughter: Theory, Research and Applications.* (pp.11-36). London/N.Y: Wiley and Sons.

[55] Ritchie, G. (1999). Developing the Incongruity-Resolution Theory. In: *Proceedings of the AISB'99 Symposium on Creative Language: Humour and Stories, Edinburgh.* Retrieved online June 2011; http://www.inf.ed. ac.uk/publications/online/0007.pdf.

[56] Earlywine, M. (2011). *Creativity 101.* New York: Springer Publishing Company.

[57] Attardo, S. (2008). A primer for the linguistics of humor. In V. Raskin (Ed.), *Primer of Humor Research,* (pp. 678): Mouton de Gruyter.

[58] McGhee, P. E. (1972). On the Cognitive Origins of Incongruity Humor: Fantasy Assimilation versus Reality Assimilation. In J. H. Goldstein and P. E. McGhee (Eds.), *The Psychology of Humor: Theoretical Perspectives and Empirical Issues* (pp. 61-80). New York: Academic Press.

[59] Rothbart, M. K., and Pien, D. (1977). Elephants and Marshmallows: A Theoretical Synthesis of Incongruity-Resolution and Arousal Theories of Humour. In A. Chapman and H. Foot (Eds.), *It's a Funny Thing, Humour* (pp. 37-40). New York, NY: Pergamon.

[60] Ruch, W. (2001). The perception of humor. In A. W. Kaszniak (Ed.), *Emotion, Qualia, and Consciousness* (pp. 410-425). Tokyo: Word Scientific Publisher.

[61] Oring, E. (2003). *Engaging Humor.* Chicago, IL: University of Illinois Press.

[62] Ritchie, G. (2004). *The Linguistic Analysis of Jokes.* London: Routledge.

[63] Nerhardt, G. (1970). Humor and Inclinations of Humor: Emotional Reactions to Stimuli of Different Divergence from a Range of Expectancy. *Scandinavian Journal of Psychology, 11,* 185-195.

[64] Deckers, L. (1993). On the Validity of a Weight-Judging Paradigm for the Study of Humor. *Humor: International Journal of Humor Research, 6*(1), 43-57.

[65] Attardo, S. (2002). Cognitive stylistics of humorous texts. In E. Semino and J. Culpeper (Eds.), *Cognitive Stylistics. Language and Cognition in Text Analysis.* (pp. 231-250). Amsterdam/ Philadelphia: John Benjamins.

[66] Attardo, S. (1994). *Linguistic Theories of Humor.* (Series: *Humor Research* 1). Berlin/New York: Mouton de Gruyter.

[67] Attardo, S. (1997) The semantic foundations of cognitive theories of humor. *Humor: International Journal of Humor Research, 10*(4), 395-420.

[68] Wyer, R. S., and Collins, J. E. (1992). A theory of humor elicitation. *Psychological Review, 99*(4), 663-688.

[69] Ruch, W., Attardo, S. and Raskin, V. (1993) Towards an empirical verification of the General Theory of Verbal Humor. *Humor: International Journal of Humor Research, 6*(2), 123-136.

[70] Schank, R. C. and Abelson, R. P. (1977) *Scripts, Plans, Goals and Understanding.* New York: Wiley.

[71] Davis, C. (2011). Logical mechanisms: A critique. *Humor: International Journal of Humor Research, 24*(2), 159–166.

[72]   [72] Salvatore, A., Hempelmann C. F., and Di Maio, S. (2002) Script oppositions and logical mechanisms: Modeling incongruities and their resolutions. *Humor: International Journal of Humor Research, 15*(1), 3-46.

[73]   Oring, E. (2011). Parsing the joke: The General Theory of Verbal Humor and appropriate incongruity. *Humor: International Journal of Humor Research, 24*(2), 203–222.

[74]   Hempelmann, C. F. (2004). Script opposition and logical mechanism in punning. *Humor: International Journal of Humor Research, 17*(4), 381–392.

[75]   Canestrari, C., and Bianchi, I. (2009). The perception of humor: From script opposition to the phenomenogical rules of contrariety. In U. Savardi (Ed.), *The Perception and Cognition of Contraries*, (pp. 225-246). Milano: McGraw-Hill.

[76]   Raskin, V., Hempelmann, C. F., and Taylor, J. M. (2009). How to Understand and Assess a Theory: The Evolution of the SSTH into the GTVH and Now into the OSTH. *Journal of Literature Theory, 3*(2), 285-312.

[77]   Ruch, W., Attardo, S. and Raskin, V. (1993). Toward an empirical verification of the General Theory of Verbal Humor. *Humor: International Journal of Humor Research, 6*(3), 123-136.

[78]   Forabosco, G. (1994). "Seriality" and appreciation of jokes. *Humor: International Journal of Humor Research, 7*(4), 351-375.

In: Humor and Health Promotion
Editor: Paola Gremigni

ISBN: 978-1-61942-657-3
© 2012 Nova Science Publishers, Inc.

Chapter 3

FUNCTIONS AND MEANINGS OF SMILE AND LAUGHTER

Luisa Bonfiglioli and Pio Enrico Ricci Bitti

Department of Psychology, University of Bologna, Italy

ABSTRACT

Smiling and laughter are extremely interesting phenomena filled with implications at intraindividual, interindividual and intercultural level, and have been studied in a variety of disciplines, such as anthropology, ethology, sociology, social psychology and clinical psychology. Smiling and laughter are two highly complex expressive manifestations that can be placed in relation to humour, but which also include and perform other types of function. Some authors have recently looked at these phenomena with a view to constructing theoretical models. In order to illustrate the breadth and complexity of laughter and smiles, they are treated by adopting a descriptive model, considering the two manifestations from the point of view of their phenomenology. After having considered the relevance of laughter and the smile in relation to social communication and interaction, the qualitative differences between smile and laughter are examined, with particular focus on the acoustic features of the vocal manifestations in laughter and presenting the main developmental stages of acquiring laughter and smiles. The theme is then treated with the intention of providing a clear and, as far as possible, thorough response to the following questions: 1) which factors give rise to laughter and smiles; 2) what do laughter and smiles convey; 3) are there intraindividual health and psychological benefits to smiling and laughing. The findings emerged from the literature enable us to affirm that, while plenty of evidence has been collected in the applicative and clinical level, unanswered questions still remain in the theoretical field that future studies will have to address. These regard the nature of the relationship between laughter and smiling, identification of the expressive indices of spontaneous and voluntary manifestations and, finally, the theme of individual differences.

INTRODUCTION

Studies conducted on non-verbal communication and on the exchange of signals and information in social interaction have highlighted in a thorough and acclaimed manner that the face is undoubtedly the most important area of the body when it comes to expression and communication, in that it is the best channel for expressing emotion, it contributes to the manifestation of interpersonal attitudes, it produces notable "dynamic" interaction signals, conversational signals and enables the externalisation of mental processes [1]. From a phylogenetic point of view, it has been found that, in mammals living in groups, the facial expression and the possibility of articulating it through the movement of the facial muscles performs an indisputable adaptive function. It is also deemed that humans have a greater ability than primates to differentiate and evolve because they can modulate their expressiveness in a more aware and skilled manner. As Ceccarelli [2] underlines, in a biosocial anthropology essay dedicated entirely to the smile and laughter, they can be defined as complex behaviours or motor schemes and, as "expressive movements", they are connected to many terms that occupy a broad semantic field including such concepts as: "ridiculous, droll, satirical, hilarious, risible, jokey, witty, amusing, funny, derisive, comical, bizarre, playful, facetious, cheerful, humorous, farcical and so on" [2: 5]. An indisputable "terminology fluctuation" can be noted here. Such fluctuation inevitably derives from two specific factors that belong to both the physical and to the social sciences. They are represented, on the one hand, by the natural indeterminateness of current language and, on the other, by the fact that the terms used to define a concept, rather than constituting a premise to a theory, derive from it. Ceccarelli therefore highlights the complexity of the expressive behaviours of laughing and smiling, at different levels: both at the level of defining the continuous or discrete nature of the relationship between laughter and smiles and at the level of the factors underlying such manifestations. For the issues associated with distinguishing between laughter and smiling and with their relationship, see the next paragraph of this chapter. With regard to the second aforementioned factor of complexity, the author notes how analyses of the smile have erroneously confused three factors that must, on the contrary, be kept separate. These are: communication, motivation and emotion. In particular, it is necessary to distinguish between the communicative, "social", aspect, and the other aspect, which Ceccarelli defines as "psychological" and which concerns the relationship between the individual's internal state, motivation and expressive manifestation. If, indeed, the smile is, in a general sense, a social signal that conveys and possesses an anti-aggressive, anti-hierarchical and cohesive connotation, the relationship between smiling and the individual's internal states may vary since the individual is able to modulate and control this expressive manifestation. Aside from the presence of certain emotions or internal states, the meaning of the message, according to Ceccarelli, is universal and cross-cultural studies conducted by Darwin [3], Eibl-Eibesfeldt [4], and Ekman and Friesen [5] have found many common elements in the way of smiling and of attributing meaning to the smile in even very different cultures. The other distinction considered by Ceccarelli [2] concerns the level of analysis of the different motivations that can lead an individual to smile. "[…] even though my smile may arise from myriad different motivations, it is nonetheless a message of friendship. Its meaning does not change according to the smiling person's internal motivation, and if the motivation is to deceive, smiling at my victim certainly does not convey 'I want to deceive you', but 'I want to be your friend', even if the hidden purpose is to deceive - which is not communicated, although it may be guessed by the receiver" [2: 19]. It is no coincidence then that psychological literature addressing the theme of authentic (or genuine) smile vs. non spontaneous smile represents an extremely broad and significant part of studies into the smile. This research, as shown in the paragraph of this chapter dedicated to the expressive aspects of smiling (cf. par. 4), has contributed considerably towards accurately finding and identifying the facial indices associated with sincere smiles and with non-genuine smiles, even though some evidence has recently been called into question and the complexity of the issue is once again underlined. Niedenthal and colleagues [6] analyse this distinction in their model of the processing of the smile to illustrate how to advance the application of theories of embodied cognition in the study of facial expression of emotion. Taking complexity into account is essential when discussing laughter. The list of different manifestations of laughter (cf. par. 4) is very extensive and articulated. Aside from this heterogeneity, it is important to state some aspects that distinguish this expressive manifestation and that relate to both its nature and its function. Laughter is essentially a phenomenon whose nature lies in a social dimension - the fact that it is a potentially "contagious" phenomenon is proof of that - and which involves the body to a considerable extent (movements and changes in posture that lead to a state of relaxation) and modifications to some physiological parameters. Finally, laughter is closely connected to breathing and, compared to smiling, has different acoustic-sound configurations or profiles (which can be analysed according to their speech rate, pitch, loudness, pitch variability, and rising or falling end) [7-9].

STRUCTURAL ASPECTS AND QUALITATIVE DIFFERENCES BETWEEN LAUGHTER AND SMILE

Darwin [3] posed the problem of differentiating between laughter and smiling and discussed the possibility of considering them as two distinct manifestations, two discrete categories or, on the contrary, of hypothesising the existence of a continuum between laughter and smiling. In his essay on the expression of emotions in man and animals, the author proposes two alternative hypotheses: firstly, laughter could be considered as the end result of a fully developed smile and, secondly (and more probably, according to the author), the smile may constitute the last trace of the reiterated habit of laughing in correspondence with pleasant affective states. Ceccarelli [2] illustrates a possible continuum between laughter and smiling by grouping the markers belonging to two expressive behaviours into three groups which represent the main areas (or observable behaviours) involved in them. The three groupings consider phenomena observable at the face, breathing (including vocalisations) and body.

Before illustrating the elements in this analytical description of the observable markers in laughter and smiles, it should be pointed out that the author also specifies the presence of physiological changes. These changes, in a continuum structured on the intensity dimension, chiefly involve an increase in blood pressure, which causes, at the circulation level, a vasodilation of the arterial system and, at the observable level, a reddening of the face, neck and, in some cases, the scalp and hands. Physiological changes may include the activation of the lacrimal glands which may cause the eyes to become brighter and even produce tears.

In the continuum elaborated by Ceccarelli, considering a sort of baseline of intensity that does not envisage the presence of particular manifestations in the face, nor specific bodily configurations or postures, the first level of intensity involves the horizontal stretching of the mouth (without showing the teeth), and the indentation and lifting of the corners of the mouth.

At this level, there is no change in the other two groups of markers. The second level involves the elevation of the upper lip and the skin below the nose with partial uncovering of the upper front teeth. The infra-nasal depression also becomes more evident. Wrinkles at the edges of the eyes and a small bag beneath the eyes appear. When laughter occurs at this level the breathing begins to change, with emissions of air caused by clonic spasms of the diaphragm and vocalisations that start out quiet and progressively increase in volume. There are no particular bodily configurations at this level. The third and final level involves the opening of the mouth, the visibility of the teeth and the jaw moving slightly downward.

The nostrils are moderately dilated and move slightly upward. The eyes protrude somewhat and appear brighter. This level can include Darwin's [3] description of uncontrolled laughter, which involves the presence of dilated veins, red face, spasmodic contraction of the muscles around the eyes and lachrymation. The breathing becomes an increasingly determining factor (cf. par. 2.1). Bodily changes involve the head and torso being progressively thrown backward until the laugher has to bend forward due to the tiring of the diaphragm and the abdominal muscles.

ACOUSTIC FEATURES OF LAUGHTER

In his essay on the expression of emotions in man and animals, Darwin [3] declares that laughter is essentially an expression of joy. Since the acoustic and vocal elements of laughter are decisive in this expressive manifestation, it seems appropriate to begin this paragraph, while maintaining a descriptive-phenomenological intention, with the words of this author who, in the aforementioned volume, provides a wonderful and precise illustration of laughter. "The sound of laughter is produced by a deep inspiration followed by short, interrupted, spasmodic contractions of the chest, and especially of the diaphragm.

Hence we hear of 'laugher holding both his sides'. From the shaking of the body, the head nods to and fro. The lower jaw often quivers up and down, as is likewise the case with some species of baboons, when they are much pleased. During laughter the mouth is opened more or less widely, with the corners drawn much backwards, as well as a little upwards; and the upper lip is somewhat raised. The drawing back of the corners is best seen in moderate laughter, and especially in a broad smile-the latter epithet showing how the mouth is widened. [3: 199] […].A bright and sparkling eye is as characteristic of a pleased or amused state of mind, as in the retraction of the corners of the mouth and upper lip with the wrinkles thus produced. [3: 205]. Darwin also underlines the repetitive nature of laughter, hypothesising that this feature has developed in order for this sound manifestation to be clearly distinguishable from screams or cries of pain which are produced by prolonged and continuous exhalation and by short and interrupted inhalation. On the contrary, the manifestations of joy typical of laughter feature short and interrupted exhalation and prolonged inhalation. Again on the subject of the vocal manifestations of laughter, Ruch and

Ekman [10], in their analysis of laughter in terms of respiration, vocalization, facial action and body movements, note how respiratory changes such as increased exhalation are at the basis of the characteristic vocalisations of laughter, to a point that the maximum voluntary exhalation limit may at times even be exceeded. Bachorowski [11], in her analysis of the acoustic features of laughter, identified certain important aspects.

According to the author, these include the existence of a sort of dictionary of laughter that distinguishes between the various manifestations of laughter, such as cackles, hisses, breathy pants, snorts, grunts, and songlike laughs. She also identifies two broad categories: voiced and unvoiced laughter. The first type concerns acoustic manifestations involving the vocal cords, which sound like songs or melodies (rising and falling) and represent an invitation to friendly interaction. The second type (which includes hisses, snorts and grunts), contrary to the first, is not associated with a pleasant affective state.

A further finding by Bachorowski in the acoustic analyses of laughter relates to the analysis of the interrelation (or laughter duets) between partners sharing laughter. Friends laughing together for a brief period of two or three seconds are joined in a sort of antiphonal laughter consisting of the sharing of the same acoustic space, just like that which occurs for the different instruments in an orchestra. Another element concerns the fact that, although the acoustic aspects of laughter are customarily written down using vowels and consonants (e.g. "ha ha ha" or "he he he"), it should be pointed out that the regions of the vocal apparatus that produce vowels and consonants are distinct from those involved in laughter.

DEVELOPMENTAL ASPECTS OF LAUGHTER AND SMILE

In the course of ontogenetic development, expressive manifestations such as laughter and smiling appear at a very early age. The smile in early dyadic interaction is an indicator of positive affective states (pleasure), just as it is an interpersonal approach invitation. It generates attention from the mother, reduces aggressiveness, induces gratification, prolongs interaction times and, finally, encourages attachment. Studies into early mother-child interaction have found that laughter appears as early as the fourth month in an infant's life. In a recent book on the illustration of mechanisms of empathy, Keltner [12] describes the dynamics of laughter by underlining, on a phenomenological level, how shared laughter involves a spontaneous shift from separate vocalisations emitted by each individual to a progressive interconnection of the laughters; he also argues for the social valence of laughter, underlining that laughter, which appears before the development of vowels and consonants, is an important part of an innate heritage that favours collaboration among human beings. Smile, on an ontogenetic level, develops and differentiates as early as the first month of life, during which time the smile (reflex smile) involves only the stretching of the lips and occurs during REM states, just as it can be provoked by gently tickling the skin, by gentle sounds or soft lights. Subsequently, the so-called social smile appears which is stimulated initially by the mother's voice, then by the moving human face and later by the unmoving face. A further stage consists in the appearance of the so-called selective social smile, which appears in response to familiar faces. It is interesting to note that these stages occur in the same sequence in all infants, and individual differences are found solely in the duration of each specific stage. This recalls the theme of the cultural or innate origin of the facial expressions of emotion, a theme that has been the subject of much debate. Relevant authors on smiling include Birdwhistell [13] who, in his studies conducted in different parts of the United States, observed a number of qualitative and quantitative differences and, from this, assumed a theoretical position that countered the hypothesis of innatism. A supporter of innatism, Eibl-Eibesfeldt [4], referring back to Darwin's extensive work, conducted numerous cross-cultural studies and studies on blind and deaf children and found interindividual and intercultural resemblances in expressive manifestations such as smiling and laughter. The two theoretical positions were reconciled by Ekman [14] who, in his theory on the facial expression of emotions called neurocultural theory, highlights and analyses the interaction between cultural and innate factors. According to this author, there is a so-called facial programme of emotions, at least in part innate, made up of a series of instructions coded at neural level that, by modulating the observable responses of the central and autonomic nervous system of the subjective experience, would explain the relationship between a given emotion and the activation of specific facial muscles. Cultural factors, on the other hand, can define both the particular events and circumstances able to activate the various emotions and the rules of exhibition, which are learned by the individual and which allow him to modulate the manifestation of emotions in different contexts. This would be possible thanks to the fact that, in the event of activating circumstances belonging to interpersonal situations, the individual's internal cognitive processes would enable him to appraise the situation.

ANTECEDENTS OF LAUGHTER AND SMILE

While admitting the complexity of the issue, Darwin [3] gave a rather detailed list of the causes of laughter, with the premise that the causes differ between adults and children. According to the author, the most common causes of laughter in adults are absurd or strange circumstances, events or phenomena that he qualifies by defining as "not too serious" and that can arouse surprise and "some sense of superiority in the laugher, who must be in a happy frame of mind" [3: 196]. Another cause of laughter is a comical idea capable of "tickling" the mind and the imagination. This idea, as in the previous case, must not be too serious and must possess an unexpected, unusual or absurd quality capable of interrupting the normal thought processes. Tickling can also cause laughter; in this case this manifestation must be considered a reflex and is very different in nature from laughter caused by a comical idea. We should add, however, that, according to Darwin, laughter caused by a comical idea and laughter caused by tickling possess a shared element represented by the fact that the individual's mind is in a pleasant mood. Being tickled by a stranger does not make a child laugh, Darwin observes. The phenomenon of tickling has still not been investigated thoroughly. In a recent study conducted with adult subjects, some authors found empirically that tickle-induced smiling can be dissociated from positive affect [15]. The authors discuss this data by considering the hypothesis according to which, in the same way as the startle, the reaction to tickling is a sort of complex reflex that, from a developmental point of view, may perform the specific function of promoting the bond between infant and adult. In this case, however, the reason for tickling arousing a feeling of aversion would still have to be explained. With regard to laughter, Darwin, in support of Spencer's thesis, hypothesised that laughter occurs in cases in which an individual has an excess of nervous energy that cannot be offloaded through new thoughts and/or emotions and that it is therefore vented in the form of muscular activity. On the subject of the antecedents of laughter, Provine [16] conducted a study of 1200 episodes of laughter recorded in real-life contexts and transcribing these episodes in narrative form. By analysing these episodes as a function of the topics arising between the interlocutors immediately prior to laughter, it emerged that humorous content preceded laughter in no more than 20% of cases. The analysis of these narratives states that 80% of the episodes of laughter came after affirmations of widely varying content, demonstrating that, when it comes to raising a laugh, conversational events unrelated to humour are not the exception but the rule. For what concerns antecedents of smile, the par. 2.2 of the chapter presents the developmental aspects. Studies on smile indicate that there are many different smiles and several antecedents; Ekman [17] classified 18 different smiles and hypothesized the possibility to extend this classification. Recently, Niedenthal and colleagues [6] indicate different antecedents dividing the correspondent smiles into three categories that consider the meaning of the smile from the view of the person doing the smiling. One could distinguish between a first type of smile produced by positive emotion, a second type of smile produced by positive social motives (affiliative smiles) and, finally, a third type of smile as a way of communicating and maintaining social status (dominance smiles).

EXPRESSIVE AND COMMUNICATIVE ASPECTS OF LAUGHTER AND SMILE

Keltner [12] sustains that laughter may be a language in itself and that the heterogeneity of its different manifestations makes theoretical formulation a very complex matter. The list of multiple expressive behaviours is extensive: "There are derisive laughs, flirtatious laughs, singsongy laughs, embarrassed groans, piercing laughs, laughs of tension, silent, head-lightening laughs of euphoria, barrel-chested laughs of strength, laughs that signal the absurdity of the shortness of life and the extent to which we care about our existence, contemptuous laughs that signal privilege and class, and laughs that are little more than grunts or growls" [12: 125]. To thoroughly understand the multiple functions of the smile, we need to consider both its expressive and its social and interactive components. With regard to the first type of components, the literature indicates the existence of smiles in correspondence with certain emotions, not all of which are related to pleasure. These are: happiness, sadness, embarrassment, shame, contempt, anger and fear [18]. As for the second type of components, it is interesting to note that, from a phylogenetic point of view, the origin of the social function of the smile may be found in the need for affiliation and appeasement. This distinction between the two types of components is also linked to some important research, stimulated by the possibility of conducting an exacting analysis of facial movements (broken down into specific Action Units or AUs) offered by F.A.C.S., Facial Action Coding System [19], which studied the differences between a sincere and spontaneous smile (linked to the emotional dimension) and a voluntary and strategic smile (indicator of social instances and functions). In addition to operationalizing this traditional distinction in terms of the activation of specific muscles (corresponding to as many AUs), this research enabled the different types of smile and their actual recognition to be analysed in more depth. Before describing this fundamental distinction, it is appropriate to point out that the two sides of the face have different expressive capacity: this emerged from a number of studies conducted as early as the 1970s [20] and was recently corroborated by studies using a three-dimensional reproduction of chimeric faces made from placing two hemifaces together [21]. Facial asymmetry, which manifests itself in the left hemiface's greater expressive intensity, may be attributed to the right hemiface's specialisation in regulating the perception and facial expression of emotion [22]. This data, connected to the results of studies that found that the two types of smile differ according to the presence vs. absence of facial asymmetry, is solid empirical evidence in support of the possibility of considering the presence of asymmetry as a factor enabling observers to distinguish a spontaneous facial expression from a voluntary one. To better understand the distinction between various types of smile in relation to their sincere character, we should specify that, while an insincere smile is produced by activating only the zygomaticus major muscle which lifts the corners of the mouth (AU 12) and is characterised by the presence of asymmetry and a duration of over 4 seconds, the genuine smile (also called the Duchenne or D-smile) simultaneously activates the zygomaticus major and the orbicularis oculi muscles (AUs 12 + 6), creating wrinkles near the eyes, facial symmetry and lasting less than 4 seconds. As some authors observe [23], the aforementioned distinction between genuine smile and voluntary smile does not correspond to the distinction between the emotional and social components of the function of a smile. There are some smiles, such as the smile of embarrassment, shame or compassion, that, while still being spontaneous and genuine, are attributed to a different emotional state than that typical of the Duchenne smile. From the point of view of AU analysis, these smiles have the AUs typical of the Duchenne smile together with the activation of other specific AUs. Furthermore, an individual may produce a smile that does not match his/her internal emotional state. The same authors [24], through several studies conducted using recognition tasks, further investigated the smile and, considering the emotional and social components of the smile, found the possibility of distinguishing between four different types of smile: a polite or "formal" smile, an enjoyment smile, an elation smile and, finally, a smile of sensorial pleasure. These four types of smile can be described using AUs, indicating that the polite or "formal" smile is produced by activation of the zygomaticus major alone, which lifts the corners of the mouth (AU 12), and corresponds to the so-called "non-enjoyment smile" described by Frank et al. [25]. The smile of enjoyment activates both the orbicularis oculi and the zygomaticus major (AUs 6+12), as well as lifting the upper eyelids (AU 5) and opening the mouth (AU 25). The third smile identified, the elation smile, simultaneously activates the orbicularis oculi (producing the so-called "crow's feet") and the zygomaticus major (lifting the corners of the mouth) (AUs 6+ 12), as well as the opening of the mouth (AU 25). The fourth and final type of smile identified, the smile of sensorial pleasure, activates the orbicularis oculi and zygomaticus major (AUs 6+12) together with the closing of the eyes (AU 43). In general terms, this distinction has identified that, in accordance with the pioneering observations of Darwin [3], opening the mouth may be significant in identifying a spontaneous or genuine smile, closing the eyes enables subjects to recognise a smile associated with sensorial pleasure, and opening the eyes is interpreted as an indicator of joyousness. The need to make distinctions within the so-called Duchenne smile is confirmed by several recent studies [26], which have found that not only is the presence of the markers of this smile (AU 6 and AU 12) verifiable even in non-spontaneous smiles and in relation to negative emotions, but also that these markers cannot be considered as necessary and sufficient signals for recognising a smile as spontaneous and happy. Other observable elements in dynamic manifestations of smiles also contribute, such as the duration of the peak of the smile and facial asymmetry. Aside from the debate about the distinctive components of a genuine smile, it seems interesting to note that some recent studies have further investigated the role of this smile in social interaction. In particular, one study found that the genuine smile, as opposed to the polite smile, has intrinsic reinforcement value even when it is not relevant for the performance of an assigned task and is not a predictive factor of a possible monetary reward [27]. The authors of the study comment on this empirical evidence by stating, in general terms, the importance of social stimuli, such as facial feedback, and in more specific terms, the value in terms of social reinforcement of genuine smiles, which seem to possess a more significant role than polite smiles in the regulation of social interaction.

FUNCTIONS OF LAUGHTER AND SMILE AND THEIR EFFECTS ON PSYCHOLOGICAL WELL-BEING AND ON HEALTH

The theme of the effects of laughter and smiles on psychological wellbeing and on health (cf. chap. Gremigni), as can be imagined, is frequently discussed both in clinical psychology and psychotherapy (see chapter X in this book) and in the context of care for hospitalised patients (see chapter XI in this book). In this chapter, we intend to underline the fact that the theme is closely linked to the relationship between emotions and health both at intraindividual and at interindividual and social level. Papa and Bonanno [28] analysed some of the mechanisms that may link smiling to well-being and highlighted intrapersonal functions of smiling (associated with self-regulation) and interpersonal functions of smiling (associated with increases in the type of social resources that promote coping with adversity). Research conducted to investigate the relationship between emotions and health now agrees on the fundamental role of strategies for regulating the emotions. In order for an individual to benefit from the adaptive value of emotional experience, he must acquire, in the course of his affective development, the ability to regulate his own emotions at intra-psychical and interindividual level. The outcome of any episode of social interaction depends largely on the regulation processes that the individuals involved put in place, which are learned and which derive from the social representations typical of every culture, which indicate which emotions are appropriate for a given situation, how to convey them verbally and how to manifest them in non-verbal communication [29]. According to Solano [30], it is possible to hypothesise that both the reduced expression and the overwhelming expression of emotions imply inadequate regulation of emotions. It should also be considered that empirical studies in the literature have now demonstrated that altering the emotional response by regulating one specific component may also affect other components. In the specific case of expressive manifestations, such as laughter and smiling which constitute the expressive-behavioural component of the emotional response, it should be pointed out that regulating this component may lead to a modification of the physiological processes, just as regulation of the latter results in a change in the subjective experience component. Studies have shown that the immediate effects of the expressive inhibition of emotional experience seem to be associated with increased sympathetic activation and that the suppression of negative emotions seems linked long-term to cardiovascular disease and to altered immune system function. It should be pointed out, however, that the literature has not yet sufficiently clarified what relationships there are between the short- and long-term consequences of different strategies of emotional regulation, which seems to be extremely interesting and significant for the relationship between styles of regulating the emotions and health. By way of example, we can observe that if inhibiting the expressive-behavioural component can be considered as an effective and functional strategy for maintaining social interaction – and therefore beneficial in the short term – we should consider that emotional experience does not disappear in the immediate term; it leaves traces that require subsequent processing after the episode that elicited them. The failure of adequate emotion processing strategies at this level may consequently play a decisive role in the occurrence of illness. A hypothesis was recently proposed according to which laughter, the little "vacation" from the conflicts of social living, brings countless benefits for individuals, at both social and at individual level [12]. Owren and Bachorowski [31] propose a hypothesis according to which laughter possesses the function of contributing to the construction of ties of cooperation required for group living. Indeed, laughter can be "catching", and some studies have demonstrated the presence of a "mirror" response in the neurons in the supplementary motor area of individuals listening to laughter. Laughter also signals appreciation and mutual understanding and induces pleasure (see the presence of laughter as a social signal in playful exchanges to induce cooperative response in others). As such, the authors hypothesise that laughter encourages the development of trusting relationships between individuals. Developing this hypothesis and re-examining the developmental studies conducted into the role of laughter in the development of the imagination in play, Keltner [12] underlines how laughter constitutes: "a portal to the world of pretence, play and imagination; it is an invitation to a nonliteral world where the truths of identities, objects, and relations are momentarily suspended, and alternatives are willingly entertained […] Laughter is a ticket to the world of pretence, it is a two-to-three-second vacation from the encumbrance, burdens, and gravity of the world of literal truths and sincere commitments "[12: 138-139].

CONCLUSION

From the analyses present in the literature, it emerges that the smile is an important component of an individual's facial signalling system and performs a multitude of functions in social behaviour. The smile generally expresses positive emotion and is also interpreted as an approach invitation, as is the case with a greeting, for example; in addition, the smile generates an exchange in which interaction is prolonged and consolidated. In general, the reinforcement function that the smile performs can be understood by considering that, starting from early dyadic mother-infant exchanges, the smile performs the basic biological function of enabling and consolidating social nearness and that, subsequently, it constitutes an important signal that increases the possibility of interaction in interpersonal situations [32]. The infant's smile is a signal that draws the attention of the adult. Ambrose [33] describes the effects of encouragement, reward and satisfaction aroused in the mother by the infant's first social smile and Bowlby [34] defines as "amorous" the maternal behaviour aroused by the infant smiling at the mother. The influence of the smile is not only immediate but long-term, since it encourages future maternal nurturing behaviours, thus performing the function of preserving the infant's survival. With regard to laughter, despite the fact that the complexity of the phenomenon has produced a number of diverse theoretical hypotheses on its nature and function, in general terms, many scholars, starting with Darwin, agree that it is caused by a contrast, a change or an unexpected contradiction and that, in order for it to manifest itself, the incongruence must be perceived within a social context. Bergson [35] argued that laughter strengthens the social relationships between individuals who laugh; recent contribution [12] highlights its strong connection with the social element, hypothesising that, by providing individuals with the possibility of finding new interpretations of reality, it can contribute to countering conflict and encouraging cooperation in social exchanges. A final fascinating question yet to be resolved concerns the relationship between laughter and smiling and the possibility of finding a continuum between the two expressive manifestations. In general, it can be noted that while laughter and smiling are closely connected and, to a certain extent, interchangeable, there remains the possibility of identifying situations in which specific causal and functional aspects occur consistent with the hypothesis of their having different origins.

REFERENCES

[1]   Ricci Bitti, P. E. (1995). Volto, personalità e comunicazione. In L. M. Lorenzetti (Ed.), *Psicologia e Personalità* (pp. 111-120). Milano: Franco Angeli.

[2]   Ceccarelli, F. (1988). *Sorriso e Riso. Saggio di Antropologia Biosociale*. Torino: Einaudi.

[3]   Darwin, C. (1872). *The expression of Emotion in Man and Animals*, London: John Murray, (3rd edition) London: Harper Collins Publishers, 1998.

[4]   Eibl-Eibesfeldt, I. (1970). *Ethology: the Biology of Behavior*. New York: Holt, Rinehart and Winston.

[5]   Ekman, P., and Friesen, W. (1969). The Repertoire of Non Verbal Behavior: Origins, Usage, Codings. *Semiotica*, *1*, 49-98.

[6]   Niedenthal, P. M., Mermillod, M., Maringer, M., and Hess, U. (2010). The Simulation of Smiles (SIMS) Model: Embodied Simulation and the Meaning of Facial Expression. *Behavioral and Brain Sciences*, *33*, 417-433.

[7]   Kipper, S., and Todt, D. (2003). The Role of Rhythm and Pitch in the Evaluation of Human Laughter. *Journal of Nonverbal Behavior, 27*(4), 255-272.

[8]   Szameitat D. P., Darwin, C. J., Szameitat, A. J., Wildgruber, D., and Alter, K. (2011). Formant characteristics of human laughter. *Journal of Voice*, *25*(1), 32-37.

[9]   Vettin, J., and Todt, D. (2004). Laughter in Conversation: Features of Occurrence and Acoustic Structure. *Journal of Nonverbal Behavior*, *28*(2), 93-115.

[10]   Ruch, W., and Ekman, P. (2001). The expressive pattern of laughter. In A. Kaszniak (Ed.), *Emotion, Qualia, and Consciousness* (pp. 426-443). Tokyo: Word Scientific Publisher.

[11]   Bachorowski, J. A., Smoski, M. J., and Owren, M. J. (2001). The acoustic features of human laughter. *Journal of Acoustical Society of America*, *110*(3), 1581-1597.

[12]   Keltner, D. (2009). *Born to be good. The Science of a Meaningful Life*. New York: W. W. Norton and Company.

[13] Birdwhistell, R. (1970). *Kinesics and Context*. Philadelphia: University of Pennsylvania Press.

[14] Ekman, P. (1972). Universal and cultural differences in facial expression of emotion. In J. R. Cole (Ed.), *Nebraska Symposium on Motivation, 1971, Vol. 19* (pp. 207-283). Lincoln, NE: Nebraska University Press.

[15] Harris, C. R., and Alvarado, N. (2005). Facial Expressions, Smile Types, and Self-report during Humor, Tickle, and Pain. *Cognition and Emotion, 19*, 655-699.

[16] Provine, R. R. (1993). Laughter Punctuates Speech: Linguistic, Social and Gender Contexts of Laughter. *Ethology, 95*, 291-298.

[17] Ekman, P. (2001). *Telling Lies: Clues to Deceit in the Marketplace, Politics, and Marriage* (3rd edition). New York: Norton.

[18] Ekman, P. (1985). *Telling Lies*. New York: Norton.

[19] Ekman, P., and Friesen, W. V. (1978). *Manual for Facial Action Coding System*. Palo Alto: Consulting Psychologist Press.

[20] Sackheim, H. A., Gur, R. C., and Saucy, M. (1978). Emotions are expressed more intensely on the left side of the face. *Science, 202*, 433- 435.

[21] Indersmitten, T., and Gur, R. C (2003). Emotion Processing in Chimeric Faces: Hemispheric Asymmetries in Expression and Recognition of Emotions. *The Journal of Neuroscience, 23*(9), 3820-3825.

[22] Làdavas, E., Umiltà, C., and Ricci-Bitti, P. E. (1980). Evidence for sex differences in right-hemisphere dominance for emotions. *Neuropsychologia, 18*(3), 361-366.

[23] Ricci Bitti, P. E., Caterina, R., and Garotti P. L. (2010). Qualità espressive del sorriso in differenti emozioni ed atteggiamenti interpersonali. In R. Galatolo, and R. Lorenzetti (Eds.), *Forme e spazi della comunicazione. Scritti in onore di Marina Mizzau* (pp. 241-250). Bologna: Clueb.

[24] Ricci Bitti, P. E., Caterina, R., and Garotti P. L. (2000). I segreti del sorriso. *Psicologia Contemporanea, 158*, 38-47.

[25] Frank, M. G., Ekman, P., and Friesen, W. V. (1993). Behavioral markers and recognizability of the smile of enjoyment. *Journal of Personality and Social Psychology, 64*(1), 83-93.

[26] Krumhuber, E., and Manstead, A. S. R. (2009). Can Duchenne Smiles Be Feigned? New Evidence on Felt and False Smiles. *Emotion, 9*(6), 807-820.

[27] Shore, D. M., and Heerey, E. A. (2011). The value of genuine and polite smiles. *Emotion, 11*(1),169-174.

[28] Papa, A., and Bonanno, G. A (2008). Smiling in the face of adversity: The interpersonal and intrapersonal functions of smiling. *Emotion, 8* (1), 1-12.

[29] Ricci Bitti, P. E., and Zani, B. (1983). *La comunicazione come Processo Sociale*. Bologna: Il Mulino.

[30] Solano, L. (2006). Emozioni e salute. In A. Mauri, and C. Tinti (Eds.), *Psicologia della Salute* (pp. 42-67). Novara: De Agostini Scuola.

[31] Owren, M. J., and Bachorowski, J. A. (2001). The evolution of emotional experience: A 'selfish-gene' account of smiling and laughter in early hominids and humans. In T. J. Mayne, and G. A. Bonanno (Eds.), *Emotions: Currrent Issues and Future Directions* (pp. 152-191). New York: Guilford Press.

[32] Ricci Bitti, P. E., and Cortesi, S. (1977). *Comportamento Non Verbale e Comunicazione*. Bologna: Il Mulino.

[33] Ambrose, J. A. (1969). The development of the smiling, response in early infancy. In B.M. Foss (Ed.), *Determinants of Infant Behaviour, Vol.I* (pp. 179-201). London: Methuen.

[34] Bowlby, J (1969). *Attacchment and Loss: I, Attacchment*. London: Hogarth Press.

[35] Bergson, H. (1900). *Le Rire. Essai sur la Signification du Comique*. Revue de Paris. (5th edition), Paris: Alcan, 1908.

In: Humor and Health Promotion
Editor: Paola Gremigni

Chapter 4

A MODEL OF HUMOR SYNTONY: FROM FAILED TO SUCCESSFUL HUMOR IN INTERACTION

Carla Canestrari

Research Centre for Psychology of Communication, University of Macerata, Macerata, Italy

ABSTRACT

In this chapter a model of syntonic and non-syntonic humorous interactions is discussed and supported by a corpus-based analysis.

The syntonic or non-syntonic dimension of a humorous interaction is due to the presence or lack of an attuning between two or more interactants which is observable on the basis of three variables that play a central role in defining a humorous interaction as syntonic or not: 1) a detectable humorous structure of the linguistic features of a verbal humorous stimulus (as specified by the General Theory of Verbal Humor); 2) the meta-communicative humorous signals used by the interlocutors to build a humorous frame (such as those outlined within the field of Conversational and Discourse Analysis), 3) the psychological implications of recognition, comprehension and appreciation of a humorous stimulus (as specified by Hay [1]) which are disclosed by the addressee of a humorous stimulus.

The analysis of the presence or lack of one or more of the three variables against a corpus of humorous dialogues is shown. As a result, the interactants' moves may range widely from failed humor to playing along. Such moves are represented by a model of syntonic and non-syntonic humorous interactions, which resulted to be organized in seven levels depending on the degree of humorous syntony reached by interlocutors.

Clearly, the model presented here may be considered as a tool to monitor an on-going communication, included the therapeutic ones.

INTRODUCTION

Among the several kinds of humorous communication, such as written (e.g. collections of jokes) or drawn humor (e.g. cartoons), the present chapter is focussed on the dialogical one.

Therefore, the attention is on the face-to face interactive dimension of conversation where at least two interlocutors are involved. The object of this chapter is humorous exchange, considered as a peculiar way to interact with other people.

When we say something is humorous our goal is, intuitively, to be funny and when someone tells us something humorous we do our best to make the attempt of being funny successful, at least in case we cooperate. During the on-going communication a humorous attempt is constantly and, more or less, unconsciously monitored by the interlocutors in order to get its gains, in terms of amusement and social appreciation, or, if it failed, to repair it. Successful and failed humorous interactions can be adduced on the basis of communicative and descriptive elements. In fact, since '70s, several scholars, interested in the pragmatics of humorous communication, have pointed out how a successful humorous interaction works, from the conversational point of view, by means of corpus-based analysis, e.g. [2-10]. In the last few years, the same methodology has been applied to the study of conversational cases of failed humor in everyday talk [11-14].

Up to now an analytic knowledge on successful and failed humorous conversations has been achieved, so it is time to fruitfully turn back to it to gain a synthetic tool which embraces both syntonic (or successful) and non-syntonic (or failed) humorous dimensions of face- to-face interactions.

Successful and failed attempts of humorous conversations can be considered as the extreme poles of a continuum. This idea was applied to the analysis of a corpus of filmic dialogues by Canestrari and Attardo [15] with the aim of micro-analytically describing how the interlocutors succeed or fail in co-constructing a humorous sequence and to macro-analytically provide a model of humorous syntony, to monitor the humorous level of a communication. In this chapter a revisited and updated model of syntonic and not-syntonic humorous interactions is shown. The aim of this paper is to generalise the model of humor syntony previously proposed [15] on the basis of a comparison of the results coming from the model to the findings of the studies on humor in spontaneous contexts. Moreover, a revisited version of it is provided on the basis of stringent methodological steps.

The model presented in this chapter is thought to monitor the humorous syntony of an interaction, generally considered, and could be useful also in the therapeutic context.

TOOLS OF ANALYSIS

From the methodological point of view, one of the first aspects to take into account is how to distinguish the humorous turns from others in a conversation. This point has been explicitly considered poorly by Conversation Analysis (CA) and Discourse Analysis (DA), which represent the main frames of reference in the study of humor in interaction. Usually, meta-communicative signals, such as laughter, have been considered as a symptom of humorous sequences, since they meta-communicate the message "this is play" [16]. The most used criterion for a collection of spontaneous humorous sequences includes all those signals, such as tone of the voice and audience reactions, on which basis it is possible to infer the speaker's intention to be funny [1, p. 56], [6, p. 8]. This criterion clearly excludes cases of unintentional humor and sequences reframed as humorous by the audience. In general, the presence in a performance of humorous signals, which are interpreted on the basis of the analyst's humor competence, results in being the most adopted tool of detection of humorous sequences. On one hand, the indexes that can occur in humorous sequences may be present also in other kinds of conversations, as in the case of laughter [17]. On the other hand, basing the analysis on the analyst's own humor competence risks affecting the reliability of the analysis. These limits can be overcome by applying the two-pronged analytical model of humorous interactions proposed by Canestrari [18]. A humorous text is supposed to contain a textual humorous structure and, sometimes, meta-communicative signals, used by the interlocutors to define the humorous frame of their conversation. On the basis of these two assumptions, such a structure should be identified according to a theory (first phase), and the presence or the lack of meta-communicative signals and their qualities can then be monitored, in agreement with the tools provided by CA and DA (second phase). As for the first phase, the incongruity-resolution approach to humor states that a humorous text is structured in an incongruity and its resolution. Several cognitive theories stress this point and belong to this general approach, such as the bisociation theory by Koestler [19], the two-stage model by Suls [20], the frame bisociation by Norrick [21], Oring's appropriate incongruity [22], the comprehension-elaboration theory of elicitation of humor by Wyer and Collins [23], the concept of delicate balance of congruity and incongruity stressed by Forabosco [24], some cognitive-perceptual studies [25-31], the linguistic theory by Raskin [32] and its evolution into the General Theory of Verbal Humor [33,34] considered as a cognitive linguistic theory [34-37], especially after the application of Giora's [38-43] graded salience theory. An exhaustive synthesis of the cited studies can be found in Chapter 2 of this book, in Dynel [44], Forabosco [24,45], and in Martin [46]. A central aspect of the studies cited so far is that a humorous text is structured in an incongruity and a resolution, which can be recognized by a hearer/reader. Among the several approaches to the analysis of the humorous structure of a text, the General Theory of Verbal Humor (GTVH) results in being the most appropriate here, given that it provides a formalization of the linguistic structure of a humorous text and that its application to the analysis of humorous interactions (conversational narratives as well as filmic dialogues) has been verified by Archakis e Tsakona [47], Brock [48], and Canestrari [18]. Among the six Knowledge Resources pointed out in the GTVH, the script opposition and the logical mechanism are the necessary ones because they correspond to the incongruity and resolution [35] and on them the perception of similarity between two humorous texts relies [49].

As for the second phase, it should be clarified what the signals indicate. According to Hay's analysis [1] of the humorous reception of a stimulus, an interlocutor crosses three scalar implicatures: the recognition of the humorous frame of the stimulus, the comprehension of the humorous content and the appreciation of the humorous attempt. The first implicature refers to the interlocutor's ability to decode the meta-communicative signals of a stimulus, in order to detect the humorous frame. The second is a *eureka* moment: when the incongruity, or script opposition, of a humorous text is resolved by means of a logical mechanism, the interlocutor gets the humorous stimulus. The third implicature occurs when the interlocutor feels amused by the humorous attempt and implies an agreement with the humorous content[1]. They are organized into a hierarchy: a humorous attempt may be

---

[1] Hay [1] posits that "agreement" is the fourth implicature of her model and that it turns out to be explicit when the humorous attempt is appreciated and followed by a negative remark on its content. For example a speaker may note that a joke is offensive after having laughed at it.

appreciated if it has been previously comprehended and, at first, recognized. Hay's analysis provides an operative definition of failed and successful humor if associated to the GTVH, as a tool to single out the humorous structure of a stimulus, and the CA, as a methodology to analyse the humorous frame of an interaction. The three implicatures of humor processing, namely recognition, comprehension, and appreciation [1], can be monitored on the basis of the presence or lack of humorous meta-communicative signals (such as those listed by Canestrari [18] on the basis of CA approach) and are justified when the supposed humorous stimulus is structured in a script opposition and a logical mechanism (pointed out by the GTVH). On the basis of the three-fold approach to the corpus described above, several levels of syntonic and non-syntonic humorous interactions were pointed out [15].

CORPUS

A characteristic of the model, which may turn out to be only apparently its main limit, is that it was based on filmic conversations, whereas it aimed at describing humorous dynamics in general and in this chapter two conversational domains, movie and everyday interactions, are merged. This limit can be easily overcame since Rossi [50-52] demonstrated that the filmic sequences performed by the Italian comic actor Totò, who is also the main character of the corpus of filmic dialogues considered to build the model, share the same structure and several conversational phenomena with everyday conversations. Moreover, Rossi [51] analysed the dialogues coming from six Italian movies of the same period but different in genre, in order to verify how distant they are from everyday conversations. Among the six movies, the one played by Totò resulted in being the closer to spontaneous interactions, since the two domains share several conversational patterns. Later on, it was demonstrated that the specific corpus considered for the model, made up of two movies performed by Totò, and shares several conversational aspects with everyday humorous conversations [53].

Moreover, mostly in the field of dubbing, it has been demonstrated that artificially written-to-be-spoken conversations can be considered as mirrors of everyday conversations: the same conversational patterns, such as discourse markers and phraseological elements, occur in dubbing and in spoken discourse, in order to make a filmic conversation as authentic as possible [54-57]. The filmic dialogues performed by Totò and everyday conversations are very close to one another. Therefore, the fact that the two domains are convergent enables us to merge the results coming from the two domains and to generalise the use of the model to the humorous verbal interactions.

RESULTS AND DISCUSSION

Cases Excluded from the Model

The application of the three tools of analysis to the corpus produced a first important result: there are some kinds of humorous interactions that cannot be taken into account while some others can.

Example (1)[2]. is drawn from the Italian comic movie "*Totò, Peppino e la malafemmina*", performed by the Italian comic actors Totò and Peppino. The humorous sequence revolves around the fact the *maître* is a very tall man and it is built on the misunderstanding introduced in line 4 and culminating in a punch line in turn 5:

(1)   1 Totò: veramente volevamo parlare con il cameriere
         1 actually we would like to speak to a waiter
         2 Maître: appunto io sono il maître (.)
         2 that's it i am a maître(.)
         3 Peppino: {a Totò} che ha detto?
         3{to Totò} what did he say?
         4 Totò: è un metro
         4 he is a meter
         5 Peppino: (.) ah un metro (.) se li porta bene i centimetri però
         5 (.) uh one meter (.) he doesn't look his centimetres
         6 Totò: {al maître} molto piacere (.) prego si accomodi
         6 {to the maître} nice to meet you (.) sit down please

The application of the GTVH to the above example should clarify the humorous structure of the text in terms of script opposition and logical mechanism. The incongruity lays on two opposite scripts, namely "tall", expressed by the physical quality of the *maître*, and "short", introduced by the word "*metro*/meter", and their resolution is possible thanks to the juxtaposition, which represents the logical mechanism, between two assonant words: "*maître*" and "*metro*/meter".

Once the humorous structure of an interaction is verified according to a theory, for example the GTVH (first phase), the analysis of the signals used by the interlocutors to build a humorous frame can be carried out (second phase). In Example (1) no signals are available. In fact, the interlocutors talk to each other as if a serious communication was going on. This phenomenon can be explained in light of the filmic nature of the dialogue: the perception of the humorous key of the sequence is completely up to the audience to whom a possible syntonic interaction is addressed. Cases like this are very common, at least in the movie "*Siamo uomini o caporali?*" performed by Totò: 57 out of 80 verbal humorous sequences contain a humorous structure but no humorous frame is built [18]. The fact that no humorous frame is built, nullifies the humorous interaction between the two interlocutors. Therefore, cases such as Example (1) are excluded from the model.

Also the following excerpt, drawn from the same movie as Example (1), makes the analysis of the syntonic humorous level impossible. The editor of a scandal magazine is trying to persuade Totò to say he is the eye witness of a crime that he had never seen.

---

[2] The transcription model employed in this chapter is based on Jefferson's model [58] with some additions:
    ?   ascending tone;
    .   descending tone;
    (.)   brief pause;
    h   audible expiration;
    :   prolonged sound;
    -       truncated word;
    [ ]   overlap;
    { }   includes important non-verbal information;
    ˘ ˘   includes laughter;
    EMPHASIS block letters.

(2) 1 editor: lei ha sentito un urlo invocante aiuto si è precipitato (.)e ha visto il cadavere (.)
     1 you heard someone calling out for help you rushed (.) and you saw the dead body (.)
     2 Totò: cadavere?
     2 dead body?
     3 editor: già
     3 that's right
     4 Totò: quale?
     4 which?
     5 editor: come lei (.) non ha visto il cadavere?
     5 what? didn't you see the dead body
     6 Totò: quale cadavere
     6 what dead body
     7 editor: ˘ehehe˘ ma che SIMPATIC˘h˘O ma che simpati-˘ ehehe˘
     7 ˘ahahah˘ how FUNN˘h˘Y how funn-˘ahah˘

In the interaction above there are no script opposition and logical mechanism, but the editor is acting as if there were by using several meta-communicative signals in line 7: he laughs loudly and says twice "how funny" with emphasis and interposing laughing. Clearly, there is no humorous syntony between the speakers because there is no humorous stimulus.

In contrast to the two examples, the analysis of the syntonic dimension of a humorous communication presented in this chapter takes into account those interactions where meta-communicative humorous signals are detectable and the stimulus is structured in an incongruity and its resolution (see Table 1). If both conditions are satisfied, inferences on humorous intention, recognition, comprehension and/or appreciation can be carried out.

In fact, cases such as Example (1) provide no humorous frame. On the contrary, examples such as Excerpt (2), where an empty frame is built, are not taken into account by the model of syntonic and non-syntonic humorous interactions presented in this chapter, because of the lack of a humorous structure.

Table 1. Synthesis of the applicability of the model depending on the presence or lack of humorous frame and content

	Humorous Frame (meta-communicative signals)	Humorous Content (script opposition and logical mechanism)
Cases excluded from the model	No	Yes
	Yes	No
Cases accounted for by the model	Yes	Yes

The examples in the last line of Table 1 are analysed in the next two paragraphs, which focus on the results pertaining to the model of syntonic and non-syntonic humorous interactions, which is organized in seven hierarchy levels. The exemplifications of these levels are clearly not exhaustive: the same level can take different forms, but maintain the peculiarities described by the model.

FAILED HUMOR AND LEVELS OF NON-SYNTONIC HUMOROUS INTERACTIONS

Non-syntonic humorous interactions are determined by failed humor and are characterized by: 1) the presence of a humorous stimulus, namely a script opposition and a logical mechanism; 2) the speaker's intention to be humorous, which is gathered on the basis of meta-communicative signals; 3) the lack of one of the three implicatures, which is inferred on the analysis of the meta-communicative aspects. Depending on which implicature is not achieved, three levels can be outlined.

Level 1

At the lowest level the humorous attempt fails due to a lack of recognition, as in the following case. Excerpt (3) is drawn from the same movie as Example (1), the scene takes place in Milan and Marisa is ironically teasing Lucia because of her strong southern Italian dialect:

(3) 1 Marisa: bell'accento milanese eh?
    1 {behind Lucia and smiling} what a nice milanese accent ah?
    2 Lucia: noi napoletani abbiamo molto orecch- (.) ci basta stare poche ore su un posto che
    3 subbito apprendiamo
    2 we neapolitans are very receptive (.) we immediately learn after few hours spent in
    3 a new place

The humorous intention of Marisa is disclosed by her smiling and changing the tone of her voice, as is typical in irony [59], besides the evident contradiction of the semantic content. Lucia replies seriously. It can be hypothesized that Lucia's reply reveals a lack in recognizing the ironic meaning, since Lucia cannot see Marisa's smile, or that it is a strategy to disregard the humorous attempt by pretending she does not bridge the ironic gap. In both cases, from the descriptive point of view a lack of recognition is detected.

Level 2

The presence of recognition by the interlocutor characterizes the second level of non-syntonic humorous interactions. At this level the humor fails on account of comprehension. In such a situation the interlocutor may pretend to have understood the humorous mechanism and disclose fake laughter or groaning [10]. Otherwise, the lack of comprehension can be overtly declared by the hearer, as in the example of the "singing telegram" provided by Norrick [8, pp. 179-180] as a case of spontaneous conversational joking.

The first two levels of non-syntonic humor resulted in being quite common in spontaneous conversations among native and non-native speakers: due to their linguistic limits, the latter may fail to recognize a humorous frame, or to process language at elocutionary level, or to understand the meaning of words or the pragmatic force of an utterance [13, pp. 430-433].

Level 3

Finally, a humorous interaction may fail on account of appreciation. This case is present in everyday conversations [11], [12] as well as in the filmic corpus. The following example is taken from the movie "*Siamo uomini o caporali?*", Totò is waiting for an interview and next to him a woman and her pretty daughter are sitting. The girl is applying for a job as a dancer and her mother is complaining about waiting so long, in spite of the beautiful daughter's legs, as if that was enough to be called immediately:

(4) 1 mother: con queste gambe {guarda le gambe della figlia} è un'ORA che stiamo facendo
     2 anticamera
     1. with her legs{looks at her daughter's legs} we have been waiting for
     2 an HOUR
     3 Totò: signora ci vuole pazienza vede anche io con QUESTE GAMBE facciol'anticamera
     4 ˘eh eh˘
     3 lady you have to be patient as you can see i have been waiting for an hour too with
     4 MY LEGS {he shows his legs} ˘ah ah˘
     5 mother: {astonished face}

The humorous stimulus is delivered and signalled by Totò in line 3, by comparing the attractive and female girl's legs to his own, with the aim of teasing the woman. The mother's surprised face in line 5 shows the lack of appreciation of the teasing and this reply makes the interaction non-syntonic from the humorous point of view. This excerpt of filmic dialogue results in being very similar to the domain of spontaneous conversations: according to Drew's study [4] teasing is rejected in the majority of the 50 cases he investigated, as in Example (5). Probably the rejection is due to the perception of teasing as a sarcastic manner to interact. Moreover, Drew [4] pointed out that teasing is a phenomenon tightly linked to the conversation where it takes place, in the sense that it occurs after an exaggeration performed by the interlocutor. In Example (5) the woman is complaining excessively.

At the third level of non-syntonic humorous interactions, appreciation is not achieved and the conversational strategies used by interlocutors to disclose a refusal of the humorous attempt can even be impolite and aggressive [11], [12]. This kind of rude responses to failed humor occurs easily when an interlocutor says intentionally a poor joke, as in the study carried out by Bell [11], [12].

The results of Bell's study fit in only the third level of non-syntonic humorous interactions, since the definition of failed humor considered by Bell is limited to those cases characterized by recognition, comprehension but not appreciation [11, p. 1827]. Examples of replies used to signal lack of amusement are: interjections (e.g., "oooh" and "mmm") performed with a falling intonation or in a sarcastic way, fake or forced laughs, ironic evaluation (e.g., "good one"), sarcasm (e.g., "are you drunk?"), topic changes, and so on [11], [12]. The results found in Bell's study are not exhaustive of non-appreciated humor responses, since the replies were elicited by canned and childish or poor jokes, performed as if they were spontaneous. A comparison to spontaneous conversational joking is advocated by the author herself [11, p. 1835].

The strategies used to repair a failed humorous attempt represent an almost unexplored aspect. An exception is Montague's study [60] aimed at investigating failed humor in the context of public speech, in particular stand-up comedy. On the basis of self-reports, 102 comedians were surveyed and it resulted that the more a stand-up comedian feels her/his humor inappropriate, on the basis of the audience's reactions, the more s/he seeks for a repair in order to restore his/her image and regain audience's approval. Moreover, the comedians reported three kinds of repair: apologizing, explaining the joke, and performing self-deprecating humor [60, pp. 22-23].

According to Song's analysis [61] a humorous communication can fail on account of recognition, understanding or appreciation: a joke recipient may miss one of the three implicatures when the joke teller violates some rules, related to the six Knowledge Resources (from now on they are indicated by the initial capital letters) put forward by the GTVH. A joke teller may fail on account of:

1. Language: the speaker is redundant or uses words not capable of an immediate switch from one script to another;
2. Narrative Strategy: the timing to deliver the punch line is violated or the joke teller discloses the funniness, especially at the end of the joke;
3. Target: the butt of the joke is not relevant to one of the two opposed scripts; for example, for a dumb joke to work, the conventional stupid group of a society should be hit, since one of the script involved is "stupidity";
4. Situation: the content of the joke is not aligned to the recipient;
5. Logical Mechanism: the humor is too easy, as in the knock-knock joke or other childish episodes, or too difficult to get;
6. Script Opposition: the opposition of two scripts does not produce a surprising effect.

According to a corpus based analysis carried out by Priego-Valverde [14], humor can fail when it is not perceived or if it is refused by the interlocutor. She explains these two phenomena by applying the Bakhtinian double voicing approach: in the first case of failed humor, the hearer misses the locutor's playful voice and takes into account only the serious one.

In the second case, the hearer chooses to consider only the serious voice and refuses the playful one. To sum up the above cited studies, it results that: cases of failed humor can occur for several reasons [13], [61]; from the conversational point of view they are signalled [11], [12]; the GTVH as well as the Bakthinian double voicing analysis fit well the analysis of failed humor respectively from the linguistic and dialogical points of view [61], [14].

SUCCESSFUL HUMOR AND LEVELS OF SYNTONIC HUMOROUS INTERACTIONS

After a humorous attempt is recognized, comprehended and also appreciated, a syntonic humorous interaction may occur. Four levels of humorous syntony were detected in the corpus, ranging from an almost full appreciation to mode adoption.

Level 4

The first three levels are exemplified in the same scene, which has been broken down into three sequences. They are reported from the lowest to the highest level of humorous syntony, even though they are placed in the scene in the exact opposed order. The original progression is revealed by the numeration assigned to the turns. Just to give a brief description of the scene, Totò is having dinner in a luxury restaurant, where a lady with her husband asks for his autograph. Totò accepts and gains knowledge of her surname, Ossobuco, and her place of origin, Naples. Totò, who probably thinks that Ossobuco is the lady's maiden name, wants to know her married name, in order to write her a dedication. In line 11 he asks for this information with an ambiguous manner, which may serve to know both married and maiden names. The lady replies that Gennaro was dead, but did not disambiguate that Gennaro was her father, therefore her maiden name, and that the man who is with her is her husband. In fact, the surprised remark by Totò in line 13 reveals the misunderstanding and refers to the man who is physically present in the scene. In line 14 the lady clarifies the situation and introduces the topic of her father's death, which lays the ground for the teasing in line 21:

```
(5)   23 Totò:     eh di?
      23            {expression meaning "wife or daughter of" }
      24 Madam: no fu gennaro
      24             no, he was the late gennaro
      25 Totò:     che strano credevo fosse stato suo marito
      25            odd i thought he was your husband
      26 Madam: no: fu gennaro papà:
      26            no: gennaro was my fa:ther
      27 Totò:     ah fu gennaro papà
      27            oh the late gennaro was your father
      28 Madam: papà è morto
      28             my father is dead
      29 Totò:     ah è morto mi dispiace
      29            oh he's dead i'm sorry
      30 Madam: povero paparino
      30             poor daddy
      31 Totò:     eh: esequie signora faccio le mie esequie
      31            my obsequies madame my obsequies³
      32 Madam: hh grazie
      32            hh thank you
      33 Totò:     poteva morire suo marito era meglio
      33            it'd've been better if your husband had died {smiling, he gently shoves her arm
                   with his hand twice}
      34 Madam: no ˘ahah˘ perché poverino [˘ah ah˘]
      34            no ˘ah ah˘ why poor thing? [˘uh uh˘]
      35 Totò:                              [io]io scherzo
      35                                    [just] kidding
      36 Madam: sì lo so
      36            yes i know
```

---

³ The assonance between the Italian words "ossequi homage" (as in "pay homage to") and "esequie obsequies" is
   enough to produce a humorous moment. From the communicative point of view, this case is analogous to
   Example (1).

The lowest level of syntonic humorous interactions is represented by Example (5), where a sequence of teasing occurs. The first pair of the sequence is in line 21. According to Alberts' definition [62], teases include a serious and a playful dimension [62, p. 158]. In Example (5) the serious message serves to create complicity with the lady at her husband's expense, husband who was introduced as a poor authoritative man at the beginning of the scene. The humorous aspect lays in the exaggeration of the content and in the playful frame, signalled Totò's smiling face and his gentle jostle of woman's arm in line 21 and by the verbal reassurance in line 23. The second pair of the sequence is made of the mixed reply provided by the woman in line 22, which reveals that the humorous attempt has not been completely appreciated or refused. In Hay's terminology [1], the lady appreciated but did not agree. Due to its ambivalent nature, this example is located approximately in the middle of the continuum of the syntonic and non-syntonic humorous interactions model.

Level 5

In the following sequence, which exemplifies the second level of syntonic humorous interactions, Totò ascertains the correct spelling of the lady's name:

```
(6)  17 Totò:     o: mi dica un po' ossobuco co- con due buchi (.) ossobbu-
     17           oh listen ossobuco wi- with two holes(.) ossobbu-
     18 Madam: no con con una b
     18        no with just one b
     19 Totò:     ah con un buco solo (.) ˇuh uhˇ ossobuco con un buco solo
     19 {serious face}ah: just one hole(.)ˇuh uhˇossobuco with just one hole
     20 Madam: [ˇha ha ha: hee hee heeˇ]
     20        [ˇhu hu hu: ha ha ha ha ha haˇ]
     21 Totò:     [{risata afona} ossob(.)uco con un bu(.)co solo (.) le risate]
     21        [{silent laughter} ossob(.)uco with one ho(.)le only what a laugh]
     22 Madam: ˇah ahˇ che simpa- ˇih ih ihˇ
     22        uh uhˇ that's funny- ˇeh eh ehˇ (.)
```

Example (6) is a case of unintentional humor: in line 19 Totò realizes the funniness of what he has just said. The letter "B" is confused with the word "*buco*/hole" (incongruity), by means of juxtaposition because "*buco*" is part of the name he is writing down (resolution). From the communicative point of view the humorous attempt is later signalled by the locutor: in lines 19 and 21 Totò laughs and also repeats the humorous words to stress their funniness in a similar way that happens in spontaneous conversations, where the echoing is performed by hearers [1,7]. The woman supports the humorous attempt in turns 20 and 22 by laughing and by a verbal appreciation.

Level 6

The next level is more syntonic than the previous one due to the speaker's intention to be humorous. This prototypic humorous sequence is exemplified by the following excerpt:

(7) 1 Totò: il suo cognome signora per cortesia
     1   your last name, madame, please
     2 Madam: ossobuco
     3 Totò: ossobuco?
     4 Madam: sì
                  yes
     5 Totò: ossobuco
     6 Madam: mhm
     7 Totò: milanese
     8 Madam: no napoletana
     8   no neapolitan
     9 Totò: e a napoli ci sono gli ossobuchi?
     9   and are there ossobuchis in naples?
     10 Madam: tanti ce ne sono eh
     10   lots of them
     11 Totò: sì: deve essere una famiglia(.) importante vero?
     11   ye:s must be an important (.) family, right?
     12 Madam: ma forse
     12   maybe
     13 Totò: gli ossobuchi sono milanesi
     13   {smiling} the ossobuchis are milanese
     14 Madam: ah sì? ˘ha ah ah˘
     14   oh is that so? ˘hu hu hu˘
     15 Totò: o meglio lombardi (.) [lombardi]
     15   or better they're lombards (.) [lombards]
     16 Madam: [˘ha ha˘]
     16 Madam: [˘hu hu˘]

Totò asks the lady her surname and, intrigued by the word "Ossobuco", he guesses she is from Milan (line 7), since "ossobuco" is a typical Milanese dish. A false reasoning allows the joker to switch from a script (a surname) to another (food). In line 13 Totò signals his intentional humorous attempt by smiling and the madam appreciates it by laughing in lines 14 and 16.

Level 7

In the previous two levels, the strategies used to support humor as described by Hay [1] are very frequent. Among them, the model presented here comprises of "playing along with the gag" not merely as a strategy of humor support, but as the highest level of achieved humorous syntony. This distinction follows the one made by Davies [63] who distinguishes between cooperation and collaboration in the joking activity. The first case comprises of those interactions where the humorous attempt performed by a locutor is supported by the interlocutor, then it can be assimilated to the first three levels of humorous syntonic model. In the second case, which corresponds to the highest level of humorous syntony, the interlocutor replies playing along with the humorous attempt of the locutor. Such a level is referred to here as mode adoption. For example, a joke-telling mode of communication takes place when "a playful, mirthful, humor mood prevails between the speakers and hearer(s)" [32, p. 141]. A mode can be adopted when the hearer replies to a speaker using the same type of implicature or mode used by the speaker herself/himself, as Attardo [64] pointed out. Mode adoption is a conversational phenomenon usually referred to as playing along, joining in the joking or in general humorous attempts, punning for instance [6], [65], that elicit further attempts of the same genre.

In the example below, taken from a naturally occurring conversation [1, p.66], the speakers are three women who are punning around the double meaning carried out by the word "pulses". In line 4 DF pretends to misunderstand the word "pulses" used by BF in line 3. DF goes on punning and teasing CF in line 4, by introducing "kidney beans". In line 8 CF goes along with the joke and adds the word "lentils". From this point on CF becomes the joker and she delivers another punch line in turn 10

(8)   1CF: i mean i've got bad feelings in my hands anyway
      2BF: have you
      3CF: like i can never feel pulses or stuff like like you know
      4DF: pulses what like beans? like beans? you mean
      5BF: NO
      6DF: pulses you mean [kidney beans] and the like
      7CF: [yeah]
      8CF: and lentils
      9BF: oh does she ˘h˘
      10CF: i find it really hard to feel lentils

The first attempt at humor, made in line 4 by DF, is an invitation to play. The other interlocutors could reply refusing the invitation and going on with the serious frame. The move made by CF is to play along with the joker, showing mode adoption: she introduces the word "lentils" in line 8 and goes on with that topic in line 10.

According to Davies' analysis [63, pp. 1366-1367], what is referred to here as mode adoption consists of confirming the joking initiator's utterance, for example by mirroring the prosodic form or repeating the same words s/he used, and adding something different within the same frame set out by the initiator or introducing a new way of playing, for example running from an initial ironic mode addressed to a third party to a self-parody. In Example (8) CF confirms DF, who is the joking initiator, by adopting the same prosody and by showing an analogous word choice (from "beans" and "kidney beans" to "lentils") in line 8, and adds something more in line 10 restructuring the utterance she has performed in line 3, so that "feel pulses" turns out as "feel lentils".

This peculiar way of interacting has also been found also in spontaneous interactions among nine-year old children, for what pertains to irony: at this age they are able to deliver ironic comments and to adopt this mode in reply [66]. In spite of the early acquisition of mode adoption, at least as for irony, it results in being the less used option to interact within a humorous frame.

According to Attardo's meta-analysis [64] of 5 different studies that investigated the pragmatic aspects of humorous spontaneous conversations on the basis of corpora of everyday talk, mode adoption results in being a rare phenomenon: only 3 out of 50 cases (6%) of teasing reported by Drew [4] can be assimilated to mode adoption; 22 out of 109 instances (20,2%) of playful insult (or "jocular abuse") analysed by Hay [67] correspond to mode adoption; Kotthoff [68] demonstrated that mode adopting is more frequent when the conversations take place in an informal context, such as dinner with friends, than in the TV debates she took into account, where only one example of mode adoption occurred; 33% of the 289 ironic occurrences reported by Gibbs [69] present mode adoption; mode adoption results to be less preferred when ironic/sarcastic interactions occur: 26 out of 395 responses to ironic/sarcastic occurrences (6,58%) are cases of mode adoption [70].

A similar result comes from the analysis of the filmic corpus described above: out of 26 humorous interactions where at least one interlocutor builds a humorous frame, only one case of mode adoption seems to take place. Interestingly, it is the only case where the humorous attempt is not performed by the character Totò.

The following example comes from the movie "*Siamo uomini o caporali?*" and the scene takes place in the police headquarters and Totò is dressed up as a woman and is supposed to be a prostitute. Totò is sitting next to real prostitutes and asks the policeman if he can speak to the police commissioner:

(9) 1 Totò: voglio parlare col commissario
     1   i want to speak to the commissioner of police
     2 policeman: vuoi parlare col commissario
     2   you want to speak to the commissioner of police
     3 Totò: dai dai dai
     3   come on come on come on
     4 policeman: adesso ti facciamo parlare col PRESIDENTE DELLA REPUBBLICA
     4   now we will let you speak to the PRESIDENT OF THE REPUBLIC
     5 prostitutes: ˇahah[ahah]ˇ
     5   ˇuhu[huh]ˇ
     6 Totò: [eh sp]iritoso
     6   [you're fu]nny
     {20 seconds of dialogue are cut}
     7 prostitute 1: ma chi sarà mai
     7   who is she
     8 prostitute2: e no la vedete (.) ava gardner
     8   don't you see it (.) ava gardner
     9 prostitutes: ˇah ah ah ahˇ
     9   ˇuh uh uhˇ

In the example above Totò is the butt of the sardonic jokes performed by the policeman in line 4 and supported by the prostitutes in line 5, and by prostitute 2 in line 8, who is again supported by the other prostitutes in line 9. The joke initiator is the policeman who pokes at fun Totò by an hyperbole performed with emphasis in a sarcastic mode in line 4. The same prosody is adopted by prostitute 2 who adds to the initiator's utterance a new aspect to laugh at, namely Totò's ugliness.

Examples (8) and (9) could be defined as a case of mode adoption, since they fit the main characteristics of playing along as identified by Davies [63], but they show two main differences. The first lays on the kind of humor involved: jocular teasing in Example (8) and sarcasm in (9). This difference confirms that the definition of mode adoption does not deal with affiliative-aggressive humor dimension: since the boundary between the two extreme poles of this dimension is not a clear-cut one, the definition of mode adoption is based on the descriptive structure of an interaction. The second difference is about timing: in Example (8) mode adoption occurs after a few turns following the joke initiator's utterance, then they behave as an adjacent pair. On the contrary, in Example (9) the initiator's utterance and the adoption are divided by several turns, not reported in the transcription, which are coherent with the whole conversation and where a ping pong of sarcastic accusations and defences between Totò and some of the interlocutors takes place. This phenomenon raises the possibility that mode adoption is a sequence which can occur as adjacency pairs or take the form of insert sequences.

CONCLUSION

A descriptive model of humorous interactions covering the entire dimension ranging from failed to successful humor up to now has not been thought up. The only exceptions are Attardo's analysis [64] and Canestrari and Attardo's model [15] which represent the starting point of the study presented in this chapter.

The model of syntonic and non-syntonic humorous interactions shown in this chapter provides a description of hierarchy organized cases of failed and successful humorous interactions, on the basis of three tools of analysis: 1)the GTVH, which serves to define a text as humorous on the basis of a peculiar linguistic structure; 2) the detection of humorous meta-communicative signals, on which basis it is possible to build a humorous frame and infer which implication is gained; 3) three cognitive implications, namely recognition of the humorous attempt, comprehension of the humorous structure of a stimulus and appreciation of it.

Given a corpus of filmic humorous dialogues the three tools were tested and their synchronic application against it produced a model of syntonic (or successful) and non-syntonic (or failed) humorous interactions. The filmic nature of the corpus taken into account may weaken the model. Then, the results obtained on the basis of the chosen corpus were compared to those of studies that investigated successful or failed humor in naturally occurring conversations. Since the findings in the two domains, filmic and natural, confirm each other, it is possible to generalize the model so that it accounts for face-to face interactions, independently from their fictional or spontaneous nature.

The potentiality of the model can be expressed by its application to an actual conversation, particularly when it is applied by the interlocutors themselves. In fact, bearing in mind which are the seven levels may help in coping with failed humor and in performing more and more syntonic humorous interactions. In particular, in the therapeutic context, where humor is advocated as a technique (see Chapter 9 of this book), the model can be used as a tool to monitor the level of syntony achieved, then possible changes toward one of the two extreme poles of the continuum can be reported.

FILMOGRAPHY

Siamo uomini o caporali? (1955) by Camillo Mastrocinque. Starring Totò (Totò Esposito), Paolo Stoppa (various corporals), Fiorella Mari (Sonia). Story by Totò. Screenplay by Vittorio Metz, Francesco Nelli, Mario Mangini, Camillo Mastrocinque and Totò. Produced by Lux Film (Ponti-De Laurentiis studios).

Totò, Peppino e la...malafemmina (1956) by Camillo Mastrocinque. Starring Totò (Antonio), Peppino De Filippo (Peppino), Dorian Gray (malafemmina). Story by Nicola Mannari. Screenplay by Camillo Mastrocinque, Eduardo Anton, Alessandro Continenza, Francesco Thellung. Produced by D.D.L. Cineriz.

REFERENCES

[1]   Hay, J. (2001). The pragmatics of humor support. *Humor: International Journal of Humor Research, 14(1),* 55-82.
[2]   Bonaiuto, M., Castellana, E., and Pierro, A. (2003). Arguing and laughing: the use of humor to negotiate in group discussions. *Humor: International Journal of Humor Research, 16(2),* 183-223.
[3]   Davies, C.E. (1984). Joint joking. Improvisational humorous episodes in conversation. In C. Brugman and M. Macauley (Eds.), *Proceedings of the Tenth Annual Meeting of the Berkeley Linguistics Society* (pp. 360-371). Berkeley: Berkeley Linguistics Society.
[4]   Drew, P. (1987). Po-faced receipts of teases. *Linguistics, 25,* 219-253.
[5]   Jefferson, G. (1979). A technique for inviting laughter and its subsequent acceptance declination. In G. Psathas (Ed.), *Everyday language* (pp.79-86). New York: Irvington Publishers.
[6]   Norrick, N. R. (1993). *Conversational Joking: Humor in Everyday Talk.* Bloomington, Indianapolis: Indiana University Press.
[7]   Norrick, N. R. (1993). Repetition in canned jokes and spontaneous conversational joking. *Humor. International Journal of Humor Research, 6(4),* 385-402.
[8]   Norrick, N. R. (2000). *Conversational Narrative. Storytelling in Everyday Conversations.* Amsterdam-Philadelphia: Benjamins.
[9]   Norrick, N. R., and Chiaro, D. (2009). *Humor in Interaction.* Amsterdam: John Benjamins.
[10] Sacks, H. (1974). An analysis of the course of a joke's telling in conversation. In R. Bauman and J. Sherzer (Eds.), *Explorations in the Ethnography of Speaking* (pp. 337-353). Cambridge: Cambridge University Press.
[11] Bell, N. (2009). Responses to failed humor. *Journal of Pragmatics, 41,* 1825-1836.
[12] Bell, N. (2009). Impolite responses to failed humor. In D. Chiaro and N. R. Norrick (Eds.), *Humor in Interaction* (pp. 143-146). Amsterdam: John Benjamins Publishing.
[13] Bell, N., and Attardo, S. (2010). Failed humor: issues in non-native speakers' appreciation and comprehension of humor. *Intercultural Pragmatics, 7(3),* 423-447.
[14] Priego-Valverde, B. (2009). Failed humor in conversation: a double voicing analysis. In D. Chiaro and N. R. Norrick (Eds.), *Humor in Interaction* (pp. 165-183). Amsterdam: John Benjamins.

[15] Canestrari, C., and Attardo, S. (2008). Humorous syntony as a metacommunicative language game. *Gestalt Theory, 30*, 337-347.

[16] Bateson, G. (1955). A theory of play and fantasy. *A.P.A. Psychiatric Research Reports, 2*, 39-51. Reprinted in G., Bateson (1972). *Steps to an Ecology of Mind* (pp. 177-193). New York: Ballantine.

[17] Provine, R.R. (1996). Laughter. *American Scientist, 84(1)*, 38-47.

[18] Canestrari, C. (2010). Meta-communicative signals and humorous verbal interchanges: a case study. *Humor. International Journal of Humor Research, 23(3)*, 327-349.

[19] Koestler, A. (1964) *The act of Creation.* London: Hutchinson.

[20] Suls, J. M. (1972). A two-stage model for the appreciation of jokes and cartoons. In G. Goldstein and P. McGhee (Eds.), *The Psychology of Humour* (pp. 81-100). London-New York: Academic Press.

[21] Norrick, N. R. (1986). A frame-theoretical analysis of verbal humor: bisociation as schema conflict. *Semiotica, 60(3-4)*, 225-245.

[22] Oring, E. (1992). *Jokes and their relations.* Lexington: The University Press of Kentucky.

[23] Wyer, R.S., and Collins, J.E. (1992). A Theory of humor elicitation. *Psychological Review, 99(4)*, 663-668.

[24] Forabosco, G. (1992). Cognitive aspects of the humor process: the concept of incongruity. *Humor. International Journal of Humor Research, 5(1/2)*, 45-68.

[25] Canestrari, C., and Bianchi, I. (2009). From script opposition to the phenomenological rules of contrariety. In U. Savardi (Ed.), *The Perception and Cognition of Contraries* (pp. 225-246). Milan: McGraw-Hill.

[26] Canestrari, C., and Bianchi, I. (forthcoming). Perception of contrariety in jokes.

[27] Maier, N. R. F. (1932). A Gestalt theory of humour. *British Journal of Psychology, 23*, 69-74.

[28] Metz-Göckel, H. (1989). *Witzstrukturen.* Opladen: Westdeutscher Verlag.

[29] Metz-Göckel, H. (2008). Closure as a joke-principle. *Gestalt Theory, 30(3)*, 331-336.

[30] Russell, R. E. (1996). Understanding laughter in terms of basic perceptual and response patterns. *Humor. International Journal of Humor Research, 9(1)*, 39-55.

[31] Smith, K. (1996). Laughing t the way we see: The role of visual organization principles in cartoon humor. *Humor. International Journal of Humor Research, 9(1)*, 19-38.

[32] Raskin, V. (1985). *Semantic mechanisms of humor.* Dordrecht-Boston-Lancaster: D. Reidel.

[33] Attardo, S., and Raskin, V. (1991). Script theory revis(it)ed: joke similarity and joke representation model. *Humor. International Journal of Humor Research, 4(3/4)*, 293-347.

[34] Attardo, S. (2001). *Humorous Texts: a Semantic and Pragmatic Analysis.* Berlin New York: Mouton de Gruyter.

[35] Attardo, S. (1997). The semantic foundations of cognitive theories of humor. *Humor. International Journal of Humor Research, 10(4)*, 395-420.

[36] Attardo, S., Hempelmann, C. F., and Di Maio, S. (2002). Script opposition and logical mechanisms: Modelling incongruity and their resolutions. *Humor. International Journal of Humor Research, 15(1)*, 3-46.

[37] Pickering, L., Corduas, M., Eisterhold, J., Seifried, B., Eggleston, A., and Attardo, S. (2009). Prosodic markers of saliency in humorous narratives. *Discourse Processes, 46,* 517-540.

[38] Giora, R. (1988). On the informativeness requirement. *Journal of Pragmatics, 12(5/6),* 547-565.

[39] Giora, R. (1991). On the cognitive aspects of the joke. *Journal of Pragmatics, 16(5),* 465-485.

[40] Giora, R. (1997). Understanding figurative language: the graded salience hypothesis. *Cognitive Linguistics, 7,* 183-206.

[41] Giora, R. (2003). *On our Mind: Salience, Context, and Figurative Language.* New York: Oxford University Press.

[42] Giora, R., and Fein, O. (2007). Irony: Context and Salience. In R. W. Jr. Gibbs, and H. L. Colston (Eds.), *Irony in Language and Thought. A Cognitive Science Reader* (pp. 201-217). New York: LEA.

[43] Peleg, O., Giora, R., and Fein, O. (2008). Resisting contextual information: You can't put a salient meaning down. *Lodz Papers in Pragmatics, 4(1),* 13-44.

[44] Dynel, M. (2009). *Humorous Garden-Path. A Pragmatic-Cognitive Study.* Newcastle: Cambridge Scholars Publishing.

[45] Forabosco, G. (2008). Is the concept of incongruity still a useful construct for the advancement in humor research? *Lodz Papers in Pragmatics, 4(1),* 45-62.

[46] Martin, R. (2007). *The Psychology of Humor. An Integrative Approach.* Burlington, MA: Elsevier Academic Press.

[47] Archakis, A., and Tsakona, V. (2005). Analyzing conversational data in *GTVH* terms: A new approach to the issue of identity construction via humor. *Humor. International Journal of Humor Research, 18(1),* 41-68.

[48] Brock, A. (2004). Analyzing scripts in humorous communication. *Humor: International Journal of Humor Research, 17(4),* 353-360.

[49] Ruch, W., Attardo, S., and Raskin, V. (1993). Towards an empirical verification of the General Theory of Verbal Humor. *Humor. International Journal of Humor Research, 6(2),* 123-136.

[50] Rossi, F. (1999). *Le Parole dello Schermo.* Roma: Bulzoni.

[51] Rossi, F. (2002). *La Lingua in Gioco.* Roma: Bulzoni.

[52] Rossi, F. (2002). Il dialogo nel parlato filmico. In C. Bazzanella (Ed.), *Sul Dialogo, Contesti e Forme d'Interazione Verbale* (pp.161-75). Milano: Guerini Associati.

[53] Canestrari, C., Bongelli, R., Riccioni, I., and Zuczkowski, A. (in press). Representations of humorous dialogues. *Proceedings of the 13th IADA Conference,* Montreal, Canada, April, 26-30, 2011.

[54] Forchini, P. (2010). 'Well, uh no. I mean, you know'. Discourse Markers in Movie Conversation. *Perspectives on Audiovisual Translation, Lódz Studies in Language, 20,* 45-59.

[55] Freddi, M. (2008). Continuity and variation across translations: phraseology in the 'Pavia corpus of film dialogue'. In C. Taylor (Ed.), *Ecolingua. The Role of E-corpora in Translation and Language Learning* (pp 52-70). Trieste, EUT.

[56] Pavesi, M. (2008). Spoken language in film dubbing. Target language norms, interference and translation routines. In D. Chiaro, C. Heiss, and C. Bucaria (Eds.), *Between Text and Image: Updating Research in Screen Translation* (pp.79-97), Amsterdam, John Benjamins Publishing.

[57] Taylor C. (2000) Look who's talking. An analysis of film dialogue as a variety of spoken discourse. In L. Lombardo, L. Haarenan, and J. Morley (Eds.), *Massed Medias: Linguistic Tools for Interpreting Media Discourse* (pp.247-278). Milano: LED.

[58] Jefferson, G. (1984). Transcription Notation. In J. Atkinson. and J. Heritage (Eds.), *Structures of Social Interaction.* New York: Cambridge University Press.

[59] Attardo, S., Eisterhold, J., Hay, J., and Poggi, I. (2003). Multimodal markers of irony and sarcasm. *Humor. International Journal of Humor Research, 16(2),* 243-260.

[60] Montague, R. (2009). Joker's remorse: an examination of failed humor and recovery strategies. *Conference Papers-National Communication Association,* 1-33.

[61] Song, J. (2010). A pragmatic approach for the failure of verbal humor. *US-China Foreign Language, 8(5),* 14-19.

[62] Alberts, J.K. (1992). An inferential/strategical explanation for the social explanation of teases. *Journal of Language and Social Psychology, 11(3),* 153-177.

[63] Davies, C.E. (2003). How English-learners joke with native speakers: an interactional sociolinguistic perspective on humor as collaborative discourse across cultures. *Journal of Pragmatics, 35,* 1361-1385.

[64] Attardo, S. (2001). Humor and irony in interaction: from mode adoption to failure of detection. In: L. Anolli, R. Ciceri, and G. Riva (Eds.), *Say Not to Say: New Perspectives on Miscommunication* (pp. 165-185). Amsterdam: Ios.

[65] Chiaro, D. (1992). *The language of jokes. Analysing verbal play.* London: Routledge.

[66] Kotthoff, H. (2009). An interactional approach to irony development. In D. Chiaro, and N. R. Norrick (Eds.), *Humor in Interaction* (pp. 49-77). Amsterdam, John Benjamins Publishing.

[67] Hay, J. (1994). Jocular abuse patterns in mixed-group interaction. *Wellington Working Papers.*

[68] Kotthoff, H. (2003). Responding to irony in different contexts: on cognition in conversation. *Journal of Pragmatics, 35,* 1387-1411.

[69] Gibbs, R. (2000). Irony in talk among friends. *Metaphors and Symbols, 15,* 5-27.

[70] Eisterhold, J., Attardo, S., and Boxer, D. (2006). Reactions to irony in discourse: evidence for the least disruption principle. *Journal of Pragmatics, 38,* 1239-1256.

In: Humor and Health Promotion
Editor: Paola Gremigni

ISBN: 978-1-61942-657-3
© 2012 Nova Science Publishers, Inc.

Chapter 5

A TEMPERAMENT APPROACH TO HUMOR

Willibald Ruch and Jennifer Hofmann

Institute for Psychology, Personality and Assessment, University of Zurich, Switzerland

ABSTRACT

Due to the shortcomings in understanding humor, a state-trait model of cheerfulness, seriousness and bad mood was introduced to describe the temperamental basis of the sense of humor [1-4]. This chapter sketches the development and characteristics of the postulated state-trait model and presents its relationship to different models of the sense of humor. Literature will be reviewed that shows that trait cheerfulness accounts for most variation in existing self-report assessment tools of the sense of humor. Further, the relation of trait cheerfulness to health and well-being related variables (e.g., flourishing [5]; coping [6] and life satisfaction, [7]) will be discussed. Attention is given to experimental and correlational evidence, which shows that trait cheerfulness is positively related to adaptive coping mechanisms, positive experience and well-being. This is particularly interesting for cheerfulness interventions to fostering well-being and overcoming adversities. Finally, implications for the study of positive traits and respective interventions will be discussed.

INTRODUCTION: WHY A TEMPERAMENTAL APPROACH TO THE SENSE OF HUMOR?

As previously noted, at a formal level, the expression "sense of humor" refers to a personality characteristic aimed at describing habitual individual differences in humor-related behavior [8]. Like any personality trait, the sense of humor is a descriptive hypothetical construct. It is an invention of the human mind, not an existing entity. The sense of humor cannot be observed directly but is inferred via indicators, such as observed behavior or reported experience. It refers to a disposition for humor-related behavior not to the behavior itself. Thus the sense of humor is a hypothetical disposition referring to individual differences that correlate with observed humor behaviors. So, what then is "humor"?

Outside of psychology, "humor" may also refer to artifacts and products (like humorous stories, comedies, films, jokes) but in psychology it is relating to individuals and their feelings, thoughts and actions. There are many facets of humor behavior and experience (e.g., comprehension, enjoyment, creation, initiation, entertainment), and they involve many domains of psychological functioning (e.g., perception, cognition, emotion, motivation, attitudes, performance). Individuals differ in these feelings, thoughts and actions not only in one situation but habitually, and if some or all of these are intercorrelated they might be accounted for by a personality concept, such as the "sense of humor." However, the phenomena listed above are very diverse and it is unlikely that they can be traced back to a single dimension of low vs. high sense of humor. As Craik, Lampert and Nelson [9] demonstrated, the concept of "sense of humor" only covers some of everyday humorous conduct (in their view it is the socially warm and competent humor styles). Hence, a comprehensive approach to the sense of humor, meaning one that is aimed at representing all humor-related behavior, will most likely arrive at a multidimensional concept. This has not yet been undertaken and one can state that the "sense of humor" is still more of a folk-concept that has not been explicitly converted into a scientific construct so far.

The same humor-related feelings, thoughts and actions can be accounted for by personality traits other than the sense of humor. For example, elements like the tendency to laugh easily, to initiate humor, etc. were seen as components of the sense of humor [10,11]. They can also be subsumed under the higher order personality factor of extraversion. Not surprisingly, Ruch and Deckers [12] found extraversion and such defined sense of humor to be highly correlated. Sense of humor is also not the only expression that may be used; one might also speak about "trait humor," "humor styles" or use other expressions referring to the component of humor investigated (e.g., wit, nonsense, sarcasm).

Humor behaviors are often content saturated. For example, someone will laugh at lot at Monty Pythons *Life of Brian*, find sexist jokes offensive, or readily attend a carnival session and dress up as a pirate or ghost. The expression of humor may be cultural or even regional, and certain forms of amusement might be in or out of fashion. Yet, the underlying tendencies (e.g., laughing easily, enjoying to play with ideas, a robustness of positive mood, preference for true meaning compared to "as if" thoughts and acts) might be universal. Asking someone whether he or she laughs at the *life of Brian* confounds two elements: whether one likes this film or not and whether one laughs easily or more reluctantly. If we want to know whether someone enjoys *the life of Brian*, then looking at laughter in response to the film just adds a source of variance that is not needed. If we want to know whether one has an inclination to laugh in general, then it is better to just ask this and leave out the specific elements that might add noise (as some who likes to laugh a lot maybe doesn't like this film and hence won't laugh at all). Likewise, carnival is not practiced everywhere and hence people don't report dressing up in funny costumes, just for the sheer fact that it is not common there.

Ruch and colleagues [2,3,13,14] conducted a series of studies based on the observation of *interindividual* (i.e., between individuals) and *intraindividual* (i.e., across situations) variation in humor behavior. They argued that it is commonly observed that certain individuals tend to *habitually* appreciate, create, or laugh more easily/ intensively/or more often at humorous stimuli than others do. Aside of interindividual differences which are relatively stable over time, there are also *actual* dispositions for humor, varying across situations and time. Phrases like to be *in good humor*, *in the mood for laughing*, *out of humor*, *in a serious mood or frame of mind* etc. refer to such states of enhanced (or lowered) readiness to respond to humor [15].

This chapter discusses the state-trait approach of the temperamental basis relevant for the behavioral and experiential domain of humor [1,2,15,16]. This approach does not claim to be comprehensive for *all* kinds of humor-related behaviors. The state-trait model acknowledges that the disposition for humor varies intra- and interpersonally and that the utilization of the same concepts as both states and traits allows us to study the relevance of homologous actual and habitual dispositions. While the expression of humor may be culture specific and differ over time, the affective and mental foundations of humor will more likely be universal [14]. Thus, generally content-saturated humor contents and items will be largely missing in the model and its inventory, but the nature of the concepts will still allow for hypothesizing links to humor phenomena.

Rather than describing humor behaviors, thoughts, and feelings, the underlying mental state and affective basis are the focus of this approach. In short, *trait cheerfulness* is a disposition facilitating the expression of humor, while *trait seriousness* and *trait bad mood* represent dispositions for different forms of humorlessness [2]. These traits form the *temperamental basis* of humor, and their respective states represent dispositions for humor that vary within persons over time. As there is no agreement on the nature of the sense of humor yet, the study of its temperamental basis may help systematizing existing results, training the sense of humor, and developing intervention programs to foster positive health outcomes.

THE EMOTION OF EXHILARATION

The state-trait model of cheerfulness arose from the experimental study of the emotional responses to humor [13]. The emotion of exhilaration (from the Latin root *hilaris*) had been defined as either the process of making cheerful or the temporary rise and fall of a cheerful state [13]. This term is used as a technical term and it is based on its original meaning (the raise of hilarity). This emotion was also referred to as amusement, hilarity, or mirth [17]. Exhilaration most often occurs in response to humorous stimuli, but also to inhaling nitrous oxide and being tickled [18]. Among the 6 or 7 basic emotions by Ekman [19] that have a distinct and universal facial expression, exhilaration was seen to be one the facet of joy (or happiness) that is most strongly aligned with laughter.

Exhilaration can be described at the behavioral, the physiological and the experiential level [13]. Behaviorally, exhilaration is expressed in smiling and laughter. While there are about 20 types of smiles to be distinguished, only the so-called Duchenne display can be observed when people are enjoying themselves. This genuine smile of enjoyment involves the simultaneous and symmetric contraction of two muscles: the zygomatic major muscle and the orbital part of the orbicularis oculi muscle. The action of the zygomatic major pulls the lip corner obliquely up and back, and deepens the furrow running from the nostril to the lip corner. The orbicularis oculi muscle lifts the cheeks upward and draws the skin toward the eyes from the temple and cheeks. It narrows the eye opening and may cause "crow's feet" wrinkles to appear at the outer corner of the eye opening [20]. Ekman, Davidson, and Friesen [21] named this smile to honor the man who first described it, Duchenne de Boulogne (a French anatomist of the 18th /19th century).

By coding the face with the help of the Facial Action Coding System (FACS) [22], or EMG, one can distinguish between this genuine smile (and laughter) and other smiles. This includes phony and masking smiles, where nothing much is felt but one wants to appear amused and where negative emotions are felt but one wants to appear amused in the latter [19-26].

Laughter includes a Duchenne display, and the contraction of a number of further muscles, such as the m. levator labii superioris, m. risorius, m. mentalis, m. depressor anguli, and orbicularis oris muscle [27], as well as muscles relaxing/showing lower contraction during laughter (typically the m. frontalis and corrugator supercilli muscle). It typically involves a laughter sound that can be distinguished by different features (voiced, unvoiced, single sounds such as "ha", and plural sounds, e.g., "ha ha"; [28]). The sounds are extremely diverse, including all vowels and many consonants, but also voiceless laughter.

Smiling and laughter represent different levels of intensity of exhilaration [13]. Whereas laughing occurs at higher levels of exhilaration, smiling typically occurs at lower levels, with different intensity levels of smiling also representing different degrees of exhilaration. As already noted by Darwin [29] with increasing intensity of laughter, movements of the trunk and the limbs may occur as well as changes in posture.

Among the many physiological responses to humorous stimuli [13], for example, changes in heart rate and of skin conductance have already early been used as markers of intensity of responses to humor [30]. But there are more physiological changes known that are typical for exhilaration. Figure 1 gives a physiological recording of long laughter episode (consisting of many laughter bouts) of one male participant who inhaled laughing gas during trial runs prior to an experiment [18]. The term *laughter bout* was used by Ruch and Ekman [28] to refer to a whole behavioral-acoustic event, including the respiratory, vocal, and facial and skeletomuscular elements of a laugh. A laughter bout may be segmented into an onset (i.e., the pre-vocal facial part which is very short in the case of explosive laughter), an apex (i.e., the period where vocalization or forced exhalation occurs), and an offset (i.e., a post-vocalization part; often a long-lasting smile fading out smoothly). The laughter vocalization period is composed of *laugh cycles*, i.e., repetitive *laugh-pulses* interspersed with pauses. There is laughter with only one or two pulses (as in an "ha"-type "exclamation laugh"), but studies typically report that four pulses in a laugh cycle are most frequent. The upper number of pulses in a laugh cycle (a maximum of 9-12 is reported) is limited by the lung volume.

During an unusually long laughter episode, there is a joint contraction of the zygomatic major and orbicularis oculi muscle at the onset of the laughter that prevailed throughout the entire episode. It can also be seen from the recordings of respiratory movements (through an elastic band on both chest and abdomen) and the electromyographic recordings (from the diaphragm) that there is an initial forced exhalation at the onset of laughter, followed by a laugh cycle (that is visible in activity of high frequency and low amplitude). This is consequently followed by inhalatory movements, which, again, are followed by a steeper exhalatory movement and the next laughter cycle. The heart rate increases and its variability is reduced, and characteristic changes in skin conductance occur, that have been reported before [13]. Further changes are discussed [31]. Reviews of the neuroanatomical conditions of smiling, laughter, the emotion of exhilaration and the various processes are given elsewhere [32-34].

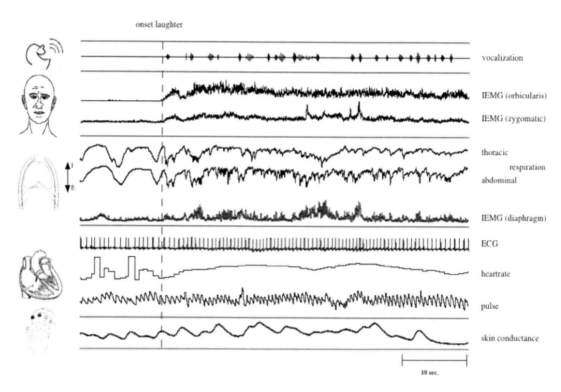

Figure 1. A laughter episode: Physiological response pattern for the emotion of exhilaration.

The experiential level of exhilaration incorporates, as with other emotions, the awareness of one's own actions and action tendencies ("I feel, I will burst out laughing"), of physiological changes ("my belly hurts of laughing"), and of the feeling structure (i.e., exhilaration may be seen as a pleasurable, relaxed excitation). Furthermore, this goes along with the awareness of the situation's meaning structure (e.g., being with friends and remembering school pranks) and the perception of stimulus properties (e.g., funniness in absurdity) of the exhilaration-inducing stimulus [13,27,32]. As exhilaration is defined as a temporary rise in a cheerful state, it is implied that the emotional experience changes over time. Typically, a sudden and intense increase in cheerfulness is expected, followed by a more or less pronounced plateau and a prolonged fading out of the emotional tone. The three levels are expected to be coordinated and indeed the relationship between facial expression and experience is quite high, given the coherence is sought for within individuals [35].

The complete model of the emotion of exhilaration includes the eliciting stimuli and conditions (the exhilarants, [36]), the consequences (social, health, etc.), and the actual and habitual (personality) moderating factors that have an impact on ones exhilaratability. The actual factors may be situative (e.g., presence of others) and organismic (e.g., mood, frame of mind) and the habitual factors relate to personality. Indeed, it is assumed that the threshold for laughter and exhilaration varies inter- and intraindividually, and this is why a state - trait model of cheerfulness, seriousness and bad mood was developed.

THE STATE-TRAIT MODEL OF CHEERFULNESS, SERIOUSNESS AND BAD MOOD

Several model implications are postulated: The state-trait model of cheerfulness, seriousness and bad mood considers humor multidimensional, meaning that people differ on more than one dimension. Secondly, it takes into account that humor is not unipolar, implying that humorlessness needs to be represented as well. Thirdly the model covers affective and mental factors relating to moods/temperaments and frames of mind. The basic structure of the model is outlined in Figure 2. Signs express the hypothesized relationship between cheerfulness, seriousness, and bad mood as states and traits and exhilaratability; i.e., the inclination to respond favorably to humor.

Figure 2 shows that exhilaratability is composed of cheerfulness, seriousness, and bad mood both as distinctive states and traits. It emphasizes that there are different degrees of how long the different states are stable, ranging from short-lived fluctuations in mood but also more tonic changes in mood level. Nevertheless, a deliberate distinction is made whether the subjects report their actual feelings (i.e., in a given moment) or their habitual feelings and behavior. Such states of seriousness, cheerfulness, and bad mood will fluctuate within individuals, but they may also be produced by experimental procedures to study causal hypotheses between states and the threshold for the release of exhilaration [2,15,37].

Cheerfulness as a mood state and cheerfulness as a personality trait were both assigned prominent roles in exhilaratability: Both should serve for controlling (i.e., predicting or explaining) individual differences. A concept of cheerfulness as an enduring disposition is necessary, since individuals differ habitually in the frequency, intensity, and duration of cheerful mood states, as well as in the ease with which exhilaration is induced [13]. As described, individuals of habitually higher levels of cheerfulness will be more susceptible to the induction of exhilaration than those of a comparable low level of cheerfulness. The reverse will be true for individuals with habitually high levels of seriousness or bad mood. They will be less readily inclined to respond positively to a given stimulus than those low in these characteristics. It was hypothesized that trait-cheerfulness can be subsumed under the higher-order temperament dimension of extraversion-introversion which is a determinant of a generalized susceptibility to positive affect [38].

Different facets of cheerfulness as mood states were distinguished [3]. A cheerful mood, which is marked by a more tranquil and composed mood state, is distinguished from hilarity, which is marked by a merry mood state (more shallow and outward). Exhilaration and state cheerfulness are conceptually different, but there is a reciprocal relationship between them: A cheerful state facilitates the induction of exhilaration, and an accumulation of exhilaration responses may lead to longer-lasting changes in the level of cheerfulness [13]. Also, if the induction of exhilaration fails, the cheerful state may be lowered. A cheerful mood lasts longer, fluctuates less and is less dependent on eliciting stimuli [13].

The operational definitions of the three concepts were defined with the help of facets or definitional components of the traits. These facets were derived on the basis of the following sources: a lexical study (e.g., definitions of the terms in encyclopedias of several languages); studies of the linguistic field (e.g., of synonyms and antonyms); study of prior related concepts; study of the German literature on cheerfulness, seriousness, sadness, and ill-humor [39]; early American studies on cheerfulness-depression [40,41]; prior factor analytic work of humor questionnaires [8]; and factor analytic studies of trait-adjectives and further research [41[1]]. Facets (or definitional components) were generated on this basis. The concept of cheerfulness (CH) comprised the following five facets: a prevalence of cheerful mood (CH1), a low threshold for smiling and laughter (CH2), a composed view of adverse life circumstances (CH3), a broad range of active elicitors of cheerfulness and smiling/laughter (CH4), and (CH5) a generally cheerful interaction style [2,15].

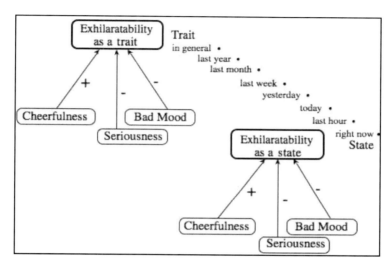

Figure 2. A state-trait model of cheerfulness, seriousness, and bad mood.

A major assumption states that cheerfulness contributes to robustness of mood, meaning that individuals high in trait cheerfulness are able to maintain a high level of state cheerfulness (and retain a low level of state bad mood) in the presence of factors prone to negative moods, while individuals low in trait cheerfulness are more likely to loose humor (get grumpy and out of cheerful mood), when facing adversity [14,37]. This assumption is very important when investigating the relationship between trait cheerfulness, health and well-being associated variables and will be specified later in this chapter. This potential of cheerfulness includes getting into state cheerfulness more easily (*threshold in*); stating that it takes less potent stimuli to induce cheerful mood. This should also be true when factors capable of inducing negative affects become active (*robustness*, or *threshold out*); i.e., it takes a more potent aversive stimulus to bring highly cheerful out of that state. Furthermore, it implies for high cheerful individuals to experience the cheerful mood more strongly (*intensity*), and remaining in that state longer (*duration*) until it fades out naturally. Finally, once a stimulus alters mood to the negative, trait cheerful individuals will rebuild the cheerful mood faster (*speed of mood recovery*); i.e., high trait cheerful people will overcome the negative affects associated with adverse situations more quickly [2,3,42,43]. While the first three relations are common to describing relationships between states and traits, the latter two are relatively new and were created to help discussing and explaining facts typically associated with the "sense of humor" within the state-trait model of cheerfulness [43].

---

[1] Young (1937) found a positive correlation between retrospectively reported cheerful mood during the last 24 hours and laughter; exemplifying the relevance of state cheerfulness.

The idea of robustness of mood is especially well compatible with the facet of cheerful composure (the cheerful-composed individual has a positive and carefree outlook of life, can unwind well, and enjoys the present moment; he/she can accept even unpleasant circumstances calmly and with composure, can look on the light side of things and is able to find something positive in them). This factor is expected to be the best predictor of robustness among all components of trait cheerfulness. So far no research has been carried out regarding the mood recovery hypotheses, but the other postulates will be discussed later in this chapter, as this notion of keeping a cheerful view on life even when facing adversity will closely relate to positive health outcome variables, such as coping with stress and maintaining life satisfaction.

In contrast, trait and state bad mood are assumed to increase the threshold for exhilaration [13]. The concept of bad mood (BM) is composed of the predominance of three mood states and their respective behaviors. These components are a generally bad mood (BM1), sadness (i.e., despondent and distressed mood; BM2), and ill humouredness (i.e., sullen and grumpy or grouchy feelings; BM4). Two further facets are specifically related to the sad (BM3) and ill-humored (BM5) individual's behavior in cheerfulness evoking situations, their attitudes toward such situations and the objects, persons, and roles involved. The role of trait bad mood has also been acknowledged by McGhee [44] who listed negative mood as one of eight defining components of *low* sense of humor. While other conceptualizations of the sense of humor do not explicitly include this affective form of humorlessness, items of scales sometimes relate to bad mood. However, bad mood might also be a disposition facilitating certain forms of humor, such as mockery, irony, cynicism, and sarcasm [14,45].

Moreover, the likelihood of a person responding to a humor stimulus with exhilaration not only depends on the predominant mood state, but also on the frame of mind (e.g., seriousness). The concept of seriousness (SE) is made up of the elements of the prevalence of serious states (SE1), a perception of even everyday happenings as important and considering them thoroughly and intensively, rather than treating them superficially (SE2), the tendency to plan ahead and set long-range goals and attaining the closest possible harmony with these goals in every action and decision (SE3), the tendency to prefer activities for which concrete, rational reasons can be produced thereby considering activities which don't have a specific goal as a waste of time and nonsense (SE4), the preference for a sober, object-oriented communication style, meaning to say exactly what one means without exaggeration or ironic/sarcastic undertones (SE5), and a "humorless" attitude about cheerfulness-related behavior, roles, persons, stimuli, situations, and actions (SE6). For people in a serious frame of mind, the threshold of exhilaratability is enhanced, and for people in low serious state (i.e., playful), this threshold is lowered [14].

As shown, the facet model also distinguishes among several forms of "humorlessness". While both serious individuals and those in a bad mood may be perceived as being humorless, they are so for different reasons. In the latter case, the generation of positive affect is impaired by the presence of a predominant negative affective state. In the former case, there is lowered interest in engaging in humorous interaction or in switching into a more playful frame of mind; i.e., a stronger aspect of volition is involved. There may be differences within the concept of bad mood as well. While an ill-humored person, like the serious person, may not want to be involved in humor, the person in a sad mood may not be able to do so. Also, while the sad person is not antagonistic to a cheerful person, the ill-humored one may be. Despite the fact that the prediction of individual differences in exhilaratability was the original motive for postulating and examining the three concepts of cheerfulness, bad mood and seriousness, it is expected that the model is not only valid for other forms of humor behavior but transcends the boundaries of humor research as well.

In sum, at least one facet (CH1, SE1, BM1, BM2, BM4) of any concept defines the postulated state-trait link, describing that the respective state occurs more often, lasts longer, and is of higher intensity than the average. Furthermore, for all constructs, at least one facet (CH5, SE6, BM3, BM5) describes the behavior of a prototypical person in a specifically cheerful environment or his/her response to exhilarating situations and stimuli, as well as the generalized attitude towards that field.

RELATIONSHIPS AMONG THE FACETS OF THE MODEL

It is expected that the facets of the three constructs are homogeneous; i.e., facets of one construct will tend to inter-correlate highly positively and there will be lower correlations with facets of other constructs. Cheerfulness and bad mood have in common that they are *affective* concepts; the hedonic tone of the former is positive and the latter negative.

As states they appear to be opposites: one can hardly be cheerful and in a bad mood simultaneously. The successful induction of a cheerful state seems to imply that it will replace the bad mood; meaning that bad mood will cease in intensity. While they may not be present at the same time as states, there will be individuals predisposed to both states (e.g., the cycloid temperament according to Kretschmer [46]). Thus, at the habitual level, the negative correlation between cheerfulness and bad mood will be lower than at the state level. While the notion of a predominant (cheerful or bad) mood already implies a negative relationship, the strength of that inter-correlation may also be depending on the facet of the trait.

As the facets CH1, SE1, BM1, BM2, and BM4 refer to prevalent states, they are more likely to produce higher correlations. Whether one is able to laugh (CH2) or entertain others (CH5) is more independent of bad mood; as it is claimed, for example, that clowns basically are sad people.

Also, an ill-humored mood may accompany the facilitated tendency of laughing at others. Dictionaries often list seriousness as an antonym of cheerfulness; thus, they are considered to be mutually exclusive terms, suggesting that the presence of seriousness excludes cheerfulness and vice versa. However, while cheerfulness refers to an affective state, seriousness denotes a quality of the *frame of mind*, allowing all combinations of both to occur. The combination of non- cheerful and serious certainly contributes to the perception of a person as being humorless, and the combination of both non-serious and cheerful would depict a playful, fun-loving person and predict a high susceptibility for that person to laugh at humorous stimuli and situations. However, the other combinations will exist, too; for instance, a cheerful temperament might go along with a serious frame of mind. In fact, there is ample reason to assume that this combination is the basis for a certain form of sense of humor [8]. Similarly, there may be the absence of both, as in nihilistic individuals characterized by pessimism/low degree of cheerfulness and low degree of seriousness. Thus, cheerfulness and seriousness will be slightly negatively correlated as traits. The correlation between cheerfulness and seriousness as states will depend on whether the state is event-related and whether the event itself is of a serious or cheerful nature.

The fact that both seriousness and bad mood represent opposites (or partial opposites) of cheerfulness limits the degrees of freedom for them being negatively correlated or orthogonal themselves. Phenomenologically, both share the elements of heaviness and darkness and lack the brightness and lightness of cheerfulness [39]. Again the fact that bad mood refers to an affective state and seriousness to a frame of mind allows them to vary more independently.

Serious people may be high and low in bad mood just as non-serious individuals. However, they react similarly negatively (albeit for different reasons and in a different manner) to humorous situations and stimuli. Thus, the facets of SE6, BM3, and BM5 (depicting the behavior of serious, sad, and ill-humored individuals in the cheerful environment) will support a positive relationship between seriousness and bad mood. As states, seriousness and bad mood will be positively associated as well.

As a prototype, during events of high negative emotionality (even flight or fight), one is concentrated and behaving seriously; meaning that energy is mobilized to be spent purposefully [2]. While bad mood situations may be associated often with a serious frame of mind, the reverse does not have to be true. States of seriousness do not have to be accompanied by a negative mood level. The inter-correlation of serious and bad mood states may increase in response to humorous events; the failure to induce exhilaration in state-serious individuals may increase their bad mood as well [2,3,14].

MEASUREMENT

Instruments were designed for the assessment of these states and traits [2,3]. The long form of the trait part of the *State-Trait Cheerfulness Inventory* (*STCI-T*) is a 106-item questionnaire in a 4-point answer format providing scores for the three traits of *cheerfulness* (STCI-T CH; 38 items), *seriousness* (STCI-T SE; 37 items), and *bad mood* (STCI-T BM; 31 items) and their 5, 6, and 5 definitional components, respectively. Because of the antithetical nature of the concepts a negatively keyed cheerfulness item, for example, could also be seen prototypical for seriousness or bad mood. While the sentence "I feel like laughing" might indicate cheerfulness, its negation "I don't feel like laughing" might well indicate sadness. Therefore, negations were only used when they represented standing expressions used in everyday language. In general, a concept-guided strategy in item reduction was preferred to a purely empirical selection of items, although indices derived from factor and item analysis, as well as indices of sensitivity to change were considered [2,3]. From the STCI-T <106>, a standard trait form with 60 items to assess the three traits with 20 items per scale was derived. This version contains items from all facets (at an equal proportion) but is not considered for scoring facets. It was constructed on the following basis: (a) the best corrected item-total correlation (citc), (b) consideration of items content, (c) roughly equal representation of the facets (where this was not possible, core facets got more weight), and (d) avoidance of very similar items as regards content or linguistic usage [2]. Ruch and Köhler [14] report high internal consistencies for the traits (CH α = .93, SE α =.88, and BM α =.94) measured by the standard forms in a sample of 600 adults. Furthermore, the one-month retest-stability was high for the traits (between .77 and .86) but low for the states (between .33 and .36), confirming the nature of enduring traits and transient states [3]. The factor structure is replicable and generalizable across samples of different nationalities and across length of the time span of the mood covered.

The state version of the STCI initially consisted of 40 items, assessing the constructs of cheerfulness, seriousness and bad mood according to their trait definitions, but with the focus of actual feeling state and with items allowing for sensitive assessment of mood alternations [3]. There is also a 4-point answer format, like in the trait version. The pilot version was tested on several German and American samples, using the technique of thought experiment, in which participants were not exposed to, or tested in state-relevant situations, but rather were provided with different scenarios (describing state-relevant prototypical situations). In the process of test construction, items were eliminated iteratively according to several pre-set criteria, based on results of the construction sample. Cheerfulness, seriousness and bad mood scales were developed with 10 items each (in a stepwise elimination procedure of items). Ruch and colleagues [3] report satisfactory internal consistencies (alpha coefficients from .85 to .94) and the test-retest correlation was low (.33-.36). Modified versions of the STCI-S (with instructions to describe predominant mood states of last week, last month, and last year) were created for the assessment of longer-lasting mood states [14].

Factor analysis of the trait STCI-T <60> and the standard form of the state STCI-S <30> revealed that homologous states and traits are separable. Correlations among heterologous states and traits yielded the expected pattern in every case and were much higher than average coefficients for heterologous pairs: All the traits where highly correlated with their respective state. Cheerfulness in state and trait was negatively related to state seriousness and state bad mood (and the latter two were positively correlated themselves).

Putting the STCI-S to the test, the items sensitively reflected changes in both imagined responses to prototypical situations and perceived own feeling state as naturally occurring or experimentally induced. The intended changes work in both directions, an uplift of state exhilaratability can be documented and so can its repression. Assessment of the three states was undertaken in states of possible altered mood covering naturally occurring mood changes (e.g., in everyday life, such as diurnal variations due to type of weather, success or failure), unobtrusively induced mood changes (e.g., exposing subjects to rooms of different "atmosphere"; experimenter's personality), more or less obtrusively induced mood changes (e.g., experimenter's social behavior; experimental treatments, presentation of humor), and chemically induced mood changes (i.e., inhalation of nitrous oxide, "laughing gas"). The values range between 10 and 40 when applying the STCI-S. For example means in state cheerfulness varied from about 19 (after exposure to situations inducing bad mood) to 35 (sober women during carnival festivities; male volunteers after inhaling nitrous oxide [subgroup of 11 smiling or laughing subjects only]; [15,18]). The level of state cheerfulness was also elevated among soccer fans before an easy to win game on TV, and after exposure to jokes and cartoons [35], a clowning experimenter [37], and an audiotape of interviews of a catching cheerful quality. State seriousness means ranged from 14 (the carnivalists) to 27 (subjects starting a two- hour mental work). Seriousness increased when listening to catching audiotapes of a serious (but also bad mood) quality and decreased in some cheerful situations. Bad mood means were typically low and ranged from 11 (the carnivalists; inhalation with nitrous oxide) to 24 (among soccer fans after their national team dropped out of the World Championships). Furthermore, It was shown that that the STCI-S is a sensitive instrument for assessing longer lasting states too: As expected, depressive patients were significantly lower in state cheerfulness, clearly higher in state seriousness and nearly twice as high in state bad mood, in comparison to the norm. Similarl results were found for schizophrenic patients compared to the norm [47,48,49,50].

Carretero-Dios, Eid and Ruch [51] applied a multi-trait multi-method method (MTMM) applying confirmatory factor analysis to data on the STCI. The MTMM approach allows separating different sources of individual differences, such as influences due to trait, method and error components. The study aimed at analyzing the convergent and discriminant validity of the trait form of STCI-T <106>. Participants completed the trait form (STCI-T<106>) in a single session and also answered the state form (STCI-S<30>) once a day at predetermined times on eight successive days. Moreover, the participants chose three close acquaintances each who rated them on the peer-evaluation form of the STCI-T<106>. The convergent validity was scrutinized using three different types of methods: self-reports, peer-reports and aggregated state ratings. With respect to the discriminant validity coefficients the authors investigated relations between cheerfulness, seriousness and bad mood. As outlined, cheerfulness and bad mood have in common that they are affective concepts, although the valence of the former is positive and the valence of the latter negative, leading to a negative correlation between the two. As seriousness refers to a frame of mind, correlations should be weaker. The results show that cheerfulness, seriousness and bad mood, as both state and traits are homogeneous factors no matter how they were measured. Aggregated states measures were clearly connected with the respective traits and self-reported traits were moderate for aggregated states (total scores across the eight days) and lower for single measurements, as expected. Furthermore, strong evidence in favor of convergent (homologous scales correlated well) and discriminant (non-homologous scales were less correlated) validity of the STCI was observed. Finally, the expected pattern of correlations between the three dimensions was confirmed in the methods sampled and the peer-evaluation data provided support for the hypothesis that traits represent the dispositions for their respective states. The coefficients of the peer ratings were all significant, and for individual states only slightly lower than for the self-reports.

BEYOND THE STCI FOR GERMAN ADULTS: GENERATION OF INTERNATIONAL AND CHILDREN VERSIONS

Since the first publication of the STCI-T in 1996 and the STCI-S in 1997 [2,3] different versions of the state and trait questionnaires have been developed and translated into various languages, mainly basing on the international version of the STCI-T <106> and the STCI-S <30>. The procedure of adapting the questionnaire to English will be exemplified next, representing the process of all translations and adaptations.

The generation of the English pilot facet form [52] of the trait STCI took place in several steps. In step 1, all 106 items were translated into English (by one German, and one native English speaker, skilled in German too). Step 2 included a comparison of both translations, discussions about linguistic peculiarities and the content of several items and ended with a first translated item list (for some items alternative versions were kept). In step 3, the list was checked by two English-speaking humor experts familiar with the state-trait model. Their corrections were examined for their correspondence regarding the items' content and taken over to a large extent.

In a final step, the modified list was discussed with further English speaking researchers, resulting in the international version STCI-T<106>. The STCI-T<106> serves as the pilot version for adaptations in different cultures and languages. Table 1 shows the different versions available. The STCI exists in 13 languages, as presented in Table 1, and can be applied in various settings, with various versions for self and peer ratings (e.g., general peer rating, for parents, at the workplace). The psychometric characteristics of these adaptations are encouraging and the instruments typically yield comparable findings, regarding their psychometric characteristics and correlational patterns. Whereas most versions are tailored to adults, a children's version has recently been developed. Ruch and colleagues [53,54] adapted the STCI to children and youth aged 10-14 years.

Table 1. Overview of the different versions of the STCI-T and STCI-S

Version		Facet structure	Languages
Trait			
STHI-T <106>	self, peer	5 cheerfulness (38 items), 6 seriousness (37 items), 5 seriousness (31 items)	German, English
STHI-T <104>		5 cheerfulness (38 items), 6 seriousness (37 items), 5 seriousness (29 items)	Spanish
STHI-T <60>	self, peer, workplace	1 facet each (20 items each)	German, English, French (Québec), Polish, Hebrew, Chinese (Hong Kong), Spanish, Italian, Romanian. Underway: Slovene, Russian, Japanese
STHI-T <30>	self, peer	3 scales (10 items each)	German, English
STHI-T <30> children	self, peer, parent, teacher	3 scales (10 items each); 2 sub-clusters each	German, Spanish
State			
STHI-S <45i>			English
STHI-S <30>		3 scales (10 items each); sub-clusters English version: cheerful, hilarity, earnest, pensive, sober, sad, ill-humored	German, English
STHI-S <20>		3 scales (8 items for cheerfulness, 6 seriousness, 6 bad mood)	English
STHI-S <18>		3 scales (6 items each)	German, English, Hebrew
STHI-S <20> children	self, peer	3 scales (8 items for cheerfulness, 6 seriousness, 6 bad mood)	German

Note. Further information on the different versions and authors involved in translation and adaptation can be obtained from the authors.

After reformulating the items of the German standard STCI-T <60> and STCI-S <30> to a language adequate to children, their comprehensibility was checked by 10 kids aged 10-14 years. Next, the two pilot forms were filled in by 400 German speaking school children (age M = 12.04; SD = 1.37). To testing the sensitivity for mood changes and differences, the state versions were given in a control condition, as well as mood induction experiments with factual (giving scenarios) and actual induction of cheerfulness, seriousness and bad mood. Trait and state cheerfulness, seriousness and bad mood could be distinguished, but a simplified facet structure (two sub-clusters each) was adequate. The inter-correlations between the trait facets emerged as expected (CH to SE r = -.04; CH to BM r = -.36; BM to SE r = .12; [53]).

It needs to be considered that these correlations might be underestimated, as the reliabilities in the children's samples were lower as compared to the adults (due to the restricted variance in the sample). The correspondence between self- and peer-evaluations of traits turned out to be sufficiently high, ranging from r = .36 for trait bad mood to r = .41 for trait seriousness, and r = .47 for trait cheerfulness. To conclude, the overall psychometric characteristics of the scales proofed satisfactory (Cronbach's α ranged from .70 to .79 in the trait, and from .76 to .86 in the state version). The children's version was so far applied in a classroom setting and to investigating its relations to orientations to happiness [55] and life satisfaction [56] among Swiss school kids [57].

THE STATE-TRAIT MODEL OF CHEERFULNESS, SERIOUSNESS, AND BAD MOOD AND ITS RELATIONS TO HUMOR

The crucial question yet remains to be answered: Do the traits claimed to be the temperamental basis of humor indeed predict the sense of humor and humor behaviors sufficiently well? What behaviors, thoughts, and actions related to humor can the three temperamental traits forming the basis of humor actually predict? As they were designed to account for the inter- and intraindividual differences in the readiness to respond to humor with positive affect it is necessary to examine whether they actually do so.

Several studies have been carried out to test the model assumptions [3,15] and there are also studies examining the three traits in the context of the nomological net of humor variables. These studies involved predicting humor behavior in experiments by the three traits, the examination of the convergent validity (i.e., the correlation with other humor questionnaires), and the joint factor analysis of the STCI-T scales and other humor instruments.

Table 2 presents the main results of experiments that aimed at testing different model assumptions. The scope is restricted to results relating to trait cheerfulness. Results are only mentioned briefly. For more details the reader is referred to the original sources.

The results of the studies in Table 2 can be clustered in two categories: Experimental evidence dependent *or* independent of amusement/exhilaration eliciting stimuli. This distinction was undertaken because it was necessary to show that trait cheerfulness also predisposes individuals to more state cheerfulness without being linked to a stimulus. Only then it could be concluded to be a temperamental factor, tailoring individual's behavior independent of elicitors. Trait cheerfulness represents the disposition to both state cheerfulness and exhilaration (smiling and laughter) irrespective of the eliciting condition or stimulus. As expected, trait cheerful individuals show more Duchenne displays in response to a clowning experimenter and to "bloopers" [37,59]. As cheerful individuals are extraverted [14] results might have been confounded with extraversion. It is known that extraverts smile and laugh more often than introverts, independent of stimuli. However, the smiles shown in the studies were not social smiles but involved the Duchenne display. To further exclude this possible sociability confound, exhilaration was elicited chemically (through inhalation of nitrous oxide, i.e., the "laughing gas") and individuals were tested in solitude.

**Table 2. State and trait cheerfulness and the experimental induction
of exhilaration and cheerful mood**

Individuals high in trait cheerfulness ...
... laugh more often and have higher increases in state cheerfulness after inhaling nitrous oxide [18]
... have higher rises in state cheerfulness after consuming kava extract [58]
... show more smiling and laughter (higher contraction of the zygomatic major muscle) when looking at video clips of simple news or news speaker's slips of the tongues [59]
... show facial signs of exhilaration more frequent and intense, when interacting with a clowning experimenter for 10 minutes [37]
... display higher increases in cheerfulness after listening to funny tapes (in comparisons to tapes containing neutral contents [37]
... report less need for structure [60]
... display BOLD activation in the inferior parietal lobule of the right hemisphere. This might be associated with a general readiness/tendency to be amused by jokes. Regions previously shown to be activated in humor appreciation studies seem more likely to be related to the understanding of individual jokes and the momentary emotion and the momentary emotional reaction of exhilaration [61]

In a psychpharmacological experiment, Ruch and Stevens [18] found that trait cheerfulness moderated the impact of nitrous oxide on state-cheerfulness, compared to placebo (inhaling pure oxygen) and baseline measures. The latter two did not differ from each other, indicating that the placebo control was successful. No mood-enhancing effect could be observed for low trait cheerful individuals. Trait cheerful individuals also smiled and laughed more often after inhaling nitrous oxide. Conversely, low trait cheerful individuals did not experience exhilaration; they just felt the numbing effect of nitrous oxide. In this respect, a definite neurological reaction could be seen in the high trait cheerful individuals that made them experience more exhilaration. A first fMRI study suggested involvement of brain structures sensitive to differences in trait cheerfulness [61]. Thus, trait cheerfulness indeed seems to predispose people to react more readily with smiling, laughter, and exhilaration/amusement; without it being tied to a humor stimulus. Similar effects were found for kava-kava extract; cheerful individuals had a higher increase in state cheerfulness indicating that trait cheerfulness moderates the drug-induced increase in cheerful mood [58]. Further, Table 2 confirms that state cheerfulness is a predictor of smiling and laughter. Ruch [35] reported that participants in a cheerful mood showed facial responses of exhilaration to cartoons and jokes at lower minimal levels of rated funniness than did less cheerful subjects. This implies that subjects high or low in cheerfulness differed with respect to the frequency and intensity of facial behavior shown, but not in terms of their judgments of funniness. This phenomenon was labeled facial hyper-expressivity [35]. State cheerfulness also predicted the frequency and intensity of exhilation, and, in turn, the intensity and duration of laughter then predicted the raise in state cheerfulness [37]. This confirms the reciprocal relationship between state cheerfulness and exhilaration. However, no study has been done yet to show that there is an upward spiral of cheerful mood facilitating smiling and laughter, that, in turn, boosts a cheerful state.

Further, there is evidence that state cheerfulness is a moderator of elicitors of smiling and laughter. A laughing experimenter [37] is only contagious for individuals that are already in a cheerful mood but not for ones that are not. Similarly, EMG-recorded smiling in response to jokes and cartoons is enhanced by mere presence (i.e., the mere presence of an else passive person) only for individuals in a cheerful state [32]. Robustness of cheerful mood, or "keeping humor," is a further parameter in the relationship between state and trait cheerfulness that deserves separate attention. Trait cheerfulness not only predicts the threshold for the induction of a cheerful mood state, its intensity and duration, but also the resistance against worsening of the mood. It was postulated and found in a rating study that it takes more adverse stimuli to impair the cheerful mood among trait cheerful individuals compared to the low cheerful ones [15]. The results of subsequent experiments are summarized in Table 3. Table 3 shows that trait cheerfulness is also a predictor of robustness of cheerful mood. In a variety of settings, individuals high in trait cheerfulness (especially in facet CH3 "cheerful composure") maintained their good mood when facing adversity but low trait cheerful individuals did not. In some of these studies the adverse situation was generated quite unobtrusively; for example, by placing the participants in a depressing room (vs. cheerful room) with poor illumination, black walls, a dried out plant on the table and a pessimistic poster on the wall facing the participant [15] or asking participants to explain misanthropic (vs. cheerful) proverbs [62]. These studies confirm that trait cheerfulness represents the tendency to maintain in cheerful mood, even when facing adversity. Their cheerful mood is more robust against inductions of negative mood and emotions. However, no study was conducted so far that actually tested the limits of trait cheerful people.

Table 3. Trait cheerfulness and robustness of cheerful mood

Trait cheerful individuals
… stay in a cheerful mood when having to elaborate proverbs with negative, misanthropic contents [62]
… show more smiling and laughter when being confronted with one's own grimaced face unexpectedly [63]
… keep a cheerful state, even when having to sit in a depressing room while working on several tasks [15]
… show more Duchenne smiling in response to seeing distorted photographs of themselves [64,65]
… report more positive emotions and less negative emotions when confronted with a distorted photograph of themselves [65]

When trait cheerful individuals keep humor in face of adversity, are they also able to laugh at themselves? Recently, an experimental paradigm for the study of "laughing at oneself" was developed [65,66]. The Distorted Photograph Task (DPT; [66]) is a computer based task aimed at eliciting situations where laughing at oneself is possible. First, a cover story is told to participants, which justified the taking of photos of the participant's face. Then these photos are electronically distorted (e.g., flattening or bowing the face) without the knowledge of the participant. In the main part of the experiment, the participants are instructed to look at 12 distorted photographs on a computer screen and to rate the degree of appreciation (funniness and aversiveness), unaware that their own photographs had been inserted into the presented series. The photos are presented randomly and the participants are unexpectedly confronted with their own distorted photo. During this task, participants are alone in a room [62] and secretly filmed and the facial responses are FACS-coded. As expected, trait cheerfulness predicts the level of positive affect (and of low negative affect) when people either laugh at themselves rather than being upset. In detail, trait cheerful individuals found their own distorted photographs funnier and reported more positive emotions (e.g., joy and serenity) and less negative emotions (e.g., discomfort, anger, fear) than low trait cheerful individuals. Furthermore, they showed more intense Duchenne smiling and laughter and reported a higher increase in state cheerfulness and a stronger decrease in state seriousness from before to after the experiment. Also, low trait bad mood individuals reported high degrees of negative emotions when looking at their distorted photograph and less positive emotions than high trait bad mood individuals [65]. Thus, trait cheerful individuals can deal with being the butt of a joke and even see the positive side of it. This ability to distance oneself from being the target of a joke, or experiencing an embarrassing situation or mishap, can actually help to gain perspectives and overcome negative feelings [44]. By laughing at the mishap or the joke, one has taken the first step in mastering the situation.

In a conceptually related study [64] participants were instructed to pose different facial expressions (among them also a silly face) and then visual feedback was given. Although laughing at oneself was not explicitly investigated, it was shown that more smiling and laughter occurred in high trait cheerful individuals when being confronted with one's own grimaced face unexpectedly. Also, habitually cheerful individuals reported no decrease in cheerful mood while low the trait cheerful did.

Taken together, trait cheerfulness represents a disposition for exhilaration and the induction and robustness of cheerful mood. In this sense, trait cheerfulness underlies humor, as typically in everyday conversations a "good sense of humor" would be used to explain these behaviors to occur in some people but not in others. While this is good support it should be mentioned that this is not unique to trait cheerfulness, as extraversion has also been shown to predict frequency and intensity of humor-induced smiling and laughter [8,12]. Hence, one might argue that trait cheerfulness is a redundant concept. Therefore, extraversion was examined in most of these studies as well and its predictive power typically turned out to be lower than the one for trait cheerfulness [37]. Likewise, the predictive power of state cheerfulness compared to the one of more general mood states, such as elation or positive affectivity, was controlled in two studies [32]. It turned out that an index of cheerful mood was a better predictor compared to all scales of positive mood used. Thus, state and trait cheerfulness are superior in accounting for humor induced positive affect than more general personality traits and broader mood states, respectively.

If trait cheerfulness predicts humor behavior in experiments (i.e., a single situation), it should also predict humor related habits, as typically reported in humor questionnaires. Above, selected humor behaviors were studied that stem from the state-trait theory of cheerfulness. Trait conceptualizations of humor, such as the "sense of humor" often draw on those behaviors (such as being able to laugh at oneself) and hence an overlap between sense of humor and trait cheerfulness can be expected.

However, humor is a multifaceted phenomenon and there will be aspects of humor that are not based to trait cheerfulness (e.g., ridiculing others, having a "dry wit", or liking bathroom humor). The STCI was administered together with many humor questionnaires and the results are given in Table 4. Furthermore, when a broad selection of humor instruments was administered a joint factor analysis was performed to see where cheerfulness (and seriousness and bad mood) is in the factor space derived.

Table 4 confirms that trait cheerfulness predicts most facets of sense of humor conceptualized, like *coping humor* (measured by the Situational Humor Response Questionnaire, SHRQ, [11]; or the Coping Humor Scale, CHS, [71]), *humor styles* (measured by the Humor Styles Questionnaire, HSQ, [67]), the *facets of the sense of humor* (Sense of Humor Scale, SHS, McGhee, [10,44]), and *styles of everyday humor conduct* (e.g., Humorous Behavior Q-Sort Deck, HBQD, [72]; and the Humor Use in Multiple Ongoing Relationships, HUMOR, [73]), as well as various other models [42].

Ruch and colleagues [43] investigated the relationship between the trait cheerfulness, bad mood and seriousness on the one hand, and humor styles and uses of humor on the other. The HSQ [67] claims to measure potentially adaptive and maladaptive styles of humor in four distinct dimensions, namely affiliative, self-enhancing, aggressive, and self-defeating humor. Styles of everyday humor conduct were assessed by the HBQD [9,71] which measures 10 styles located along five bipolar dimensions: socially warm vs. cool, reflective vs. boorish, competent vs. inept, earthy vs. restrained, and benign vs. mean-spirited humor. The STCI-T traits predicted the contents of the HSQ and the HBQD well: Trait cheerfulness was strongly correlated with the socially warm, affiliative, self-enhancing humor style and use of humor in everyday life, and was also predictive of competent, earthy, and self-defeating humor. The HSQ concept of affiliative humor refers to the tendency to joke around with others, say witty things, tell amusing stories, laugh with others, and amuse others. In this sense it strongly resembles facet CH5 (a generally cheerful interaction style) of trait cheerfulness. Indeed, trait cheerfulness was a very potent predictor of affiliative humor ($r = .69$, $p < .001$) and CH5 was the facets that correlated almost interchangeably with affiliative humor ($r = .80$, $p < .001$). The self-enhancing humor scale contains items relating to perspective-taking humor, the tendency to maintain a humorous outlook on life, and the use of humor in emotion regulation and coping and thus also overlaps with facet CH3 (a composed view of adverse life circumstances) of trait cheerfulness. Indeed, trait cheerfulness predicted self-enhancing humor ($r = .58$, $p < .001$) and both CH3 ($\beta = .24$) and CH4 ($\beta = .44$) predicted self-enhancing humor in a step-wise regression analysis (R = .65, $F_{(2,165)} = 55.667$, $p < .001$). The items of the aggressive humor scale relate to sarcasm, teasing, use of humor to criticize or manipulate others, and compulsive expressions of humor without regard for the effects on others. This sounds perhaps a bit too serious as, after all, it is a playful expression of aggression. Indeed the "aggressive" humor style mostly indicated lack of seriousness: Low trait seriousness was involved in the prediction of socially cold, earthy and repressed humor styles, and in affiliative ($r = -.45$, $p < .001$), self-enhancing and aggressive humor ($r = -.34$, $p < .001$).

Finally, self-defeating humor comprises tendencies to use humor in an excessively self-disparaging and ingratiating way, to allow oneself to be the butt of others' jokes, and to use humor as a form of defensive denial to hide underlying negative feelings. Trait bad mood was a potent predictor of the socially cold and inept humor styles and was negatively correlated with benign, earthy, affiliative and self-enhancing humor styles, as well as having incremental validity in the prediction of self-defeating humor.

The study also investigated the HUMOR [72], which highly correlated with trait seriousness ($r = -.54$, $p <.001$) and with cheerfulness ($r = .45$, $p <.001$). Some items correlated more highly with trait cheerfulness (e.g., "I laugh at TV or radio programs that I think are funny"), but more individual items were primarily representing low seriousness (e.g., "I laugh about upsetting things that have happened to me"). Taken together, these results support the view that traits forming the temperamental basis of humor are able to predict everyday humorous behavior. They demonstrate their utility as a valid alternative to the folk concept of the sense of humor.

Several studies applied factor analyses to the intercorrelation of the STCI and a variety of self-report humor instruments. Generally, studies repeatedly resulted in factors related to cheerfulness and (low) seriousness (e.g., [8,42]), but also bad mood [52].

Table 4. Correlations between trait cheerfulness and various measures of the sense of humor

High trait cheerful individuals...
... are higher in socially warm, competent, earthy humor of the HBQD [4]
... are higher in affiliative and self-enhancing humor styles, report less self-defeating humor of the HSQ [4,67]
... score higher on all to the sense of humor facets measured by the SHS [52,68]
... report more humor behavior [4]
... report using humor as a coping strategy [69]
... report less fear of being laughed at (gelotophobia, e.g., Ruch and Proyer [70]), and report more gelotophilia, the joy of being laughed at [65]

For example, Ruch and Carrell [52] assessed the STCI and the facets of the sense of humor as proposed by McGhee and measured by the SHS [10,44] in two samples (American and German). The SHS assesses eight facets of the sense of humor (e.g., finding humor in everyday life, using humor under stress), which are related to McGhee's humor training program. The Scree test of the joint factor analysis of the subscales of the SHS and STCI-T suggested in both samples the retention of three factors (explained variance US: 64.5%; German: 61.1%). Factor 1 (cheerfulness/sense of humor) was loaded by the SHS scales and the facets of trait cheerfulness. Thus, this factor merged elements like enjoying humorous stimuli (SHS-1, STCI-T CH4), enjoying cheerful interactions (STCI-T H5) and telling jokes (SHS-5), finding humor in everyday life (SHS-6) and in one's own mishaps (SHS-7), a tendency to laugh (SHS-4, STCI-T CH2), prevalence of cheerful mood (STCI-T, CH1), and the use of humor under stress (SHS-8). Factor 2 (seriousness) and 3 (bad mood) was loaded by the respective facets in the STCI-T and the scales of the SHS (SHS-2: seriousness and negative mood, and SHS-3: playfulness and positive mood) and were negatively correlated with the factor of cheerfulness/sense of humor.

The discussed studies typically report that trait cheerfulness accounts for most variance in sense of humor assessment tools. However, these findings [43,52] can be criticized to largely overestimate the role of cheerfulness in "the sense of humor". This is due to the fact that the recent conceptualizations of the sense of humor give too much weight to the affective-expressive and social qualities, and hence, there is much conceptual overlap with cheerfulness. Thus, it is no surprise that cheerfulness predicts humor operationalized via its affective and behavioral qualities. A sense of humor conceptualized as an attitude or worldview should not be so strongly related to affect, thus leaving room for additional, moderating variables to be involved [15,43,52]. Indeed, being able to laugh at oneself (a core facet of the sense of humor) correlated to $r = .50$ with trait cheerfulness. Two seriousness facets had incremental validity: SE5 entered the regression equation with a negative and SE2 with a positive weight [52]. Thus, 'laughing at oneself' is highest among those cheerful individuals who do face things seriously, but also communicate humorously.

STCI AND HEALTH AND WELL-BEING OUTCOME VARIABLES

Many promoters of humor and also researchers claim that humor and laughter are beneficial to health and well-being, although empirical evidence is still scarce [31]. The lack of accumulative research in this area is due to many reasons. One is that too little time and effort has been spend on building solid foundations for applied research. For example, if one assumes that laughter is relaxing, does this apply to all types of laughs? Obviously, the question of how many types of laughter exist needs to be solved first before we ask whether they would all be beneficial. Likewise, humor research has spent way too little effort in working on solid conceptualizations of the sense of humor, but rushed into looking whether they are beneficial or detrimental. As a consequence, research knowledge is a bit of a patchwork, rather than a solid field of knowledge. In the present chapter it was decided to present findings on trait cheerfulness only, as it overlaps greatly with many other conceptualizations of the sense of humor.

Generally speaking, health is not solely the absence of negative affect and physical symptoms, but a *"complex state of complete physical, mental, and social well-being and not merely the absence of disease or infirmity"* [74: 100]. Well-being is a complex construct that concerns optimal experience and functioning (e.g., [75,76]). Ryan and Deci [76] claim that well-being is derived from two general perspectives: The first one is the hedonic approach, which focuses on happiness and defines well-being in terms of pleasure attainment and pain avoidance. The second one is the eudamonic approach, which focuses on meaning and self-realization and defines well-being in terms of the degree to which a person is fully-functioning. Seligman [77] presented three basic orientations to happiness, namely life of pleasure (i.e., hedonism), life of engagement, and life of meaning (relating to eudemonia) and indeed all three were found to happiness [55]. Recently, Seligman [78] has redefined what constitutes human's thriving in life and this brought a shift from life satisfaction to *flourishing*. Flourishing goes beyond being happy with one's life and life circumstances and constitutes five elements. Flourishing includes human's needs to find meaning, achievement and being engaged too. Flourishing can be reached through a combination of *positive experience/emotions*, *engagement, relationships to others, meaning and accomplishment*, leading to well-being and summed under the acronym *PERMA* (see Seligman, [78]). Seligman [78] reports less health problems and more productivity for flourishing individuals. In the next sections, the relations of trait cheerfulness to health, life satisfaction and the relevant elements of PERMA will be discussed.

HEALTH

Good health and well-being relate to satisfaction with life. Life satisfaction gained much attention in research during the past decades, mostly due to the growing interest in Positive Psychology [55]. Correlations between cheerfulness and life satisfaction were established for both adults [43,79] and children [54] reporting that trait cheerful individuals are more satisfied with their lives.

Table 5 brings together further relevant findings on trait cheerfulness and its relation to health variables. Zweyer, Velker and Ruch [80] reported higher pain tolerance (in the cold pressure test) for trait cheerful individuals. This occurred after watching a funny film and producing humor to it, or smiling and laughing voluntarily at it. The moderating effect of exhilaration and trait cheerfulness on pain perception should be considered, for example in post-operative care. Milder pain killers might be partly substituted by exhilaration (e.g., through humor interventions, hospital clowns etc.), leading to less cost and physical and psychological side effects.

Also, stress causes physiological reactions, and maladaptive strategies dealing with stress can decrease health [81,82]. Coping can be defined as dealing with a negative situation and its feelings in different ways [83,84]. Adaptive coping is an important variable in dealing with stressful life events, overcoming problems, and in a long-term perspective life satisfaction. In 2004, Diener and Seligman [75] found adaptive coping to be positively related to life satisfaction. Ruch and Zweyer [69] showed that trait cheerful individuals use more constructive and adaptive stress coping mechanisms (e.g., positive self-instruction, relaxation) as measured by the SVF 120 [6]. Especially the facet "cheerful composure" (i.e., CH3) predicted positive coping strategies. Furthermore, for habitually cheerful individuals, state cheerfulness stays high, and no more physical symptoms were reported in retrospect, even when having faced negative life events and stress [15,69].

As seen in the study of Ruch and Carrell [52], trait cheerfulness predicts various facets of the sense of humor in the model of McGhee. Interestingly, some of McGhee's facets are closely related to *coping*, namely the facet humor under stress and laughing at oneself. McGhee [88] views the sense of humor as an accumulation of facets, which can be trained and fostered to contribute to stress-resistance and resilience. Displaying a cheerfully composed view on life can help mastering difficult life-events and negative mental states. As trait cheerfulness accounted for most variance in the SHS, it can be concluded that cheerfulness plays a crucial role in humor facets related to coping too.

Hehlmann [89] stated that a humorous worldview is a sign of human maturity, an attitude akin to wisdom, and developed on prior suffering, pain, and exposure to an imperfect world. Applying this to a more clinical focus, it can be concluded that the humorous world view enables what clinicians would call "post-traumatic growth" [77,90,91]. While some individuals response to tragedy with depression, PTSD, rumination and learned helplessness, others actually take something away from it: they grow in response to the tragedy.

Table 5. Experimental and correlational evidence to trait cheerfulness and health and well-being outcome variables

Individuals high in trait cheerfulness...
Health
Physical
... report higher state cheerfulness, and no more physical symptoms, even when facing negative life events and stress [15,69,85,86]
... have a higher pain tolerance (in the cold pressure test) after watching a funny film and producing humor to it, or smiling and laughing voluntarily at it [80]
Mental/Robustness of mood (see also Table 3)
... report using humor as a coping strategy [69]
... use more constructive and adaptive stress coping mechanisms, like positive self-instruction and relaxation [69]
Well-being: Person Factors
... experience more positive affect and report less negative affect [42]
... report more quality of life [79]
... report more life satisfaction [45]
... score lower in neuroticism, higher on extraversion, and higher on agreeableness [8,15,36,87]
... score lower on Eysenck's psychoticism [87]
... report less fear of being laughed at (gelotophobia, e.g., [70], and report more gelotophilia, the joy of being laughed at [65]
... report higher need for play, affiliation, exhibition, dominance and nurturance [42]
Well-being: Social
... Highly trait cheerful are emotionally intelligent and possess high interpersonal competence [87]
... High trait cheerful experience more social closeness [14]

Notably, the maintaining a cheerful outlook on life and not loosing humor in the face of adversity refers to the robustness of mood postulate of the facet model. This cheerful outlook is different from the view of humor as a coping strategy [92]. Such as trait cheerfulness is the *underlying* trait and better coping the overt behavior shown, not the mechanism behind. Furthermore, the facets CH2 (low threshold for smiling and laughter) and CH4 (having a broad range of active elicitors of cheerfulness, smiling and laughter) may explain possible relations between cheerfulness and stress, as stress reactivity studies have shown that smiling through stressful tasks in the laboratory lead to faster recovery. Also, the decrease of positive affect was smaller throughout the whole experimental session in participants showing smiles. Therefore, trait cheerful individuals who can laugh and smile easily also do this when completing stressful tasks in an experimental setting and consequently recover faster.

POSITIVE EXPERIENCE (PERMA) AND LIFE OF PLEASURE (AUTHENTIC HAPPINESS)

The most obvious relation between trait cheerfulness and well-being is found in the fact that cheerfulness facilitates positive experiences (like state cheerfulness, exhilaration) and prevents negative experience (i.e, the "keeping humor", or "robustness of positive mood" effect). Where as the former part is most purely incorporated in the positive experience element of PERMA, the combination of both (presence of positive and absence of negative affect) is an element of the life of pleasure, one element of authentic happiness. Indeed, like humor, trait cheerfulness is significantly correlated with all three orientations to happiness. However, it is more highly correlated to life of pleasure than to engagement and meaning in both children and adults [4,43,54]. The life of pleasure, as an orientation to happiness relates to the principle of maximizing pleasure and minimizing pain, again relating to establishing positive feelings and avoiding negative.

Meehl [93] developed the concept of *hedonic capacity*. Hedonic capacity is a disposition, which is (to different degrees) inherent in all individuals, enabling the experience of positive affect. This accumulation of positive affect directly contributes to well-being. This converges with the view that trait cheerfulness is a habitual trait fostering positive experience. The hilarity component of cheerfulness (e.g., facet CH2: *low threshold for smiling and laughter*) might be the ones representing the induction of positive affect and the cheerful composedness component (e.g., CH3: a *composed view of adverse life circumstances*) represents the tendency to be immune negative states and more quickly overcome them [2,15].

Experimental evidence for these two effects have already been given in Tables 2 and 3. Moreover, Köhler and Ruch [42] report that high trait cheerful individuals experience more positive affect and report less negative affect as measured by the Positive Affect Negative Affect Scale (PANAS [94]). Trait cheerful individuals have the ability to laugh at themselves and therefore overcome aversive situations and happenings more easily [66]. While the results presented suggest that trait cheerfulness entails *resilience* against the induction of negative affect, it has to be said that higher levels of adversity have not been studied so far. It is safe to assume that trait cheerful individuals will eventually get grumpy and grouchy when being confronted with highly adverse circumstances. Generally, distal effects of being more resilient to negative events might be the rare occurrence of the health effects of predominant negative affect. Hence fostering the appearance of exhilaration may help to mitigate, suppress, interrupt, or even permanently replace a variety of negative states [13].

TRAIT CHEERFULNESS AND RELATIONSHIPS TO OTHERS

Trait cheerfulness not only represents a disposition to positive mood, it incorporates the sharing of fun with others. This is expressed most clearly in facet CH5 ("a generally cheerful interaction style"). Cheerfulness enables individuals to engage easily in playful and cheerful interactions and therefore fosters interpersonal bonds. This may not be the core element of positive relationship with others and relations based on shred fun might miss important elements. However, laughter has been seen as a social lubricant and as such it will help the individual to establish relationships (everything else held constant). Persons scoring high in cheerfulness report to be more satisfied with their lives compared to less cheerful people. This may be due to their ability to initiate humorous behavior in social situations, larger social networks and better-developed social skills. Trait cheerfulness generally goes along with a cheerful interaction style, and perceived social closeness [14]. Consequently, it could be leading to a higher level of social support. Yip and Martin [95] showed that trait cheerful individuals generally scored higher in an ability test for emotional intelligence (measured by the Mayer-Savoley-Caruso Emotional Intelligence Scale; MSCEIT [96]) and possess high interpersonal competence: They initiate relationships more easily, disclose personal information to significant others, provide emotional support to others, and manage conflicts in relationships constructive [95]. Last but not least, research on cheerfulness and domain specific satisfaction among children has shown that trait cheerfulness relates most strongly to satisfaction with friends (compared to family, self, or school) [53].

CHEERFULNESS, ENGAGEMENT AND MEANING

Research on adults and children have shown that trait cheerfulness, like humor, correlates modestly and positively with meaning and engagement; i.e., the more potent predictors of enduring happiness (compared to the life of pleasure). The meaningful life suggests that happiness can be achieved by using ones skills and talents in the service of greater goods. Cheerfulness contributes to life of meaning, as maintaining a positive view on the world, even when facing adversities may help seeing the meaning in life-events.

The engaged life is influenced by Csikszentmihalyi's works on flow. Life of engagement is supported by state and trait cheerfulness, as cheerful individuals don't get grumpy or sad easily and may be able to quest for their aims and goals longer. Although the concept of flow is not an affective one, Csikszentmihalyi [97] did claim that positive moods do usually occur after getting out of flow, at the end of an activity or in moments of distraction within it.

Accomplishment, the last element of PERMA will not be related to cheerfulness, but to seriousness. Trait seriousness predicts several accomplishment-related variables [14] including satisfaction with school experiences. Trait seriousness, together with cheerfulness, has been seen as an element in a more profound, philosophical sense of humor.

FURTHER RELATIONS

In even broader terms, cheerfulness is related to extraversion and emotional stability (low neuroticism, see [8,15,87,97]). For extraversion and neuroticism, it was found that the former is positively correlated to well-being, whereas the later is negatively related to it (e.g., [98,99]).

Furthermore, trait cheerful individuals report less fear of being laughed at and ridiculed by others (gelotophobia, the fear of being laughed at; [70]) and more gelotophilia (the joy of being laughed at [100]). This indicates that they are generally easy going in laughter and humor related situations. They can deal with being the butt of a joke and even enjoying this. This is in turn likely to be beneficial in establishing and maintaining friendships and acquaintances, for example in leisure or at the work place.

INTERVENTIONS TO ENHANCING CHEERFULNESS

Scientifically grounded training programs were established and empirically evaluated to enhance cheerfulness [48,88,101]. Brutsche and colleagues [102] showed that state cheerfulness significantly increased after humor interventions with a clown in severe refractory chronic obstructive pulmonary disease patients (COPD) and they also observed a reduction in hyperinflation. Papousek and Schulter [101] discuss that enhancing cheerfulness may improve coping with future adversities, which may promote enhancement of psychological well-being. Their cheerfulness training follows a behavioral therapy approach. The core of the training program is to learn and practice a technique to efficiently self-induce cheerful moods. This entails the imagination and voluntary production of motor and vocal expressions of cheerfulness. The authors assumed that voluntary expressions of emotions can trigger genuine feelings of these emotions (e.g., [21]). By repeating the newly learned behaviors, imaginations of subjective weaknesses and unpleasant situations are coupled with the positive moods through conditioning mechanisms. A fundamental postulate of the training is, that participants actively practice to self-induce cheerful moods, instead of just passively appreciating an instructor's jokes or humorous material. It is expected that imaginations of adversities and later real situations, automatically trigger a cheerful mood after having undergone the training. Results indicated enhanced cheerfulness levels due to the training program [100]. Mood changes were not only present during or shortly after the training sessions, but also two days after the training period, without further emotional stimulation. There was also a more general improvement of psychological well-being (more good-humored, calm, fresh, and less anxious mood). Feelings of stress and tenseness were reduced.

Hirsch and colleagues [48,49] evaluated humor therapy groups in elderly depressed patients in residential care settings. Two groups were formed. The control group participated the therapeutic program as usual. The other group attended group humor therapy session twice a week, on top of the usual range of activities. Both group's depression scores, suicidal tendency, life satisfaction, subjective general health and state cheerfulness improved over time, as well as state bad mood decreased. This shows that the general therapeutic program helped all the patients. On top of that, the humor therapy led to improvement in resilience, trait cheerfulness and a decrease in state seriousness. Here, an interaction effect was found: State seriousness decreased in both groups, but more so in the humor therapy group. Most importantly, in a yet unpublished study individuals underwent a training of the sense of humor based on the model by McGhee [10]. Not only sense of humor increased, but even more so trait cheerfulness, while trait seriousness and bad mood decreased. This confirms how closely sense of humor and trait cheerfulness, seriousness and bad mood are interconnected [88].

CONCLUSION

The results, obtained so far, provide evidence that cheerfulness, seriousness, and bad mood as states and traits are relevant to the study of humor. They account for a variety of phenomena, such as appreciation of types of humor, wit, keeping or losing humor when facing adversity, or readiness for exhilaration and laughter. There is also support for the view that these more narrow concepts are better predictors of humor phenomena than global personality concepts (like extraversion). To conclude, a few open questions for further research should be addressed. One issue is to study the state-trait model of cheerfulness in relation to other areas of humor not covered so far. For example, Schmidt-Hidding [103] summarized that humor (in the narrow sense) was based on a sympathetic heart, while wit would be based on a superior spirit, and mock/ridicule on moral sense or even haughtiness/maliciousness. Schmidt-Hidding [103] considered fun to be an expression of vitality/high spirits. Trait cheerfulness relates to the fun and humor parts of his model, but will be blind to others or need to be supplemented by others. For example, low seriousness is a predictor of wit, but the literature showed that the ability to create humor is primarily correlated with intelligence and creativity [104]. Here, the combined effects should be studied. Likewise, bad mood (and low seriousness) predicted scores in the comic styles of satire, cynicism, and sarcasm [105] but it does not account for much of the variance. Furthermore, longitudinal studies and studies that consider moderating and enabling factors are needed. The historic literature assigned cheerfulness a special role in the development of humor in the narrow sense. It was suggested that a humorous attitude or worldview is the product of a cheerful temperament and certain enabling factors, like negative life experiences and acquired insights into the human nature and human existence [39]. A person with a humorous attitude is someone who understands the insufficiencies and shortcomings of life and fellow humans but also tolerates and forgives them. In this sense, humor is considered to be serious and contains the wisdom that nothing earthly and human is perfect. In this respect, humor is different from merriment or hilarity. The former is contemplative, pensive, and profound, the latter thoughtless, superficial, and shallow. In a partial support of this hypothesis, Ruch and Carrell [52] found a mid-size correlation between trait cheerfulness and a questionnaire measure of "laughing at yourself" with components of seriousness showing incremental validity in predicting this indicator of humor in the more narrow sense. However, the total score of the SHS [10,44] and trait cheerfulness were almost indistinguishable. Similarly, in a study of temperamental predictors of comic styles it turned out that trait cheerfulness was positively related to humor (in the narrow sense), but also fun and nonsense [106]. Thus, the nature of the preferred comic style is based on one's prevalent mood. However, more studies are needed for proving that at least two factors are necessary for a humorous attitude to develop - a cheerful temperament and prior successfully mastered adverse life experiences. Thus, at best, a longitudinal study were trait cheerfulness is assessed prior to the life events (so that it is not itself affected by them) and humor is assessed after these life events should be conducted. Until now, the positive effects of cheerfulness were reported. But Friedman and colleagues [107] even reported a negative relationship between their factor cheerfulness/optimism in childhood and longevity when investigating participants of the Tearman life cycle study. They found (by applying factor analysis) cheerfulness consisting of two items: cheerfulness/optimism and sense of humor. This factor went along with earlier deaths. Martin and colleagues [108] reanalyzed these data trying to find the specific moderators of this correlation, but could not explain the relation of cheerfulness to earlier deaths via more risk behavior and such. Nevertheless, it seems important to also to consider potential negative effects of cheerfulness.

McNulty and Fincham [109] consider traits which contribute to well-being not as inherently positive. As Schwartz and Sharpe [110] already stated, the context is of utmost importance. It was suggested that well-being is not solely determined by certain psychological characteristics, but by the interplay between those characteristics and environmental factors of the person. The research further suggests that certain circumstances may lead to a decrease in life satisfaction, well-being and increase in maladaptive behaviors, when using so called beneficial traits in the wrong context or to the wrong extent (see e.g., the example of forgiveness; [111]). For example optimism can lead to an optimistic bias [112], where people underestimate health risks and miss on getting regular check-ups at the doctor's. According to McNulty and Fincham [109], three factors should be considered when fostering positive traits: It should be studied when, to whom, and to what extend well-being can be promoted, instead of examining the main effects of traits and processes on average. In the case of trait cheerfulness, coaches would need to consider that trait cheerful individuals respond differently compared to non-trait cheerful individuals when being confronted with a cheerfulness intervention. Maybe these interventions would need to look different for either high or low trait cheerful individuals, because there should be a fit between the individuals' habitual dispositions and the training offered. For example, it might be more suitable to start with less intense stimuli in low trait cheerful individuals, as not to overwhelm them. Consequently prolonging the training may help, as low trait cheerful individuals might need longer to get their cheerfulness heightened and may profit from a less intense, gradual approach. High trait cheerful individuals are easily brought into a cheerful state and that is why they might like engaging in cheerful evoking interventions more often and easily. They might also not need long interventions, as they have an inherent capacity for establishing and maintaining cheerful states. Perhaps they only need some training on polishing their cheerfulness skills. This links to the notion, whether it is possible to have too much cheerfulness. Especially the combination of high cheerfulness and low seriousness should be discussed. Somebody highly cheerful and not serious at all might find it difficult to engage in any sober and practical thinking. Then, it might be adequate to train these people in when to moderate their cheerfulness in order to concentrate on problem solving and all-day tasks. Or maybe high trait cheerful individuals would find it difficult to emphasize with somebody who cannot get him-or herself out of a grumpy or sad mood (e.g., clinically depressed individuals).

It is questionable whether high trait cheerful individuals need training at all. Going back to McNulty and Fincham [109], their next consideration states that psychological concepts need to be studied in the context of happy and unhappy people. Perhaps some traits benefit people in optimal circumstances, but can harm people in suboptimal circumstance; for example being more suitable for people in therapy. Then, approaches like the one Papousek and Schulter [101] used could be applied to the therapy of clinically depressed persons [113]. To conclude, as trait cheerful people generally experience more cheerful and happy moods, they might not need to be trained.

Thinking of evaluation studies, one should consider the matching of the control and intervention groups according to their cheerfulness levels. Responses to cheerfulness trainings might be different for low and high trait cheerful, independent from its relative success for the groups. When measuring for example facial displays of amusement and joy, one will find that cheerful individuals smile more easily, and more often. Therefore, it might be that low trait cheerful individuals already enjoy something, but not express this facially yet. Finally, implications of psychological characteristics should be studied over a long period of time. So far, it is not known whether short term benefits (which are most often investigated in positive intervention studies so far) do remain stable for medium or long time frames, or whether their quality changes. The same is true for the cheerfulness interventions conducted so far. Most of these thoughts discussed remain assumptions. The effects of cheerfulness and its training on individuals needs further consideration and research and also Friedman and colleagues' [107] counter-intuitive finding of cheerful individuals living shorter needs explaining. While the direct pathways of cheerfulness to the life of pleasure and hedonic well-being were discussed, it remains unclear how cheerfulness could relate to the other pathways, the life of engagement and the life of meaning, as well as the eudamonic well-being, which focuses on meaning and self-realization and defines well-being in terms of the degree to which a person is fully-functioning [76]. Studies focusing on these more complex relations would help finding out how cheerfulness can support people in reaching their full potential and finally bringing more light in the relation of the temperamental basis of humor to health and well-being. "*A laugh a day keeps the doctor away*" might not be as easily proven, but the results found so far are promising need continuation.

ACKNOWLEDGMENTS

The research leading to these results has received funding from the European Union Seventh Framework Programme (FP7/2007-2013) under grant agreement n 270780 (ILHAIRE project).

REFERENCES

[1]   Ruch, W. (in press). Cheerfulness. In A. C. Michalos (Ed.), *Encyclopedia of Quality of Life Research*. Berlin: Springer.
[2]   Ruch, W., Köhler, G., and van Thriel, C. (1996). Assessing the "humorous temperament": Construction of the facet and standard trait forms of the State-Trait-Cheerfulness-Inventory — STCI. *Humor: International Journal of Humor Research, 9*, 303-339.
[3]   Ruch, W., Köhler, G., and van Thriel, C. (1997). To be in good or bad humor: Construction of the state form of the State-Trait-Cheerfulness-Inventory — STCI. *Personality and Individual Differences, 22*, 477-491.
[4]   Ruch, W., Proyer, R. P., Esser, C., and Mitrache, O. (2011). Cheerfulness and everyday humorous conduct. In Romanian Academy, "George Barit" Institute of History, Department of Social Research (Ed.), *Studies and Researches in Social Sciences* (Vol. 18, pp. 67-87). Cluj-Napoca: Argonaut Press.
[5]   Seligman, M. E. P. and Csikszentmihihalyi, M. (2000). Positive Psychology: An introduction. *American Psychologist, 55*, 5-14.
[6]   Janke, W. and Erdmann, G. (1997). *Der Stressverarbeitungsfragebogen (SVF 120). Kurzbeschreibung und grundlegende Kennwerte* [The stress coping questionnaire. Short description and basic characteristics]. Göttingen: Hogrefe.
[7]   Diener, E., Emmons, R. A., Larsen, R. J., and Griffin, S. (1985). The satisfaction with life scale. *Journal of Personality Assessment, 49*, 71-75.
[8]   Ruch, W. (1994). Temperament, Eysenck's PEN system, and humor-related traits. *Humor: International Journal of Humor Research, 7*, 209-244.

[9]   Craik, K. H., Lampert, M. D., and Nelson, A. J. (1996). Sense of humor and styles of everyday humorous conduct. *Humor: International Journal of Humor Research, 9,* 273-302.

[10] McGhee, P. E. (1999). *Health, Healing and the Amuse System* (3rd edition.). Dubuque: Kendall/Hunt Publishing Company.

[11] Martin, R. A. and Lefcourt, H. M. (1984). Situational Humor Response Questionnaire: Quantitative measure of sense of humor. *Journal of Social and Personality Psychology, 47,* 145-155.

[12] Ruch, W. and Deckers, L. (1993). Do extraverts "like to laugh": An analysis of the Situational Humour Response Questionnaire (SHRQ). *European Journal of Personality 7,* 211-220.

[13] Ruch, W. (1993). Exhilaration and humor. In M. Lewis and J. M. Haviland (Eds.), *The Handbook of Emotions* (p. 605-616). New York: Guilford Publications.

[14] Ruch, W. and Köhler, G. (2007). A temperament approach to humor. In W. Ruch (Ed.), *The Sense of Humor: Explorations of a Personality Characteristic* (pp. 203-230). Berlin: Mouton de Gruyter.

[15] Ruch, W. and Köhler, G. (1999). The measurement of state and trait cheerfulness. In I. Mervielde, I. Deary, F. De Fruyt, and F. Ostendorf (Eds.), *Personality Psychology in Europe* (pp. 67-83), Tilburg: University Press.

[16] Sommer, K. and Ruch, W. (2009). Cheerfulness. In S. J. Lopez (Ed.*), The Encyclopedia of Positive Psychology* (pp. 144-148). Massachusetts: Blackwell Publishing.

[17] Ruch, W. (2009). Amusement. In D. Sander and K. Scherer (Eds.), *The Oxford Companion to the Affective Sciences* (pp. 27-28). Oxford: Oxford University Press.

[18] Ruch, W. and Stevens, M. (1995). *The differential effects of nitrous oxide on mood level: The role of trait-cheerfulness.* 7th Meeting of the International Society for the Study of Individual Differences - ISSID, July 15-19, 1995, Warsaw, Poland.

[19] Ekman, P. (1999). Basic emotions. In T. Dalgleish and M. Power (Eds.), *Handbook of Cognition and Emotion* (pp. 45-60). Sussex: John Wiley and Sons Ltd.

[20] Ekman, P. and Friesen, W. V. (1982). Felt, false and miserable smiles. *Journal of Nonverbal Behavior, 6,* 238-252.

[21] Ekman, P., Davidson, R. J., and Friesen, W. V. (1990). The Duchenne smile: Emotional expression and brain physiology II. *Journal of Personality and Social Psychology, 58,* 342-353.

[22] Ekman, P., Friesen, W. V., and Hager, J. C. (2002). *Facial Action Coding System: A Technique for the Measurement of Facial Movement.* Palo Alto: Consulting Psychologists Press.

[23] Ambadar, Z., Cohn, J. F., and Reed, L. I. (2009). All smiles are not created equal: Morphology and timing of smiles perceived as amused, polite, and embarrassed/nervous. *Journal of Nonverbal Behaviour, 33,* 17-34.

[24] Ekman, P., Friesen, W. V., and Ancoli, S. (1980). Facial signs of emotional experience. *Journal of Personality and Social Psychology, 39,* 1125-1134.

[25] Keltner, D. (1995). Signs of appeasement: Evidence for the distinct displays of embarrassment, amusement, and shame. *Journal of Personality and Social Psychology, 68,* 441-454.

[26] Papa, A. and Bonanno, G. A. (2008). Smiling in the face of adversity: The interpersonal and intrapersonal functions of smiling. *Emotion, 8,* 1-12.

[27] Ruch, W. (2000). Erheiterung und Heiterkeit [Exhilaration and cheerfulness]. In J. Otto, H. A. Euler and H. Mandl (Eds.), *Emotionspsychologie. Ein Handbuch in Schlüsselbegriffen* (pp. 231-238). Stuttgart: Psychologische Verlagsunion.

[28] Ruch, W. and Ekman, P. (2001). The expressive pattern of laughter. In A. W. Kaszniak (Ed.), *Emotion, Qualia, and Consciousness* (pp. 426-443). Tokyo: Word Scientific Publisher.

[29] Darwin, C. (1998). The expression of the emotions in man and animals. In C. Darwin and P. Ekman (Eds.), *The Expression of the Emotions in Man and Animals* (3rd edition). New York: Oxford University Press.

[30] Goldstein, J. H., Harmon, J., McGhee, P. E., and Karasik, R. (1975). Test of an information-processing model of humor: Physiological response changes during problem- and riddle solving. *Journal of General Psychology, 92,* 59-68.

[31] Martin, R. A. (2007). *The Psychology of Humor: An integrative approach.* Burlington: Elsevier Academic Press.

[32] Ruch, W. (1990). *Die Emotion Erheiterung: Ausdrucksformen und Bedingungen* [The emotion of exhilaration: Forms of expression and conditions.] Unpublished habilitation thesis, University of Düsseldorf, Germany.

[33] Wild, B., Rodden, F. A., Grodd, W., and Ruch, W. (2003). Neural correlates of laughter and humour: A review. *Brain, 126,* 2121-2138.

[34] Wild, B., Rodden, F. A., Rapp, A., Erb, M., Grodd, W., and Ruch, W. (2006). Humor and smiling: Cortical areas selective for cognitive, affective and volitional components. *Neurology, 66,* 887-893.

[35] Ruch, W. (1995). Will the real relationship between facial expression and affective experience please stand up: The case of exhilaration. *Cognition and Emotion, 9,* 33-58.

[36] Ruch, W. (1998). Exhilaration, exhilaratability and the exhilarants. In A. Fischer (Ed.), *Proceedings of the 10th conference of the International Society for Research on Emotions* (pp. 122-126). Würzburg: ISRE.

[37] Ruch, W. (1997). State and trait cheerfulness and the induction of exhilaration: A FACS study. *European Psychologist, 2,* 328-341.

[38] Eysenck, H.–J. and Eysenck, M. W. (1985). *Personality and Individual Differences: A Natural Science Approach.* New York: Plenum Press.

[39] Lersch, P. (1962). *Aufbau der Person* [Personality]. München: Barth.

[40] Washburn, M. F., Booth, M. E., Stocker, S., and Glicksmann, E. (1926). A comparison of directed and free recalls of pleasant experiences, as tests of cheerful and depressed temperaments. *American Journal of Psychology, 37,* 278- 280.

[41] Young, P. T. (1937). Is cheerfulness-depression a general temperamental trait? *Psychological Review, 44,* 313-319.

[42] Köhler, G. and Ruch, W. (1996). Sources of variance in current sense of humor inventories: How much substance, how much method variance? *Humor: International Journal of Humor Research, 9,* 363-397.

[43] Ruch, W. and Müller, L. (2010). Wenn Heiterkeit zur Therapie wird [When cheerfulness turns into a therapy]. *Geriatrie Praxis Österreich, 3,* 22-24.

[44] McGhee, P. E. (1996). *Humor, Healing, and the Amuse System: Humor as Survival Training* (2nd edition). Dubuque: Kendall/Hunt Publishing.

[45] Dworkin, E. S. and Efran, J. S. (1967). The angered: Their susceptibility to varieties of humor. *Journal of Personality and Social Psychology, 6,* 233-236.

[46] Kretschmer, E. (1961). *Körperbau und Charakter* [Body build and character]. Berlin: Springer.

[47] Falkenberg, I., Jarmuzek, J., Bartels, M., and Wild, B. (2011). Do depressed patients lose their sense of humor? *Psychopathology, 44,* 98-105.

[48] Hirsch, R. D., Junglas, K., Konradt, B., and Jonitz, M. F. (2010). Humortherapie bei alten Menschen mit einer Depression. Ergebnisse einer empirischen Untersuchung [Humortherapy in elderly depressed patients: Empirical results]. *Zeitschrift für Gerontologie und Geriatrie, 43,* 42-52.

[49] Krantzhoff, E. U. and Hirsch, R. D. (2001). Humor in der Gerontopsychiatrischen Klinik: Ergebnisse einer therapiebegleitenden Studie [Humor in geriatric psychiatric hospitals: Results of a therapy evaluation study]. In R. D. Hirsch, J. Bruder, and H. Radebold (Eds.), *Heiterkeit und Humor im Alter* (pp. 139-162). Kassel: Chudeck Druck.

[50] Falkenberg, I., Klügel, K., Bartels, M., and Wild, B. (2007). Sense of humor in patients with schizophrenia. *Schizophrenia Research, 95,* 259–261.

[51] Carretero-Dios. H., Eid, M., and Ruch. W. (2011). Temperamental basis of sense of humor: A multilevel confirmatory factor analysis of multitrait-multimethod data. *Journal of Research in Personality, 45,* 153–164.

[52] Ruch, W. and Carrell, A. (1997). Trait cheerfulness and the sense of humor. *Personality and Individual Differences, 24,* 551-558.

[53] Hösli, K., Sommer, K., and Ruch, W. (2006). Development and validation of a children and youth version of the State-Trait Cheerfulness Inventory. Poster presented at the *Fifth International Positive Psychology Summit, October 5- 7 2006,* Washington.

[54] Ruch, W., Auerbach, S., Sommer, K., and Hösli, K. (2011). The humorous temperament of children and youth: Development of a children's version of the State-Trait Cheerfulness Inventory (STCI-C). Poster presented at the *11th European Conference on psychological Assessment (ECPA),* Riga, Latvia.

[55] Peterson, C., Park, N., and Seligman, M. E. P. (2005). Orientations to happiness and life satisfaction: The full life versus the empty life. *Journal of Happiness Studies, 6,* 25-41.

[56] Huebner, E. S. (1997). Brief Multidimensional Students' Life Satisfaction Scale. Retrieved online June 2011: http://www.psych.sc.edu/facdocs/hueblifesat.html.

[57] Sommer, K., Hösli, K., and Ruch, W. (2006). Predictors of life satisfaction in children and youth: Cheerfulness and the good life. Poster presented at the *Fifth International Positive Psychology Summit, October 5- 7, 2006,* Washington.

[58] Thompson, R., Hasenöhrl, R., and Ruch, W. (2004). Enhanced cognitive performance and cheerful mood by standardized extracts of piper methysticum (Kava-kava). *Human Psychopharmacology: Clinical and Experimental, 19,* 243-250.

[59] Beyler, M. (1999). *Ist Erheiterung entspannend?* [Is exhilaration relaxing?] Unpublished Master Thesis, Department of Psychology, University of Düsseldorf, Düsseldorf, Germany.

[60] Hodson, G., MacInnis, C. C., and Rusch, J. (2010). Prejudice-relevant correlates of humor temperaments and humor styles. *Personality and Individual Differences, 49,* 546-549.

[61] Rapp, A. M., Wild, B., Erb, M., Rodden, F. A., Ruch, W., and Grodd, W. (2007). Trait cheerfulness modulates BOLD-response in lateral cortical but not limbic brain areas - a pilot fMRI study. *Neuroscience Letters, 445,* 242–245.

[62] Wancke, C. U. (1996). *Der Einfluss unterschiedlicher emotionaler Qualitäten von Sinnsprüchen und des Umgangs mit dem Material auf die aktuelle Befindlichkeit von Probanden* [The influence of sayings of different emotional qualities and the handling of the material on the mood of participants]. Unpublished Master Thesis, Department of Psychology, University of Düsseldorf.

[63] Korpela, K. and Hartig, T. (1996). Restorative qualities of favorite places. *Journal of Environmental Psychology, 16,* 221-233.

[64] Beermann, U. and Ruch, W. (2011). Can people ever "laugh at themselves"? Experimental and correlational evidence. *Emotion, 11,* 492-501.

[65] Hofmann, J., Beermann, U., and Ruch, W. (2010). Laughing at oneself (?!). A FACS study. Poster presented at the *International Summer School and Symposium on Humor and Laughter (ISS), July 5-10, 2010,* Boldern-Männedorf, Switzerland.

[66] Hofmann, J., Beermann, U., and Ruch, W. (2010). *Distorted Picture Task (DPT).* Unpublished Research Instrument. Department of Psychology, University of Zurich.

[67] Martin, R. A., Puhlik-Doris, P., Larsen, G., Gray, J., and Weir, K. (2003). Individual differences in uses of humor and their relation to psychological well-being: Development of the Humor Styles Questionnaire. *Journal of Research in Personality, 37,* 48-75.

[68] Ruch, W., Beermann, U., and Proyer, R. T. (2009). Investigating the humor of gelotophobes: Does feeling ridiculous equal being humorless? *Humor: International Journal of Humor Research, 22,* 111-143.

[69] Ruch, W. and Zweyer, K. (2001). Heiterkeit und Humor: Ergebnisse der Forschung [Cheerfulness and humor: Empirical evidence]. In R. D. Hirsch, J. Bruder, and H. Radebold (Eds.). *Heiterkeit und Humor im Alter* (pp. 9-43). Bornheim-Sechtem: Chudeck-Druck.

[70] Ruch, W. and Proyer, R. T. (2008). The fear of being laughed at: Individual and group differences in Gelotophobia. *Humor: International Journal of Humor Research, 21,* 47-67.

[71] Martin, R. A. and Lefcourt, H. M. (1983). Sense of humor as a moderator of the relation between stressors and moods. *Journal of Personality and Social Psychology, 45,* 1313-1324.

[72] Craik, K. H., Lampert, M. D., and Nelson, A. J. (1993). *Research Manual for the Humorous Behavior Q-sort Deck.* Berkeley: University of California, Institute of Personality and Social Research.

[73] Manke, B. (2007). Genetic and environmental contributions to children's interpersonal humor. In W. Ruch (Ed.), *The Sense of Humor: Explorations of a Personality Characteristic* (pp. 361–384). Berlin: Mouton de Gruyter.

[74] World Health Organization (WHO) (1946). Preamble to the Constitution of the World Health Organization as adopted by the International Health Conference, New York, 19–22 June 1946. Retrieved online June 2011: www.who.int/bulletin/archives/80 (12)981.pdf.

[75] Diener, E. and Seligman, M. E. P. (2004). Beyond money: Toward an economy of well-being. *Psychological Science in the Public Interest, 5,* 1-31.

[76] Ryan, R. M. and Deci, E. L. (2001). To be happy or to be self-fulfilled. A review of research on hedonic and eudemonic well-being. In S. Fiske (Ed.), *Annual Review of Psychology* (Vol. 52, pp. 141-166). Palo Alto: Annual Reviews/Inc.

[77] Seligman, M. E. P. (2002). *Authentic happiness: Using the new positive psychology to realize your potential for lasting fullfilment.* New York: Free Press.

[78] Seligman, M. E. P. (2011). *Flourishing. A visionary new understanding of happiness and well-being.* New York: Free Press.

[79] Gorovoy, I. (2009). *Best predictors of quality of life (QOL) based on character strengths of gratitude, curiosity and cheerfulness.* Unpublished Master Thesis, Victoria University, Melbourne, Australia.

[80] Zweyer, K., Velker, B., and Ruch. W. (2004). Do cheerfulness, exhilaration and humor production moderate pain tolerance? A FACS study. *Humor: International Journal of Humor Research, 17,* 67-84.

[81] De Longis, A., Folkman, S., and Lazarus, R. S. (1988). The impact of daily stress on health and mood: Psychological and social resources as mediators. *Journal of Personality and Social Psychology, 54,* 486–495.

[82] Lazarus, R. S. and Folkman, S. (1984). *Stress, appraisal and coping.* New York: Springer.

[83] Eppel, H. (2007). *Stress als Risiko und Chance* [Stress as risk and opportunity]. Stuttgart: Kohlhammer.

[84] Kaluza, G. (2005). *Stressbewältigung. Trainingsmanual zur psychologischen Gesundheitsförderung* [Stress coping. Training manual to psychologically foster health]. Heidelberg: Springer.

[85] Hausser, S. (1999). *Heiterkeit, kritische Lebensereignisse und Wohlbefinden* [Cheerfulness, critical life events and well-being]. Unpublished Master Thesis, Department of Psychology, Heinrich-Heine University, Düsseldorf.

[86] Jackson, D. N. (1974). *Personality Research Form manual, revised.* Port Huron: Research Psychologists Press.

[87] Wrench, J. S. and McCroskey, J. C. (2001). A temperamental understanding of humor communication and exhilaratability. *Communication Quarterly, 49,* 142-159.

[88] McGhee, P. E. (1979). *Humor, its Origin and Development.* San Francisco: W. H. Freeman.

[89] Hehlmann, W. (1968). *Wörterbuch der Psychologie* [Dictionary of psychology]. Stuttgart: Kröner.

[90] Linley, P. A. (2002). Can traumatic experiences provide a positive pathway? *Traumatic Stress Points, 14,* 5.

[91] Tedeschi, R. G., Park, C. L., and Calhoun, L. G. (Eds.) (1998). *Posttraumatic Growth: Positive Changes in the Aftermath of Crisis.* Mahwah: Lawrence Erlbaum.

[92] Kuiper, N. A. and R. A. Martin (1998). Is sense of humor a positive personality characteristic? In W. Ruch (Ed.), *The Sense of Humor: Explorations of a Personality Characteristic* (pp. 159–178). New York: Mouton de Gruyter.

[93] Meehl, P. (1975). Hedonic capacity: Some conjectures. *Bulletin of Menninger Clinic, 39,* 295-307.

[94] Watson, D., Clark, L. A., and Tellegen, A. (1988). Development and validation of brief measures of positive and negative affect: The PANAS scales. *Journal of Personality and Social Psychology, 54,* 1063-1070.

[95] Yip, J. A. and Martin, R. A. (2006). Sense of humor, emotional intelligence, and social competence. *Journal of Research in Personality, 40,* 1202-1208.

[96] Mayer, J. D., Salovey, P., and Caruso, D. R. (2002). *Mayer-Salovey-Caruso Emotional Intelligence Test (MSCEIT): User's Manual.* Toronto: Multi-Health Systems, Inc.

[97] Csikszentmihalyi, M. (1997). *Finding flow: The Psychology of Engagement with Everyday Life.* New York: Basic Books.

[98] Diener, E., Suh, M., Lucas, E., and Smith, H. (1999). Subjective well-being: Three decades of progress. *Psychological Bulletin, 125,* 276-302.

[99] McCrae, R. R. and Costa, P. T., Jr. (1991). Adding *liebe* and *arbeit*: The full five-factor model and well-being. *Personality and Social Psychology Bulletin, 17,* 227-232.

[100] Ruch, W. and Proyer, R. T. (2009). Extending the study of gelotophobia: On gelotophiles and katagelasticists. *Humor: International Journal of Humor Research, 22,* 183-212.

[101] Papousek, I. and Schulter, G. (2008). Effects of a mood-enhancing intervention on subjective well-being and cardiovascular parameters. *International Journal of Behavioral Medicine, 15,* 293-302.

[102] Brutsche, M. H., Grossman, P., Müller, R. E., Wiegand, J., Pello, Baty, F., and Ruch, W. (2008). Impact of laughter on air trapping in severe chronic obstructive lung disease. *International Journal of COPD, 3,* 1–8.

[103] Schmidt-Hidding, W. (1963). Europäische Schlüsselwörter. Band I: Humor und Witz [European key terms. Volume I: Humor and Wit]. Munich: Huber.

[104] Feingold, A. and Mazzella, R. (1991). Psychometric intelligence and verbal humor ability. *Personality and Individual Differences, 12,* 427-435.

[105] Ruch, W. (2001). The perception of humor. In A. W. Kaszniak (Ed.), *Emotion, qualia, and consciousness* (p. 410-425). Tokyo: Word Scientific Publisher.

[106] Ruch, W. (2004). Humor. In C. P. Peterson and M. E. P. Seligman (Eds.), *Character Strengths and Virtues: A Handbook and Classification* (p. 583-598). Washington: Oxford University Press.

[107] Friedman, H. S., Tucker, J. S., Tomlinson-Keasey, C., Schwartz, J. E., Wingard, D. L., and Criqui, M. (1993). Does childhood personality predict longevity? *Journal of Personality and Social Psychology, 65,* 175-185.

[108] Martin, L. R., Friedman, H. S., Tucker, J. S., Tomlinson-Keasey, C., Criqui, M. H., and Schwartz, J. E. (2002). A life course perspective on childhood cheerfulness and its relation to mortality risk. *Personality and Social Psychology Bulletin, 28,* 1155-1165.

[109] McNulty, J. K. and Fincham, F. D. (2011). Beyond positive psychology? Toward a contextual view of psychological processes and well-being. *American Psychologist.* doi: 10.1037/a0024572.

[110] Schwartz, B. and Sharpe, K. (2006). Practical wisdom: Aristotle meets positive psychology. *Journal of Happiness Studies, 7,* 377-395.

[111] McNulty, J. K. (2002). The dark side of forgiveness: The tendency to forgive predicts continued psychological and physical aggression in marriage. *Personality and Social Psychology Bulletin, 37,* 770-783.

[112] Weinstein, N. D. (1987). Unrealistic optimism about susceptibility to health problems: Conclusions from a community-wide sample. *Journal of Behavioral Medicine, 10,* 481-500.

[113] Papousek, I., Ruch, W., Freudenthaler, H. H., Kogler, E., Lang, B., and Schulter, G. (2009). Gelotophobia, emotion-related skills and responses to the affective states of others. *Personality and Individual Differences, 47,* 58-63.

In: Humor and Health Promotion
Editor: Paola Gremigni

ISBN: 978-1-61942-657-3
© 2012 Nova Science Publishers, Inc.

Chapter 6

IRONY, SURPRISE AND HUMOR

Roberto Caterina and Iolanda Incasa
Department of Psychology, University of Bologna, Italy

"The secret to humor is surprise"
Aristotle

ABSTRACT

In this chapter we describe humor and the main humor theories outside of their natural linguistic context. Non-verbal elements and body involvement in humor expressions are taken into consideration following Darwin's tradition and hypothesis. Aspects of humor communication and miscommunication are then examined considering that humor can be presented as a special case of expectancy violation where surprise, irony and other emotions play an important role.

A passage from a situation characterized by pretending to communicate – such as seduction – to another characterized by communicating to pretend, as in irony, is described as part of a general communicative process in which surprise and emotional regulations are the two main aspects. Some analogies may be made between the cognitive and emotional process of humor and the process of art fruition, especially listening to music. In both cases subjective experiences and surprise are determinant elements to solve cognitive incongruity and regulate emotional outputs.

A general model in which surprise and social sharing of emotion are both taken into account is presented in relation to humor expression and art fruition. The latest discoveries in the field of neurosciences are discussed, proposing some new suggestions that may be useful for a less reductive vision of the complex relationship between body, brain and mind.

Finally, a clinical and experimental study on autistic and normal children is presented in order to stress the role of surprise in individual creativity and empathy. Potentialities in emotional expressions and discoveries are presented as important steps of adult mental life. Some facial expressions, in particular smiles, may be seen as representative of emotional potentialities where humor, irony and surprise are important factors of human growth.

INTRODUCTION

Although there is no univocal definition of humor, and humor theories have often covered single aspects of too large a topic, it is nevertheless worthwhile to consider humor not only as a product of cultural standards but as a very basic instance in human life and development.

Of course it may be difficult to talk about humor outside of the linguistic realm and a specific cultural context: metaphors, puns, conversational strategies that make up the essential root of humor cannot really be understood in the absence of social interaction and shared social rules, but nonverbal signs may also occur and play a significant role in the expression and communication of humor.

Furthermore humor may be represented as a cognitive process which in some way involves body activation: laughing and relaxation from tension are in fact evident signs of some body involvement. Humor – the witty way of approaching life problems – is the final part of a long and complex process that begins where the body is alerted and where thinking and playing take place. Various humor theories actually make reference to different moments of this process: incongruity may be either the brilliant conclusion of cognitive achievements, as studied in the linguistic realm and particularly in metaphors [1-4] and the resolution of incongruity in the realm of conflict [5-8], or the very first situation of surprise in our infant life where we realize that things do not always go as we wish (see Scherer's "novelty check" [9,10]); emotions seem to be deeply involved in humor: surprise, relaxation are emotional words that show how nonverbal behavior is important in the expression of humor, but it is hard to say which emotions are clearly expressed in humor. Positive emotions clearly go towards some sort of sensory satisfaction, but also negative emotions may be present in irony, sarcasm and mild forms of contempt; emotional aspects of humor seem to come after that very basic form of incongruity mentioned above, which is a very primitive form of surprise. We would like to talk about that in this chapter, since surprise, as Aristotle first remarked, is the secret to humor definitions and functions.

The search for the source of humor can go beyond the boundaries of the human world. Although there are only a very few not systematic evidences that non-human animals have a sense of humor there are many observations – far removed from an anthropomorphic point of view – concerning non-human animal activities that have no biologic scope, but that are done just for the sake of an inner pleasure; other observations concern miscommunication, playing, empathy, all activities that may have something in common with the "misleading" qualities of humor.

Alongside the classical theories concerning humor, Freudian theory [11,12], although often criticized as mentalistic and not supported by scientific evidences, has still in our view a considerable value insofar as it presents humor not only as a "defense mechanism" but also as a valid instrument to reduce aggressiveness and ambiguity.

According to Freud insight and knowledge are present in humor: in particular, clarity of insight, let us say even truth, may be reached if violation of expectations and predictions are somehow enacted. In this respect Freudian analysis of humor is not far from Gestalt theory and Wertheimer's idea of "productive thinking" [13]: a different display and arrangement of things with which we are familiar may produce humor, cut aggressiveness, reduce incongruity and create new things and new instruments of thinking.

In this chapter we would like to suggest that one might think about humor as a sort of story to tell where aggressiveness, negative emotions are transformed into safer entities, harmless contents where love, humor and thinking may be joined together.

It may seem rather odd that humor comes from surprise and love, but most of our communicative tools are indeed deeply linked with these emotional instances. Humor comes from mental life that, according to many authors, develops very early in the first months or even days of our existence: on the other hand our mental life is made up of many "eurekas" where we fulfill our wishes, find what we need, meet the unexpected. In one of those "eurekas" we find humor, but not only: creativity, art products, playing, social and emotional sharing, empathy may all come along the same path.

DARWIN'S TRADITION: FROM TICKLING TO THE ORIGIN OF DENIGRATION AND SARCASM

Three points in Darwin's famous book *The expression of emotions in man and animals* [14] are connected more or less directly with our topic concerning humor.

When speaking of tickling and laughing, Darwin somehow linked the two activities and speculated that something similar to the tickling-laughing reaction happens when we laugh at a joke or a pun. He talks about tickling of the mind. This hypothesis, later known as the Darwin-Hecker hypothesis (named after Charles Darwin and the physiologist Ewald Hecker) predicted that humor and tickling are interrelated because they are effective only when the person being tickled is in a pleasurable condition. A child who is tickled by a stranger would scream because of fear instead of laughing. Evidences about this hypothesis are controversial even if Friedlund and Loftis [15] seem to support it. Anyhow, besides the value of the Darwin-Hecker hypothesis it is interesting to remark how both tickling and humor need an unexpected situation in order to elicit laughing. Darwin quotes the example of a child who tries to tickle himself-herself: he/she may laugh as a consequence of that action, but that happens not so frequently in comparison with a situation in which someone else tickles the child who does not know where he-she is going to be tickled. Of course the link between humor and tickling pinpoints other "links": the link between human and non-human animal, since the tickling-laughing reaction applies not only to humans, or the relationship between humor and body, since humor and tickling seem to elicit the same body reactions.

In talking about smiling, laughing and surprise Darwin stresses how different expressive patterns are involved in such instances. In surprise the mouth is wide open and the eyebrows are raised in order to hear and see better what is going to happen outside. In laughing the mouth is still open, the muscle *zygomaticus major* is activated (in order to produce a smile), the eyebrows are normal and the eyes "smaller", so to speak, as the cheeks are raised up by *zygomaticus major* causing the activation of the muscle *orbicularis oculi*. In laughing the activation of sound can be interpreted as a positive reaction to a harmless environment. The expressive pattern of smiling is similar to that of laughing, but less intense: the mouth may be closed, *orbicularis oculi* activation may be absent and there is no sound production. Darwin's observations on surprise, laughing and smiling were very important as they described the facial muscles involved in these expressions and postulated the continuity between human and non-human animal mimic. The works of the French anatomist Duchenne de Boulogne were quoted by Darwin to verify the extent to which it was correct to link surprise, laughing and smiling to emotional outputs and to check the value of single facial movements in the expression of different emotions. According to Duchenne it was possible to differentiate a genuine smile of joy from a non-emotional smile because only in the smile of joy is there the activation of the muscle *orbicularis oculi* together with the muscle *zygomaticus major*. About one century later Ekman and Friesen [16] rediscovered Darwin's and Duchenne's ideas and proposed a well-known scoring system of the main facial actions (the FACS, Facial Action Coding System). Scoring systems of facial movements on the other hand were not new: we may recall the pioneering works ranging from the painter Le Brun in the 17th century to Hjortsjo [17] of which Ekman and Friesen [16] were informed. However we would like to follow Darwin's ideas concerning the interaction with the environment that surprise, laughing and smiling somehow seem to predict: surprise is linked to the organism's alertness, we do not know yet if something pleasant or unpleasant is going to happen; in laughing some relaxation comes, the situation is evaluated as not dangerous; in smiling we may tell other people of our peaceful intentions. We can see that in this model humor comes between surprise and laughing: surprise need not necessarily be a good surprise; the acknowledgment of non-pleasant contents may be transformed into a harmless and socially acceptable situation. It is not very easy to follow this process, but it is important to grasp the point that humor may come from emotional transformation and regulation, as Freud's ideas would later suggest.

One of the most interesting Darwinian ideas is that transformation processes concerning the value attributed to some nonverbal signs are not limited to the human world, but may trespass from non-human animal behaviors to human expressions. For example the unilateral upper lip raising at the corner of mouth so that the canine tooth is exhibited is a sign that Darwin found in some expressions of contempt, scorn, disdain and especially in sardonic or derisive smiles: according to his observations this expression is very similar to that of a snarling dog (the same word sneer probably comes from snarl). This curious expression – whether that of a playful sneer or ferocious snarl – clearly comes from our non-human animal descent, and the large size of the canine teeth of anthropomorphous apes would give some support to this thesis. Originally linked to rage and fight this expression is transformed into a new situation where contempt seems to play a prevalent role: we do not fear a person who deserves our contempt, his or her threats just make us laugh. Denigration or sarcasm share some aspects with humor insofar as humor may coexist with irony, superiority, cold anger and even mild forms of contempt; its facial expression may be a smile, different from the smile of enjoyment. The element of surprise in this context goes together with the use of misleading strategies in order to avoid a direct attack towards people. Miscommunication, lying are elements belonging to irony; they represent a reaction to negative feelings and come after surprise. Irony, in this model of humor, comes at the end of a long process of emotional transformations and regulations.

Darwin's observations on vocal utterances of non-human animals are not only oriented to describe the biological functions of those signals such as reproductive, flight and fight behavioral patterns, but also give us many suggestions concerning the value of the single vocal outputs independently from their functions. Birds, and some apes like gibbons, sing in order to be more attractive towards their sexual partners, but they sing also for the pleasure of doing that activity. According to Darwin there is a primitive form of pleasure that may be later used for social aims. Biological functions, for example, cannot explain why some songs are chosen and others not. This primitive form of pleasure is strictly connected with the aesthetical qualities of a signal. In other words a signal may be beautiful or ugly. Our attraction towards beauty is instinctual and immediate: it may of course be connected with reproductive aims (beautiful people are more apt to ensure good and healthy descendants) but there is much more. In many courtship rituals males attract female partners through exhibitions of some expressive patterns (colors, sounds, movements, and so on): exhibitions are made in order to catch the partner's attention, to create a situation of surprise and astonishment. Some seductive qualities of humor probably come from this context and humor is sometimes used to attract people, keep a conversation alive or share the pleasure of amusing ourselves.

From Darwin's ideas therefore we may elicit and add something to our knowledge about humor. Humor comes from a situation of surprise: this surprise is directly driven by the body's reactions (tickling) or may evoke different emotions that have somehow to be kept under control or may be communicated to other people. In this respect humor may be seen as an instrument to attract people's attention. Three different aspects of humor (linked to body reactions, emotional regulation and communicative processes) can be generated from the incongruity provoked by a surprise situation: in all these situations body and mind cooperate to create a sort of narrative frame in which the time perspective is organized and communication among the members belonging to the same group can be deeply transformed and arranged in a step by step process.

BETWEEN DECEIT AND DISILLUSION: COMMUNICATIVE ASPECTS OF HUMOR, IRONY AND SARCASM

The case of humor could be seen as emblematic in understanding how communication and miscommunication belong to the same interactive system [18]. If we look at communication as a constructive activity which involves two or more people and create a bond between them, we could easily assume that deceptive attitudes should be banned, being a serious disruptive attack to the communicative bonds among people. On the other hand lying is a complex activity: there are different forms of lies, different social standards and different contexts in which lying may be differently disapproved or even approved. Lying in a situation of seduction is different to lying in order to harm people seriously. The so called "white lies" belong to everyday life. Furthermore lying is not always connected with verbal language. We may tell lies using nonverbal signs; it is more difficult, but not impossible as all actors know and as Ekman wrote in his classical book *Telling lies* [19]. Even non-human animals lie or, rather, may use deceptive strategies to escape potential threats and attacks using mimetic behaviors either pretending to be dead or harmful, poisonous creatures. In nature as in human life the truth is not always the best choice in some moments. In their works Sigmund Freud [20] and his daughter Anna [21] showed us how in mental life lying and deception are quite normal: all the so called "defensive mechanisms" of the Ego, first and foremost "repression", are to be considered as lying strategies – where we lie to ourselves – which are not always useless, as they have an important adaptive value in some moments of life, while of course a maladaptive use of "defensive mechanisms" leads to neurotic or psychotic outcomes. Coming back to our topic we can suggest that sometimes constructive interactions are the result of miscommunication and deception (including self-deception). Anolli and colleagues [18] differentiate some situations in which people "pretend to communicate", such as deception and seduction, from others in which people "communicate to pretend", such as irony and humor. In these different levels we can almost see a sort of passage from miscommunication to communication to meta-communication. In humor "pretending" is almost at a meta-communicative level: when humor comes we seem to say we are joking, that what we are saying is not serious and we are not to be worried about anything. Humor induces relaxation and enjoyment. Somewhat different is the reaction to irony. Irony may be sometimes so mild (as humor is) not to cause any particular distress; at other times irony may be made up of a series of subtle but sharp attacks so that the context, although playful, is not relaxed. That of course applies even more so to sarcasm where attacks are more robust and direct. The situation of "pretending to communicate" is based on illusion. This is particularly true when we consider seduction. In seduction everything – lying strategies, paradoxical exhibition, and discursive obliquity – is designed towards creating a context in which communication is ambiguous, not clearly defined and illusions are offered to whoever wants to be deluded. Illusions, surprise, astonishment come together. Verbal and nonverbal signals are both used to create a dreamy atmosphere where "a trap" may successfully be prepared, where playing is allowed and fantasy occurs. This situation recalls what goes on between a mother and her baby during the first months of life: the famous psychoanalyst Donald Winnicott [22] described the situation simply in terms of illusion. Mother first supports her baby's illusion of being omnipotent, and then little by little she gives her son or daughter some elements of reality. When the illusion is set up, interpersonal boundaries are not so fixed: mother and baby are not clearly two separate people and what belongs to one belongs to the other too. The mother-infant relation becomes potential: it may be created and recreated here and now. Illusion is strictly connected to that potentiality. Something similar happens in seduction where illusions are functional to the construction of an emotional bond between two people.

Just as in the mother-infant interaction illusion is later substituted by reality, seduction may be transformed into a more stable relationship. Seduction may, at least partially, be seen as a playful activity where lying and deception are useful tools for mental activity and life. In this respect dreams, artistic products, fantasies belong to a similar group of activities where illusion come first.

The passage from seduction to humor – previously described as from "pretending to communicate" to "communicating to pretend" [18] – may also be seen as a transition from illusion to the awareness of having been deluded. A certain amount of awareness – far removed from a dreamlike context – is present both in humor and irony: not always does awareness mean a bitter awareness that reality is so different from fantasy, more often it means a witty detachment where surprise is still present. In other words, surprise in humor is created by the incongruity of data and by the audience's expectations. In humor, somewhat like in music, there is a balance between the tension that incongruity may cause and the resolution of tension, i.e. relaxation that occurs when humoristic contents are finally produced. In the next section we will examine the comparison between music and humor in more detail just to see how humor does not belong exclusively to human verbal language but can be found in many nonverbal languages and behaviors.

Some other considerations may be made here about the communicative aspects of humor. In humor communicative aims are not separated from the search for what is unfamiliar, less obvious, even uncanny [23] creating first tension or suspense in the audience (the people who are listening to the humoristic considerations) and then relaxation. This type of communication is an emotional one. In telling a joke we communicate our emotions to some people and in return we get some emotions from those people. Therefore the communication of humor, irony, even sarcasm to other people does not concern only cognitive aspects, but is deeply involved in the communication and regulation of emotions. The passage from dreams to reality, as we said before, may be realized because when we interact with other people we need to modulate our emotions. Our ideas, our thoughts come from our capacity to express and regulate our emotions. Cognitive evaluation in the emotional process follows some steps or controls as Scherer [9,10] suggested. The first check, the "novelty check" concerns the familiarity or unfamiliarity of what is going on around us. Surprise, as we have already said, fits this first check. The second step regards how emotional stimuli may be considered either pleasant or unpleasant. A humorous situation, and the tension-relaxation movements that define it, seems to go along with novelty check - intrinsic pleasantness check progression: humor, we might say, is a cognitive-emotional evaluation of a physical and social environment where two or more people communicate.

Surprise is generally considered an emotion of short duration and neutral valence (neither positive nor negative), and is usually included within the category of basic-emotions thanks to certain characteristics, mentioned later, that identify such emotions and that are shared by surprise. According to Izard [24], emotions are basic because of their hypothesized role in evolution (i.e. their ability to facilitate adaptive responses to the vast array of demands of the environment), biological and social function and primacy in ontogenetic development. Besides, it has been suggested that each basic emotion can be associated with distinct facial signals that are common to cultures throughout the world [25].

Research on surprise has, in the past, been mainly represented within the psychological literature on emotions [14,25-27], but, in relatively recent times, specific attention has been devoted to surprise as such [28-32].

Our particular interest in this emotion comes from the general assumption that surprise may be considered as a complex evolutionary process, with manifold implications in different fields, ranging from neurological − aspecific correlates of surprise exist more or less at every level of neuronal processes [33] − to behavioral − our ability to quickly evaluate/assess, recognize and learn from surprising events are be regarded as critical for survival [34].

HUMOR AS EXPECTANCY VIOLATION

The famous musicologist Leonard Meyer [35] postulated that the relationship between music and emotion comes from the particular structure of musical language made up of moments of tension and relaxation which can create precise expectations in the listeners. According to Meyer, music may induce emotions when those expectations are somehow unattended. What happens in music is extraordinarily similar to what happens in humor and surprise. Furthermore in music surprise effects (such as the introduction of new instruments, musical ideas, and particular cadences) may cause funny and hilarious reactions in the listeners. A famous example may be the second movement of the Symphony n.94 in G major (nicknamed "the surprise") by Haydn where a series of passages make the musical phrases unpredictable causing surprise, but also a mild fear and amusement; this example shows quite clearly how surprise is a situation – more than an emotion – which creates different emotional outputs. Let us now make some considerations and speculations about the following question: if expectancy violations are so important in music as in humor and in some emotional situations, could we say that amusement and pleasure resulting from humor come only if something entirely new is presented to our attention? The answer to this question is yes and no at the same time. Yes because if we have heard a joke many times we get bored instead of amused, no because even if we know the "solution" of a joke we may still admire the ingenuity of construction, we may still have the pleasure to communicate a joke to people who do not know it and enjoy their genuine reaction of amusement. In other words in talking about surprise we have not only to consider the cognitive aspects (if something is not new we cannot be surprised), but also the emotional ones (living an experience is always different to having memory of it: in the present realm, in the here and now context, we may be surprised even if we, paradoxically, know what is going to happen). A certain amount of expectations may belong to what is called implicit memory [36,37] which is difficult to describe verbally, difficult to recall, but somehow fixed in our body's physiological responses. Therefore surprise may be partially lived as "new" when our body experiences are reactivated. In music body arousal has been studied referring to "shivers" [37,38] that sometimes accompany musical listening: those shivers may anticipate either a very pleasant experience or unpleasant feelings (which applies for example to a very sharp sound). Both in music and humor expectancies, anticipations are somehow created: to be more precise we often have the expectancy of the unexpected. In other words we manage to create surprise. Insofar as surprise may be created, it can thus be kept under control: we can avoid the harmful effects of undesirable events. On the other hand if surprise is a violation of expectations we have to create both expectancies and surprise. In a way it is just what a good joke does: create an easy, natural, even boring solution to which listeners' expectancies can be addressed and at the same time build an alternative, often unconventional output that is mostly enjoyed. However this process is never so objective and automatic: subjective elements are essential. The person who enjoys a joke is different from another person who enjoys the same joke: different elements could have been picked up by different people. So that even if amusement reaction towards humor can be general and universal, there are many individual differences in the choice of the details which according to people's experience may be significant. Just as incongruity – which belongs to humor as well as to surprise – tends to be solved through the search for a congruent pattern, people's reaction to humoristic situations is often that of giving congruity to incongruent materials. In this cognitive effort people may choose some details, some elements in order to understand better the whole situation. On this matter we may recall that the psychoanalyst Wilfred Bion [39], in his attempt to explain the connections between cognitive and emotional aspects of human life, introduced the concept of the so called "chosen fact" in order to mean that specific and particular elements may be important for some people and not for other people in their construction of reality. The "chosen facts" belong to individual emotional experiences, regard body and physical reactions and concern personal differences in the interaction with their environment. The psychoanalyst Graziella Magherini [40] linked Bion's concept of "chosen fact" to Freud's concept of "uncanny" or unfamiliar to explain our emotional reactions towards an artistic masterpiece. In the art fruition process people look at masterpieces in different ways: some details may be important for one person but not for another, and this is a good example of how Bion's "chosen fact" hypothesis is applied. Something similar belongs to humor and comic situations: in the caricature, for example, some details (or "chosen facts", so to speak) are selected to describe a public person (for example stressing some physiognomic traits) or an event. In caricature and in comic situations the "chosen facts" belong to the creative process: designers select some details and offer them to the public, while in art fruition the "chosen facts" could be the individual way of grasping the emotional meaning that a masterpiece may communicate. In both cases however a situation of surprise is stimulated or created in order to produce the pleasure that belongs to art fruition. There are many links between humor, art and playing: reactions to humor are very subjective just as they are to music and art. Not all people like the same jokes, cultural context differences are very wide, but humor in itself is a universal phenomenon that concerns some basic aspects of our life. Coming back to the relationship between humor and surprise we may say that humor meets people's emotional experiences: that is why the surprise element is so strong and powerful. Therefore considering what we have just said concerning the personal aspects and reactions to humor situations we should try to see if we can find also in the emotional context those elements which can be either universal or more attuned to personal traits and behaviors. In the realm of music (and therefore in an artistic context) the difference between universal and individual value of emotional stimulations has been carefully considered: some researches [41] pose the problem of the existence of specific emotions that have no utilitarian purpose (such as basic emotions like the fight-flight mechanisms) but are somehow linked to the music we like or dislike. These emotions could be called aesthetical emotions and refer to nine major factors according to Geneva Emotional Music Scale (GEM) [41]: wonder, transcendence, power, tenderness, nostalgia, peacefulness, joyful activity, sadness and tension. As you can see, wonder and tension that somehow describe a "surprise" situation are among the main factors and are linked to expectative violations. Some recent researches in the field of neurosciences [42] using the fMRI technique showed that only favorite music was able to activate the limbic and paralimbic neural systems, in particular, the cingulate cortex, the ventral medial prefrontal cortex and the ventral striatum. On the other hand the evaluation of happiness and sadness in music mainly activated temporal lobe structures. This means that aesthetical emotions induced by musical listening activate different areas in the brain and involve subjective evaluations in comparison with emotions that can be only recognized in the music without a personal involvement of the listeners. From our point of view personal involvement in an emotional experience (such as in music listening and more in general in the art fruition process) is due to body arousal and surprise mechanism activation. In the field of neurosciences revolutionary studies have been done in the last decades concerning the role of the so called "mirror neurons" [43] which gave a more robust evidence to a rather speculative concept, that of "empathy" [44-46]. All these researches are well known in the scientific community. The discovery of mirror neurons and of a variety of mirroring mechanisms in our brain shows that the same neural structures activated by the actual execution of actions or by the subjective experience of emotions and sensations are also active when we see others acting or expressing the same emotions and sensations. These mirroring mechanism have been interpreted as constituting a basic functional mechanism in social cognition, defined as embodied simulation. Embodied simulation is engaged also when actions, emotions and sensations are displayed as static images. One of the most productive applications of these studies concerns the art fruition process or neuroaesthetic [47,48]: a fundamental element of aesthetic response to works of art consists of the activation of embodied mechanisms encompassing the simulation of actions, emotions, and corporeal sensations. Mirroring mechanisms and embodied simulation can empirically ground the fundamental role of empathy in aesthetic experience. Two important acquisitions in the realm of understanding the art fruition process seem to come from studies on mirroring mechanisms: the first aspect concerns the fact that when we see a work of art an emotional communicative process starts within the observer from his/her body to his/her brain to his/her mind. It refers to an external object (such as a picture, a sculpture, a piece of music, and so on) but it has to do with a sort of self-reflexive communication where body, brain and mind are deeply interrelated. Secondly the notion that communicative process within art fruition is potential rather than real. Potentiality in art fruition is deeply linked to the nature of emotional experience and process described by Frijda as "action tendency" [49], as well as to cognitive abilities of self-representation as in the so called "theory of mind (TOM)" [50] where the relationship between simulation and interaction are carefully examined (see also our experience with autistic children in the next pages), and to some psychoanalytical concepts such as that of "potential space" in Winnicott [22] or the already mentioned hypothesis of "chosen facts" by Bion [39]. Although empathy and mirroring mechanisms are very important in the description of the art fruition process, there is still another part of the story that should be told: that concerning surprise and expectancy violations. This part belongs to artistic experience as well as to humor.

THE RELATIONSHIP BETWEEN HUMOR AND AESTHETIC EMOTION: FROM SURPRISE TO POTENTIALITY

If we look carefully at the art fruition process and at its intra-communicative aspects as previously described, we may see that that process is not so different from what happens in meditation and contemplation techniques. Art fruition deeply involves observers who find in a painting or in a piece of music the emotions they like: even more, a sense of a magic and dreamy unity comes between observers and particular art products. We can describe this situation in terms of "regression" if we wish to use a psychoanalytical concept. The process however does not refer only to a regressive experience, but needs something else, a new analysis or a new point of view from where to continue. In analogy with what happens when we listen to music, where moments of tension are followed by moments of relaxation, in art fruition regressive and constructive situations come one after the other. A general schema relaxation-arousal-relaxation seems to go along with the natural rhythms of life and seems to be applied in the emotional regulation process when we are in contact with certain art products. The moments of arousal where tension arrives are linked to expectancy violations. As we have said before here we encounter surprise and, to a certain extent, also humor. As the schema of these two movements is intra individual and refers to an experience of simulation, the correct passage goes from arousal to exploration to potential communication. The passage between these moments of tension and relaxation in both directions may be marked by facial expressions. Smiling as we have said before and will discuss again later, is one of the most important mimic indicators. Speaking in general terms, we may consider surprise as a main emotional response that directs attention towards an unexpected or incongruent event. We suppose, in agreement with several authors (see for example Reisenzein's theory of surprise) that this kind of reaction has important effects in evoking and mobilizing resources for processing unfamiliar information and also for coping with potential "threats". Following Reisenzein's model [30,51], surprise could ensure an effective monitoring and prediction of our surroundings, and therefore optimal transactions between the individual and the environment. In the research we present here, we have analyzed the expression and comprehension of surprise as a good indicator of some kind of emotional timing, and, from this point of view, as a specifically impaired mechanism in pathological conditions like autism. The reference to autism while talking about art and humor is not casual. In fact artistic expressions in autism are often reported and sometimes an extraordinary sense of humor has also been observed. Nevertheless interest in art and humor in autistic people is rather peculiar due to their disorders in empathy and emotional communication. An autistic person for example may laugh at other people coughing if he/she finds that activity funny without realizing the danger of the situation when choking symptoms appear. Art expressions and also humor reactions may be taken as elements which can be important for a therapeutic approach to autistic syndrome. In the realms of art and humor expectations are built in advance, novelty may be seen not as dangerous as it appears in reality. The need for order in autistic patients may be somehow fulfilled with artistic expressions, often repetitive. "The world of children with autism is not one of confusion and baffling behaviors, but involves a different way of ordering their world. The metaphor of an inner mirror that cannot reflect may help describe their experience"[52: 144]. The therapeutic approach should therefore be addressed to transforming those mirrors into reflecting mirrors and sharing little by little some emotional contents belonging to artistic language.

AUTISM, SMILE AND SURPRISE: AN EXPERIMENTAL STUDY

Autism is a developmental disorder characterized by impairments in social reciprocity and communication, and by restricted and stereotyped patterns of interest and behavior. Kanner [53] originally defined autism as "an innate inability to form the usual, biologically provided affective contact with people". In a new study of genetics that links autism to timing mechanism, reported in *Molecular Psychiatry* [54], the authors claim that timing is typical of normal infant development and that the autistic child's inability to engage in several interactions has been clinically described as social timing difficulty [55]. Social timing consists of interactive turn-taking, shifting attention, gaze switching, during communications and other types of interaction. In the first few months of life an unaffected infant can take part in social exchanges, sharing eye contact and babbling by means of 'natural' communication patterns. It is through preverbal communication that the baby anticipates and predicts the behavior of others, progressing to increasingly sophisticate social participation, like mutually enjoyable preverbal teasing games (e.g. 'peep-bo!') that are timing-dependent and appear at an early stage in the development of empathy and social pretense. Considering all the components of autism, there apparently exists an inability to achieve object constancy in early development. Behaviors that seem obsessive-compulsive, repetitive, and generally abnormal in relating to people, objects, and events may be the method by which children with autistic symptoms attempt to satisfy their need for object constancy. Children who have autism cannot order and keep their relationship with objects in their inner world constant as other children do throughout their development. "Children with autism continually insist on sameness; behavioral rigidity and specialized interests may be explained by their intense need for order and object constancy" [52: 144]. Empathy and pretending are among the life-long difficulties for individuals with autistic disorder. These may be developmentally linked to early difficulties in synchronizing with the inbuilt rhythms of communication [54]. Among other things, our study also looks at the possible link existing between surprise and smile. The smile is a facial expression widely studied, both at developmental level [56] and in adults [57]. Human smiling has a broad variety of meanings: it can be a sign of well-being, but also of embarrassment or politeness. Besides its emotional value smiling can be the expression of interactional and communicative functions. In this respect empirical studies concerning the autistic deficit suggest a poor coordination of affective response; for example these children are less able to combine smiles with eye contacts or to response to their mother's approach with smiles [58] according to a generally shared meaning of smile as a good indicator of the ability to share attention and affect. From this point of view, we have considered smile as a particular orienting reflex, in agreement with an original suggestion that smile is a sort of "soft" laughter, in response to a threat followed by a harmless situation (or a situation followed by a trivial consequence), as when a child reacts to tickling [59]. Ramachandran, moreover, argues that smile evolved from a threat grimace (as we have said before in relation to Darwin's considerations) "I find great irony in the fact that every time someone smiles at you, she is in fact producing a half threat by flashing her canines…" [59: 237]. For example, we can consider smile as a response to a potential threat, for instance if a stranger is coming towards us, but we do not immediately realize who it is, and only later do we see he/she is a friend of ours.

On the basis of this particular proposition, smiling could be seen as an emotional adjustment subsequent to a surprise that does not cause any further emotional reaction, a sort of interlocutory (temporary) reorganization, able to hold the attention suspended. Bearing in mind these theoretical proposals, we see that autistic children may have a specific problem when they are processing a new situation (a surprising situation) as they usually avoid new stimuli. Therefore it would be quite interesting to investigate whether smiles should be considered as a sort of primitive sign of a successful orienting response, as well as a good marker of affective response. Following this theoretical insight we wondered if smile may have a particular connection with surprise, representing a primitive form of focus of attention through a request for sharing. In autism there is a particular form of neurophysiological evidence – the slow habituation of the orienting response – so we could consider that the lack of smiles in autistic patients might not be only a sign of emotional-interactive deficits but also a specific difficulty to orient towards a new situation and then to direct attention towards such a situation.

THE EXPERIMENTAL HYPOTHESIS AND METHODS

On this basis we performed an experiment in which a sample of 21 children with pervasive developmental disorders (PDD) was compared with a sample of 35 children without developmental problems (control group) – whose age ranged from 3 to 12 years – on the assumption that comprehension and expression of surprise could be different in the two groups and that smile responses – associated with surprise situations – would be more frequent in the control group [60].

Five different tasks were performed by participants in our experiment:

A) After the usual preliminary approach to put the child at ease, an experimenter and an accomplice showed three boxes of nuts, easily distinguished from each other because of their different colors.

B) Then, working together with the child, the contents of one of the boxes was replaced and a different material (macaroni, pebbles) was put in the box for the purpose of preparing a surprise for someone.

C) At this stage, the accomplice excused him/herself and left, and the experimenter suggested to the child that he prepare another surprise, replacing the contents in the second box.

D) When the accomplice came back, the child was asked to give him/her a surprise by picking out the box that the child considered suitable for the purpose.

E) At the end of the task the accomplice, unbeknown to the child, changed the content of one of the boxes with candies, and asked the child to open the box. It was then possible to check if the child reacted by showing surprise (and perhaps smile) to the unexpected event.

RESULTS AND DISCUSSION

The results show a significant difference between the autistic and control group, in all tests concerning the comprehension and expression of surprise (see figs 1 and 2).

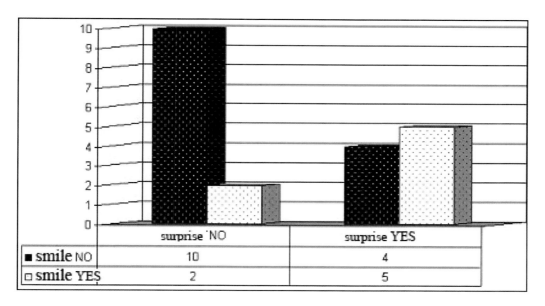

	surprise NO	surprise YES
■ smile NO	10	4
□ smile YES	2	5

Figure 1. Autistic Group.

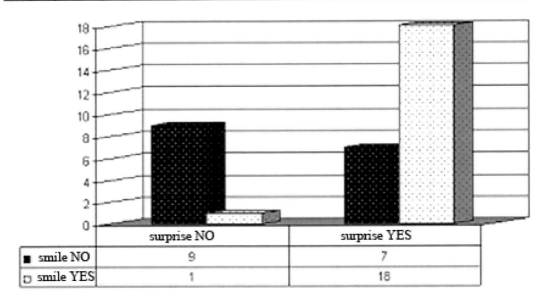

	surprise NO	surprise YES
■ smile NO	9	7
▢ smile YES	1	18

Figure 2. Control Group.

The presence of surprise was significantly lower in the autistic group than in the control group. The smile response was expressed together with surprise. More precisely, there is no statistical difference in the number of smiles between the two groups, but the normal children who succeeded in selecting the correct box to induce surprise (test D), were the ones who showed a greater number of smiles. Moreover, our results show a significant relation of co-occurrence between surprise and smile in the control group (children who were surprised did smile; children who were not surprised did not smile). In the autistic group, even if the trend was the same, there was no significant relation between surprise and smile. Our results concerning the understanding of surprise can, in our opinion, be interpreted in the light of recent theories which consider the understanding of false belief as the outcome of an innate and implicit mechanism [61,62]. In addition, the significant difference in the appearance of the expression of surprise in the two groups (we are fully aware of the limits due to the absence of a video recording of the expression) could well suggest a topic for further investigation. Co-occurrence of surprise and smile in the control group could correspond to a particular relationship between surprise and smile, which is not present in the case of a pathological condition like autism. In specific conditions in which the smile matches the test, as in the control group, it may represent a sudden insight, the Aha-Erlebnis concept coined by the German psychologist Karl Buhler that corresponds to a sort of emotion of conclusiveness.

In our research, however, there is not so much clear evidence of any explicit awareness, while, in our opinion, the children smiling in this situation may most likely represent a type of emotional rearrangement attained after having been surprised, independently of the obtained result. Clearly this is only a speculative hypothesis, which has essentially attracted our attention and which requires closer examination and more robust evidence.

CONCLUSION

Autism may be something more than a well-known developmental syndrome. Philosophers have been quite interested in this matter [63], since in the past the research on the perception of ourselves and of our environment has often been, so to speak, "autistic". It could therefore be appropriate to talk about an "autistic philosophy" insofar as thought has been separated, following Descartes' tradition, not only from its body, but also from other people's minds.

In this chapter we have tried to say that surprise, although it is an emotion, is in some ways a situation where many people's minds meet, where what we call the "meaning" (in the broadest possible sense) of our actions and behaviors comes from a continuous interaction with other people: in this respect we may talk about a "participatory sense making" activity which takes into account a flexible relationship between the bodies, brains and minds of many people. Surprise is the expectancy that our predictions may be unattended. The tolerance of a certain amount of incongruity is in some way necessary in order to build a social and, to a certain extent, collective meaning. Surprise, tension and wonder are the basic ingredients of creativity insofar as they can ensure contacts between our own body, brain and mind as well as among other people's emotional experiences. The possibility to share our emotions with other people [64], to express and regulate our emotions is strictly linked to certain transformational processes: our emotions may become our thoughts, as some psychoanalysts [39] suggest, insofar as a "potential space" [22] between ourselves and other people can be created. That potential space is where surprise and irony may arrive, where illusions and delusions may deftly come and go.

Over the last years, thanks to the progress in the field of neurosciences, some new disciplines such as neuroaesthetics have given us new possibilities to discover the links between body, brain and mind of which we have spoken and that in some way concern surprise, art, irony, emotions and mind theory as mentioned in this chapter. On the other hand a new reductionism seems to be emerging: up to what point, one might ask oneself, is it correct to say that neuronal activity can explain the complex processes of the mind? Using a metaphor or a joke we could say that an "amazing neuronal activity" [65] instead of just a simple neuronal activity could explain better the complicated link between brain and mind. In this metaphor we can see once again that surprise, amazement and wonder come to modulate our worldly experience.

Finally, one may wonder if it is just a metaphor, a joke or even a quasi-serious suggestion that neurosciences may be interested in the study of an "amazing neuronal activity". As we have said before, the role of smiling (in humans and in non-human animals) as a connection between surprise, emotions, social interaction and cognitive abilities may offer some hints in that direction.

REFERENCES

[1]   Attardo, S., and Raskin, V. (1991). Script theory revis(it)ed: joke similarity and joke representation model. *Humor: International Journal of Humor Research*, *4*, 293-347.

[2]   Attardo, S., Hempelmann, C. F., and Di Maio, S. (2002). Script oppositions and logical mechanisms: Modeling incongruities and their resolutions. *Humor: International Journal of Humor Research*, 15, 3-46.

[3]   Ruch, W., Attardo, S., and Raskin, V. (1993). Towards an empirical verification of the General Theory of Verbal Humor. *Humor: International Journal of Humor Research*, 6, 123-136.

[4]   Stame, S., and Lorenzetti, R. (2004), L'umorismo: punti di vista e punti di svolta. In R. Lorenzetti, and S. Stame (Eds.), *Narrazione e Identità. Aspetti Cognitivi e Interpersonali* (pp. 43-64). Roma-Bari: Laterza.

[5]   Berlyne, D. E. (1954). A theory of human curiosity. *British Journal of Psychology*, 45, 180-191.

[6]   Berlyne, D. E. (1960). *Conflict, Arousal, and Curiosity*. New York: McGraw Hill.

[7]   Berlyne, D.E. (1971). *Aesthetics and Psychobiology*. New York: Appleton-Century-Crofts.

[8]   Bonaiuto, P., Biasi, V., Giannini, A. M., Bartoli, G., and Bonaiuto, M. (1992). Stress, comfort and self-appraisal: A panoramic investigation of the dynamics of cognitive processes. In D. G. Forgays, T. Sosnowski, and K. Wrzesniewski (Eds.), *Anxiety: Recent Developments in Cognitive, Psychophysiological and Health Research* (pp. 75-107). Washington: Hemisphere.

[9]   Scherer, K. R. (1987). Toward a dynamic theory of emotion: The component process model of affective states. *Geneva Studies in Emotion and Communication, 1*, 1–98.

[10] Scherer, K. R. (2001). Appraisal considered as a process of multilevel sequential checking. In K. Scherer, A. Schorr, and T. Johnston (Eds.), *Appraisal Processes in Emotions: Theory, Methods, Research: Series in Affective Science* (pp. 92–120). New York: Oxford University Press.

[11] Freud, S. (1960). Jokes and their relation to the Unconscious. In J. Strachey (Ed. and Trans.), *The Standard Edition of the Complete Psychological Works of Sigmund Freud* (Vol. 8). London: Hogarth Press and the Institute of Psychoanalysis. (original work published in 1905).

[12] Freud, S. (1960). An Outline of Psycho-Analysis. In J. Strachey (Ed. and Trans.), *The Standard Edition of the Complete Psychological Works of Sigmund Freud* (Vol. 23). London: Hogarth Press and the Institute of Psychoanalysis. (original work published in 1940).

[13] Wertheimer, M. (1959). *Productive thinking (Enlarged Ed.)*. New York: Harper and Row.

[14] Darwin, C. (1872). *The Expression of Emotions in Man and Animals*. London: Murray.

[15] Fridlund, A. J., and Loftis J. M. (1990). Relations between tickling and humorous laughter: preliminary support for the Darwin-Hecker hypothesis. *Biological Psychology, 30*, 141-150.

[16] Ekman, P., and Friesen, W. V. (1978). *Manual for Facial Action Coding System*. Palo Alto: Consulting Psychologists Press.

[17] Hjorstjo, C. H. (1970). *Man's Face and Mimic Language*, Lund: Studentlitterature.

[18] Anolli, L., Balconi, M., and Ciceri, R. (2002). Deceptive miscommunication theory (DeMiT): A new model for the analysis of deceptive communication. In L. Anolli, R. Ciceri, and G. Riva (Eds), *Say Not to Say: New Perspectives on Miscommunication* (pp. 73-100). Amsterdam: IOS Press.

[19] Ekman, P. (1985). *Telling Lies*. New York: Norton.

[20] Freud, S. (1960). The Ego and the Id. In J. Strachey (Ed. and Trans.), *The Standard Edition of the Complete Psychological Works of Sigmund Freud* (Vol. 9, pp. 3-66). London: Hogarth Press and the Institute of Psychoanalysis. (original work published in 1923).

[21] Freud, A. (1966). The Ego and the mechanisms of defense. In *The Writings of Anna Freud, Vol. 2*, Revised edition. New York: International University Press. (original work published in 1936).

[22] Winnicott, D. W. (1971). *Playing and Reality*, London: Tavistock.

[23] Freud, S. (1960). The Uncanny. In J. Strachey (Ed. and Trans.), *The Standard Edition of the Complete Psychological Works of Sigmund Freud* (Vol. 17). London: Hogarth Press and the Institute of Psychoanalysis. (original work published in 1919).

[24] Izard, C. E. (1991). *The Psychology of Emotions*. New York: Plenum Press.

[25] Ekman, P. (1992). An argument for basic emotions. *Cognition and Emotion*, 6, 169-200.

[26] Izard, C. E. (1977). *Human Emotions*. New York: Plenum Press.

[27] Plutchik, R. (1980). *Emotion: A Psychoevolutionary Syntesis*. New York: Harper and Row.

[28] Meyer, W. U., Niepel, M., Rudolph, U., and Schutzwohl, A. (1991). An experimental analysis of surprise. *Cognition and Emotion*, 5, 295-311.

[29] Steinsmeier-Pelster, J., Martini, A., and Reisenzein, R. (1995). The role of surprise in the attribution process. *Cognition and Emotion*, 9, 5-31.

[30] Reisenzein, R., Meyer, W. U., and Schutzwohl, A. (1996). Reactions to surprising events: A paradigm for emotion research. In T. N. Frijda, (Ed.), *Proceedings of the 9th conference of the International Society for Research on Emotions* (pp. 292–296). Toronto: ISRE.

[31] Meyer, W. U, Reisenzein, R., and Schützwoh, A. (1997). Towards a process analysis of emotions: The case of surprise. *Motivation and Emotion*, 21, 251-274.

[32] Schützwohl, A. (1998). Surprise and schema strength. *Journal of Experimental Psychology: Learning, Memory, and Cognition*, 24, 1182-1199.

[33] Rao, R. P., and Ballard, D. H. (1999). Predictive coding in the visual cortex: a functional interpretation of some extra-classical receptive-field effects. *Nature Neuroscience*, 2, 79-87.

[34] Ranganath, C., and Rainer, G. (2003). Neural mechanisms for detecting and remembering novel events. *Nature Reviews Neuroscience*, 4, 193-202.

[35] Meyer, L. B. (1956). *Emotion and meaning in music*. Chicago: Chicago University Press.

[36] Thompson, W. F., Balkwill, L. L., and Vernescu, R. (2000). Expectancies generated by recent exposure to melodic sequences. *Memory and Cognition*. 28, 547-555

[37] Huron, D. (2006). *Sweet Anticipation: Music and the Psychology of Expectation*. Cambridge: MIT Press.

[38] Sloboda, J. A. (1991). Music structure and emotional response: Some empirical findings. *Psychology of Music, 19*, 110-120.

[39] Bion, W. R. (1962). *Learning from Experience*. London: Heinemann.

[40] Magherini, G. (2007). *Mi sono innamorato di una statua: Oltre la sindrome di Stendhal*. Firenze: Nicomp.

[41] Zentner, M., Grandjean, D., and Scherer, K. R. (2008). Emotions evoked by the sound of music: Differentiation, classification, and measurement. *Emotion, 8*, 494-521.

[42] Brattico, E., and Jacobsen, T. (2009). Subjective appraisal of music: Neuroimaging evidence. *Annals of The New York Academy of Sciences, 1169*, 308-317.

[43] Rizzolatti, G., Camarda, R., Fogassi, L., Gentilucci, M., Luppino, G., and Matelli, M. (1988). Functional organization of inferior area 6 in the macaque monkey. II. Area F5 and the control of distal movements. *Experimental Brain Research, 71*, 491-507.

[44] Gallese, V., and Goldman, A. I. (1998). Mirror neurons and the simulation theory. *Trends in Cognitive Sciences, 2*, 493–501.

[45] Gallese, V. (2001). The "Shared Manifold" hypothesis: from mirror neurons to empathy. *Journal of Consciousness Studies, 8*, 33–50.

[46] Gallese, V (2006). Corpo vivo, simulazione incarnata e intersoggettività: Una prospettiva neurofenomenologica. In M. Cappuccio (Ed), *Neurofenomenologia: La scienza della Mente e la Sfida dell'Esperienza Cosciente* (pp. 293-326). Milano: Mondadori.

[47] Freedberg, D., and Gallese, V. (2007). Motion, emotion and empathy in aesthetic experience. *Trends in Cognitive Sciences, 11*, 197-203.

[48] Zeki, S. (2009). *Splendors and Miseries of the Brain: Love, Creativity and the Quest for Human Happiness*. Blackwell: Wiley.

[49] Frijda, N. H. (1986). *The Emotions*. Cambridge: Cambridge University Press.

[50] Gallagher, S. (2001). The practice of mind: Theory, simulation or interaction? *Journal of Consciousness Studies, 8*, 83-108.

[51] Reisenzein, R. (2000). Exploring the strength of association between the components of emotion syndrome: the case of surprise. *Cognition and Emotion, 14*, 1-38.

[52] Emery, M. J. (2004). Art Therapy as an intervention for autism. *Art Therapy: Journal of the American Art Therapy Association, 21*, 143-147.

[53] Kanner, L. (1943). Autistic disturbances of affective contact, *Nervous Child, 2*, 217-250.

[54] Nicholas, B., Rudrasingham, V., Nash, S., Kirov, G., Owen, M. J., and Wimpory, D. C. (2007). Association of Per1 and Npas2 with autistic disorder: support for the clock genes/social timing hypothesis. *Molecular Psychiatry, 12*, 581-592.

[55] Newson, E. (1984). *The Social Development of the Young Autistic Child. National Autistic Child*. Paper presented at the National Autistic Society Conference, Bath, UK.

[56] Messinger, D. S., Fogel, A., and Dickson, K. L. (1999). What's in a smile? *Developmental Psychology, 35*, 701-708.

[57] Ekman, P., Davidson, R. J., and Friesen, W. V. (1990). The Duchenne smile: Emotional expression and brain physiology II. *Journal of Personality and Social Psychology, 58*, 342-353.

[58] Kasari, C., Sigman, M., Mundy, P., and Yirmiya, N. (1990). Affective sharing in the context of joint attention interactions of normal, autistic and mentally retarded children. *Journal of Autism and Developmental Disorders, 20*, 87-100.

[59] Ramachandran, V. S., and Blakeslee, S. (2003). *La Donna che Morì dal Ridere*. Milano: Mondadori.

[60] Incasa, I. (2008). *Surprise as Indicative Critical Factor of Emotional Tuning in Normal Children and in Children with Pervasive Developmental Disorders* (Unpublished Ph.D. thesis). University of Bologna, Bologna, I.

[61] Ruffman, T., Garnham, W., Import, A., and Connolly, D. (2001). Does eye direction indicate implicit sensitivity to false belief?: Charting transitions in knowledge. *Journal of Experimental Child Psychology, 80*, 201-224.

[62] Onishi, K. H., and Baillargeon, R. (2005). Do 15-month-old infants understand false beliefs? *Science, 308*, 255-258.

[63] Gallagher, S. (2009). Two problems of intersubjectivity. *Journal of Consciousness Studies, 16*, 289-308.

[64] Rimé, B. (1994, May). The social sharing of emotional experiences as a sorce for the social knowledge on emotion. Paper presented at the NATO-Workshop *"Everyday Conceptions of Emotion"*, Almagro, Spain.

[65] Giorgi, R. (2011). *Che Farò senza il Mio Ben? Cervello, Filosofia, Mistica*. Battipaglia (SA): Ripostes.

In: Humor and Health Promotion
Editor: Paola Gremigni

ISBN: 978-1-61942-657-3
© 2012 Nova Science Publishers, Inc.

Chapter 7

HUMOR AND CHILDREN

Alessandra Farneti and Reinhard Tschiesner

Free University of Bozen-Bolzano, Italy

ABSTRACT

In this chapter, we intend to give a brief overview of the development of humor, especially in childhood. First of all we describe the first steps in the development of smile and then functions, different types of smiling, the period in which they appear during growth, and the difference between a smile and laugh. In addition, we describe the most relevant steps in the development of humor, beginning with early childhood, which also concerns cognitive skills, and explain the changes that affect humor in the course of the life cycle. We also explain the role of the clown and if and when children consider a clown funny through development. Another interesting topic regarding humor is its rules in the education system; thus, we show some empirical results concerning humor used by teachers and outcome results on their pupils.

INTRODUCTION: SMILE AND LAUGHTER IN THE FIRST YEARS OF LIFE

The subject of smiles and laughter has been discussed from different theoretical perspectives, as seen in previous chapters. Even if we have had, in the past, a lot of interesting studies and observations from ethology, ethnology, philosophy and anthropology about this specific human behavior, we have relatively few studies about the development of smiles and laughter throughout the life.

Smile and laughter are fundamental elements of human behavior and communication throughout the lifespan. During the course of development, the production of smile, different kinds of laughter, understanding of humor, humor production and functionality of humor, in fact, evolve. These functions are essentially determined by cognitive, verbal and social abilities. Furthermore, there are a lot of studies which underline the neurological correlation of smiles and laughter in both normal and pathological development [1,2]. Nevertheless, there isn't a common position regarding which parts of the brain are involved in processing humoristic stimuli. A lot of researches have been made in this field, but results are not definitive [3].

There are still some interesting questions open from a psychological point of view: can we consider smiles and laughter as the same response, only different in their intensity? Or are they responses qualitatively different?

The researchers supported the second hypothesis, because smiles and laughter have different phylogenetic origins and functions [4], different goals, and develop differently in the course of life.

Darwin, on the contrary, interpreted smile and laughter as expressions of internal joy or happiness, differing only in intensity, but other authors claimed that the smile is a behavior more oriented to ask or to maintain affiliation and affective proximity than the laughter [5].

The ethological studies showed that front-teeth smiling and open-mouth laughter have different origins and functions: smile appears in affiliative contexts whereas the laughter in play context [6,4].

A second question regards the quality and intentionality of smile and laughter during the development.

We can recall Berger's distinction between "to be a body" and to "have a body" [7]. During the development, we are observing a slow change from the first to the second position but still isn't clear when and why it's possible. We don't know when the child's smile or laughter or cry became conscious responses of a "thought body". When, in the third or fourth months of age, the child is laughing to an unexpected movement or to a voice or to adult laugh, he is only a "laughing body" and we can only assume that consciousness is absent. Only later when the child is laughing at a joke or he is trying out a comic gag for friends, or he is able to understand the funniness of an actor, we can assume that he is using a "thought body", therefore, using laughter consciously!

The comprehension of funny events and the intentional behavior to elicit the other's laugh are obviously submitted to the cognitive capacities and develop from birth to adult age.

Therefore after summing various theories and opinions, we can tell that the smile and laughter in children (as well as in adults) are important signals of their good reactivity, both to the environmental stimulations and to other people in the interpersonal relationship.

THE SMILE

The smile seems to be mostly a social response, which tends to induce the relationship with others and is strongly related with the child's need for care and protection by the adults. However, the smile is elicited by visual contact or an adult's smile or vocal sweet stimulations, whereas the laughter is elicited by unexpected, unfamiliar or incongruous events

There are many reasons to consider the smile a behavior response caused by human evolution to preserve the species. The child already smiles during the prenatal life, from the fifth month of pregnancy but, when the child becomes able to smile at the human face, from the second-third month of life, the interaction with the adults changes and evolves, becoming stronger and more intense. I remember my father when my son smiled at him the first time: he was so happy and proud that his grandchild chose him as the preferred partner!

In the thirties some authors found interesting results in the observation of smile and laughter. They tried to identify some preferred stimuli, which elicited them.

Later in the fifties Spitz from a psychoanalytically point of view considered the smile like an organizer of reality. The first "social smile" leads the infant at the age of 3 months to smile at every human face and this reinforces the attachment with adults. After that at 8 months the "selective smile" permits children to direct most awareness to adults, who they have a familial relationship and to distinguish familial faces from strangers. In the mother-child-relation (object relations) infants pass through an initial status of non-differentiation (pre-objectual status) who are not able to distinguish their body from the environment. In the "precursor object" the child begins to replay a smile at human faces.

Spitz thought that a response becomes a "Gestalt-signal" (or rather to common perception regarding the signal) and not yet a response at a person, which the child perceives. And therefore it is not allowed to talk about an object relation. All in all this skill to respond at a human face as a signal, causes the condition to establish, after the 8th month, a real social relationship with the mother, perceived as a person rather than a stranger. Spitz investigated 147 children from birth until a year and found that the perception of human face and the smile to that in the third month are not an object relation. Babies at this age do not perceive the person as a person or an object but only as a signal. This signal is composed of the whole human face, however Spitz experiences show that this signal does not consist of the entire face signal – it is more a favored "Gestalt". But this Gestalt is composed of eyes, front, nose and movements. In this case development is not isolated to a certain person, for instance the mother. Therefore children respond not only to the mother's smile but also at other people. However, Children do not respond to smiles if the head is turned sideways. In this case the Gestalt is modified and the children are not able to recognize this, so the object loses its quality. For this reason he gives the Gestalt the name "precursor object". Children don't find the essential qualities in the object and that's the difference to the libidinous object, which consists in the essential qualities [8,9].

Later Morton and Johnson [10] confirmed the preference of human newborn to human face stimuli. They argue that infants innately respond to the human face from birth and that their preference is an important step in the development of socialization.

More recently, in an evolutionary perspective, the qualities of the smile and laughter during the life span have been distinguished. A brief overview dealing with the development of smile is given by Sroufe and Waters [11]: The earliest smile has been called endogenous or spontaneous smile. This kind of smile appears even if there haven't been any external stimuli. A lot of results show that this endogenous smiling has nothing to do with gastric activities or with vegetative drive state, but is correlated with the spontaneous central nervous system discharge of sub cortical origin.

First elicited smile appears within the first week after that infants are asleep, but these stimuli don't elicit smiles in the waking state. The first elicited waking smiles normally appear within the first month as consequences of low level tactile or kinesthetic elicitors, for example by light touches. These first elicited smiles are low-intensity responses to a mild stimulation in fact they show this only by raising their mouth corners. In the second week the best elicitor is especially a high-pitched voice. In this period it is still important that stimulation depends on low level background excitation or activity. Around the third week the first alert smile appears. It does mean that the infant smiles in the awaking state and with focused attention. All it means is that the infants smiles in a more active way and for the first time a wrinkling and brightening of the eyes when the first "grin" appears. In the fourth week the mother's voice is the most effective elicitor. Smile can now be evoked also if stimulation interrupts feeding. Ever since smile become more independent of organismic state. Nearing the 4th and 5th week, smile can be evoked by visual stimulation, for instance a slowly moving object and a sudden movement of the hand in the infants visual field can cause a surprise smile. In the 5th week the voice seriously loses its effectiveness as an elicitor but a nodding head can become a visual stimulus to evoke smiles. Cognitive development results are more responsive reactions to the surrounding environment. During 5 to 8 weeks authors agree that infants are most responsive to dynamic visual stimulation. In due course the first stimuli become less important.

Commonly the children smile first of all at their mother and the synchronicity and the intensity of this interaction has been considered as a signal of a good or of a disturbed relationship [12,11].

If we can consider the smile overall as a social behavior, it's clear that the smile can be a response to a sense of wellbeing or a contentment in lonely situations too. In this case it's not a social response. The first physiological smile becomes social smile in the second month of life, but we have satisfaction's or wellbeing smiles in the course of all the lifespan.

Furthermore the smiles can be very different, according to different social situations: a first classification distinguishes a *closed smile*, a *broad smile* and an *upper smile* [13].

In the *closed smile* the mouth corners are drown up and out and the upper lip is raised and the teeth are covered; in the *broad smile* the lower and the upper teeth are exposed, in the *upper smile* the upper lip is raised showing only the upper teeth.

The researchers demonstrated that each kind of smile has a different social function: the upper smile has a social function more than the closed or broad smile. Cheyne, for instance, observed that the upper smile is increasing by the age and becomes more selective: the preschooler boys, by age four, smile almost to others boys and rarely to the girls; on the contrary, do the girls smile rarely to the boys [14].

More recently Ekman, Friesen and Davidson [15] differentiated between 14 types of smiles. A very important type of smile is the so called Duchenne Smile. This facial expression is the combined contraction of the zygomaticus major muscle and the orbicularis oculi. This combination occurs during the time that people feels enjoyment. They found that two types of smiling, Duchenne smile and other smiles, differ in the pattern of regional brain activity. In the Duchenne smiles activity in the left-sided anterior temporal and parietal area appears more than in other types of smiles. Of course categorization can be distinguished also by way of the elicitor. Researchers also described the appearance of "false smiles". The function of these smiles is to convince other people that enjoyment is occurring when in fact it isn't. The "masking smiles" appears if someone has to conceal something negative like negative emotions. People show "miserable smiles" if they have to do endure unpleasant circumstance.

Therefore, investigations show that different situations cause different types of smile.

Ten months old infants show more closed smile if a stranger approach, but more upper smile if the mother. In preschool age closed smiles appears more in non-social situations as well as open-mouthed smiles during social exchanges. Different types of smile were also found in monkeys and apes. The silent-bare-teeth display is grimace in which the lips are drawn back and teeth are exposed, like in form and context a human smile. The matter of this grimace is to sign appeasement to hostile animal as well as a sign of attachment [16].

THE LAUGHTER

We remember that the difference between smile and laughter is that laughter is the maximum of a positive affective expression and requires a faster build-up of tension. But it is a more complex response than the smile: the laughter is composed of cognitive and social elements.

In fact, during the first year, children develop: the first physical self-image (self-recognition in the mirror), are able to understand a lot of words, learn simple relations cause-effect, and understand the "permanence of the objects". So they can distinguish a normal from a modified scheme (motor, vocal, visual etc.) and can laugh because they think that "things should have gone differently"! There are children who laugh more frequently than others, but we don't know why. Even if the laughter is related with temperamental variables, environmental variables have to be taken into consideration too. If we take into account only the affectivity, in the first mother-infant or adult-infant interactions, the smile and the laughter have the same function as of feeling's and intimacy's emphasize. But more the mother smiles or laughs, more the child smiles or laughs [17]!

Also, the laughter, like the smile, can be interpreted as a signal of a good mother-infant interaction but also as a signal of cognitive competence.

During the first years of life the development of the laughter as well as of the smile, increases in the third or fourth months.

We found first empirical studies in thirties of 19th century. Washburn [18] investigated 15 children with a follow up. Children were tested several time in the age from the 16th to the 52nd week and found that there are no changes in the efficiency of eliciting stimuli and in the frequency of laughter. He found also that there are no connections between developmental level and frequency. Justin [19] explored laughter provoking stimuli and found that response increases until age 3 to 5 and reach another peak at year 6 and decreases thereafter. Especially incongruent situations as elicitor are more efficient. In addition to that the author found a positive correlation between IQ and a laughing-response. Already Kenderdine [20] found similar results. Ambrose [21] studied ambivalence in early childhood and found that in the age of 4 months the appearance of laughter can be explained by the developmental process of experiencing ambivalence. Therefore a mild tickling in a baby elicits loving attention, heavier tickling avoidance and moderate tickling laughter.

Later most authors confirm that laughter appears first around the third or the fourth month. For instance the researches of Sroufe and Waters demonstrate that the elicitors for laughter in the first quarter year of life are essentially intrusive tactile and auditory stimulation and evolve later basically into interesting social-visual events. Until the first 4 months physically vigorous stimulation is most effective, for example a vigorous kissing of the infant's stomach. The change in the fourth to sixth month is from a vigorous stimulation to a less vigorous to a provocative tactile and auditory way of stimulation that always are physical: for instance tickling or movements or vocalizations or "peep-po".

With 12 months infants laugh mostly at the appearance of stimuli that show elements of obvious cognitive incongruity, for example mother walking like penguin. In due course laughter like smiling become more a product of cognitive evaluation of novel experiences and makes a contribution to elaboration of novel experiences [11].

Sarra and Otta [16] investigated smiles and laughter in Brazilian preschool children. They observed children 60 minutes in different situation (playground, classroom), then they analyze data and found two types of laughter in children. They call the first dimension *playfulness-mock aggression*. This type consists of a broad smile and laughter. The second type is the *friendliness-appeasement dimension* and it consists of a closed and upper smile. Further, they found that peers and teachers identified different types of smiling in each other.

Laughter even if is an answer to funniness and to humor, can also be used to express anger, contempt and mockery towards others or even something beyond comprehension, breaching on mental or neurological pathologies. Therefore laughter has many different facets and often has opposite meaning even if there has been little research as regards.

Laughter is also been investigated indirectly in studies on children play, for instance in the *"Rough and Tumble"* play. During this kind of play brawling children seem to be angry but their laughing is friendly. In this case laughter is a social signal which permits the others to understand the intentionality [22].

During the life laughter becomes obviously more and more complex and is related to social rules. We can in fact remark that in different cultures and in different moments of history, laughter has been considered as a good response or as a very bad one. The following examples demonstrate two different cultures and the way they considered laughter:

Anzieu-Premmereur, for instance, refers to the traditional Navajo culture, where the *"First Laugh Ceremony"* existed. It marked the social birth of the child: the first member of the family, who made the baby laugh, had to provide for the festivity in honor of the child [23]. Whereas on the contrary we know that during the Middle Ages the laugh was considered work of "the Devil"! In the same way that the laughter has been considered good or bad by parents and teachers in relation with social and temperamental variables.

During the adolescence an interesting phenomenon is contagious laughter. Persistent outbreaks of laughter appear usually between 12 to 18 year old girls at school. This laughter is a social coupling process. But the reasons for contagious laughter can be conformity, peer pressure, social norms and so on. Contagious laughter as well as yawning is a powerful species-typical behavior that plays a role in social communication and behavior [24,25].

WHICH HUMOR (OR FUNNINESS?) DO CHILDREN UNDERSTAND DURING THEIR GROWTH?

Between laughter, funniness and humor there are substantial differences. Humor is complex whereas funniness could be very simple. Funniness has been defined as a capacity to elicit 'bursts of laughter' and comes from literature and theatrical comedy. Humor on the other hand has been defined as a thin intelligence and ingenious (witty) way to interpret reality underlining its unusual, bazaar and funny aspects.

We can only presume that during development funniness is understood before humor.

Psychological literature on the development of humor during infancy is insufficient.

Research stops at preschool age and has mainly analyzed the different types of smile and laugh (as mentioned before) rather than the different types of funniness and humor in children.

It is not definitely clear when humor in infants' life begins. Up to 12 until 13 months, with the appearance of the pretended play, infants for the first time have the possibility to play out a humorous scene. With 14 months they are able to produce slapstick-humor. In experimental situations researcher showed, that child can put a foot in a cardboard box and stamp around noisily. At that instant they laugh and look at their siblings.

Another kind of humor showed a two year old child riding on a hoover, using it as a lorry, imitating engine noise and driving it over the mother's feet. At the end of second year children have the necessary requirements to use incongruent labels for objects or events. As of third year after increasing expertise children are able to fool around on a broader range.

The earlier kind of humor is based on perceptions, in the later kind, humor is the imagination of reality. This later kind of humor can only appear if children have the ability to differ in manipulated imagination and reality. A step forward in the development of humor is the theory of mind. In this period children are able to deceive others [26].

The comprehension of humor depends on attention, working memory, emotional evaluation, verbal abstraction, representation of reality, and all these are possible only after the eighth-ninth years.

During the preschool age the children can appreciate the funniness if an adult or another child which does something of funny, for instance a gesture or a vocal sound or a movement different from the children's expectation.

We can interpret this capacity as a form of imitation of adult behavior, but we can also presume that children already have a theory in mind, to understand what is funny or not, for other people. If I do something, thinking what the other could or couldn't answer, with a certain kind of behavior, *I'm thinking what the other is thinking. "I'm putting myself in their shoes!"*

Therefore it was the comprehension funniness but not sense of humor!

The children's funniness is generally a *realistic funniness* or better *a corporal funny*: the children laugh if someone says "swearwords", generally relating to the body or to something dirty such as "pooh pooh" or "wee wee".

Here is an example of what has been explained above. It is a story invented by a four year old and recorded and written by a teacher. It was then chosen by the other children as one of the funniest stories.

"Giannino says swear words and poohs himself."

One day Giannino's mum told him off because he had said swearwords at school to make the others laugh.

The teacher told his mother and also told her the swearwords that had said to make his classmates laugh: stupid, potato head, sausage legs, toothy hair, big pig, pingo pallo, hungry tooth, radish head, mincemeat eater, bloated balloon, tomato hand, fat bomb."

Giannino's mum tells him off and as a punishment his friends aren't allowed to come to his house. After Giannino pooh's and wets his knickers and smells and so he becomes red with embarrassment. His mother washes him and puts on clean knickers. Giannino says sorry and his mother forgives him.

The children enjoyed this story much that every day they asked the teacher to tell them the story again [27].

A lot of information can be deduced from this story.

Overall, according to the psychoanalytic theory, the contents of the previous story are related to the developmental stage: contents oral and anal, rules to follow, relation with the adults are the "funny elements" for children. Therefore, the story demonstrates how the humor is experienced in a transgressive way.

Adults tell children off because they say swearwords to make the other children laugh, adults tell children off because they say swear words to make the others laugh!

As we can see, these so called "swearwords" are for the likes of only the children. They bring them together into a sort of complicity against the not so permissive adults!

What's with humor in school age? Wolfenstein [28] investigated children at age 6 to 11 and found that these take riddles also for jokes. They also feel that superior and smarter face to face with the listener causes them knowing the answer. From a psychoanalytical point of view they compare unconsciously sexual features. For example *"Mummy, mummy what is that hangs off Daddy like a baseball bat?" [26, p.178]*. These riddles give children the possibility to transform the own imperfection and the adults advantage into the opposite. Riddles give children a feeling of control. Empirical studies find a connection between social and communicative skills and the frequency of telling witty or funny riddles. At the end of school age the understanding for ambiguities and metaphors increases and therefore also the humor production.

From 6-7 years on, children begin to understand simple jokes and word games. In fact there are joke books for children where it is necessary to grasp the double meaning of the words or even the thought divergence.

Here are some examples:

1. *A dentist tells his patient: "this tooth is dead, do you want me to put a crown on it?" The patient: "no, thank you, I'd prefer just a simple burial without a ceremony".*
2. *At the psychiatrists: "well, Mr. Rossi, has it happened again to you walking around the streets again naked in your socks?"*
    "Unfortunately yes doctor".
    "And like the other times you didn't feel embarrassed?"
    "Yes I did this time, I had a hole in my sock."

A sense of funniness is an individual characteristic. There are children that develop it at an early stage and others that never acquire it.

I remember an episode that impressed me: I was with my son and a 5 year old friend in the mountains. I was bending over to open a packet of biscuits when I felt the boy pushing down on my shoulders. I asked him what he was doing and he answered with a mischievous smile "down with the mums". The hidden irony in this phrase is that of adults or otherwise that child demonstrated an incredible capacity to play with words and to tease.

Verbal and cognitive features as well as knowledge increases during youth. Some investigations show that topics of humor in this period are conflicts and social rules regarding developmental tasks. Humor is aimed mostly at sexual characteristics. If youth laughs together about sexual topics, they are able to reduce fears and insecurities. Reaching adulthood we found very little investigation concerning humor. In adulthood lasting partnership and parenthood become developmental tasks with a central importance. Therefore humor aims these topics. Humor often deals with scenes in a marriage. Most common themes are differences in partnership, catharsis (of negative emotions) and mutual adjustment and intimacy. Some results show that humor become also significance in marital satisfaction. Satisfaction increases if persons rate their partner more humorous. Older people appreciate humor as well as younger but with decreasing cognitive performance they get no joy in a complex humor production. The object of humor in this period usually is losses. The authors think that humor in older age becomes an important coping strategy to avoid desperation and melancholy [26,29].

IS A CLOWN FUNNY FOR CHILDREN?

The art of the clown is difficult to understand and it's impossible that a child would catch the metaphoric meaning.

Any authors defined the clown as a metaphoric representation of the Freudian *Es*, or as the Jung's "shadow", the "internal rascal" who press us to do something of transgressive or unusual [30, 31, 32, 33, 34].

In this meaning, the clown must awake in the audience the primitive parts, the hidden and refused internal child and his imaginary world. The clown isn't an innocuous joker who attracts the children. The potentiality of the clowning is, so, very interesting from a psychological point of view. The techniques used in clowning can elicit the emotive intelligence and increase the self-consciousness of human fragility, reducing the shame and the fear of failure. A clown can tumble but he is always able to get up again!

These hidden meanings are shown through refined gestural expressiveness using symbolic objects and movements. Nowadays, overall in the theatre, the expressive techniques of well-known clowns have reached the height of perfection, as regards to mime, and the contents of the pantomime.

This type of art is for a very selective audience who would appreciate it. Otherwise the collective image of the clown still remains an actor for children.

The person who springs to mind is Augusto the circus clown. The one with the red nose the bright colored costume, big shoes who looks a bit silly: in other words the stereotype of a clown.

The clown has been labeled as a comic actor whereas we know that many great cinema and theatrical clowns rarely use funniness. Their message is often a tragic metaphor of life or a sweet expression of feelings and emotions. Just think of the great Chaplin or Marcel Marceau or the most modern Slava Polunin and Charlotte Chaplin, only to mention a few. Their art can't be simply defined as a comic art. It is difficult to put them on the same level as the traditional circus clown.

We have to discredit this mistaken belief of a way to laugh and give back these great artists a dignity they merit. The road is long to take and will require the media to change their approach, which continue to talk of clowns wrongly.

The phenomenon of the so called "doctor clown", (or better *"hospital ward clown"*) has inflicted even further the difference between the real theatre clown and those who continue to "simplify the clowns image, reducing him to make children laugh". It is not a question of undermining the job of many volunteers but if we don't want to transmit the wrong idea to children at a very early age a stereotype which is far from real it is necessary make a clarification and a distinction from the beginning.

The volunteers dressed up as clowns who do their best to amuse children are often aware of how far they are from the difficult art of a real clown. They do want to make people laugh but, as the great Fo said, they often become pathetic because they don't have the artistic ability.

Children, don't always appreciate this stereotype: the youngest ones, up to three four years old are often afraid. The heavy makeup, red nose, oversized clothes and brusque gestural expressiveness, could scare the small children. So if the clown is unable to adapt his art to the younger audience, he could even create situations of real psychological uneasiness. Their mental schemes are too rigid to embrace a new incredible novelty.

However, as we have already mentioned before, children appreciate funniness at an early age if related to concrete events in their lives and are in tune with their stage of development.

I worked two years in a preschool, with the clown André Casaca and I observed the children (four and five years) playing with the clown, who was normally dressed and without clown-makeup but he used extraordinary gesture and nonverbal communication.

The children laughed loudly and imitated the clown to elicit the other children's laughter. Children are great actors: they used the red nose, roly polies, somersaulted, and the "audience" burst out with laughter! Therefore, the clowns' stupidity (an adult brought up badly) can be appreciated by the infants up until the age of three or four because the way they fall over and get dirty is nearer to their world. Roly polies, cart wheels and silly facial expressions excite laughs even in the first two years of life. The youngest ones wouldn't be able to comprehend metaphors, self-irony nor the desecrating message of the "revolutionary" clown. Only later at school age do children seem to understand at least in part, what we call "the clown philosophy". In fact maybe because of the mirror like image they seem to recognize their transgressive self.

A research was done on 319 children from the 3rd, 4th and 5th years of elementary school, ranging from seven to nine years of age. We asked them to describe a clown. We used essays, drawings a questionnaire, and a semantic differential.

The semantic differential included 34 adjectives (17 couples) like pretty-ugly, dirty-clean, intelligent-stupid, obedient-disobedient, good-jack-ass, good smell-smelly etc. We asked the children to choose one of the adjectives to define clown, mother, father and teacher.

The answers to the questionnaire confirmed that the majority of children love clowns and they represent them in a stereotype way: *strange clothes, silly, funny, colorful, makeup faces, red nose, often playing around, does magic etc.; does strange and stupid things, sometimes even rude like blowing raspberries. He wants to show off doing difficult things but messes it up to make the others laugh. He loves children who he does his shows for.* The children's drawings and essays confirmed all these things. The results of the semantic differential clearly confirm that Augusto is seen as the opposite to parents and teachers; a transgressive character who embodies all the irrational and childish aspects which make up the key elements for socialization and interiorization of the social norms [35].

HUMOR IN EDUCATION

I think that everyone has experimented that school is the most serious and least funny environments in the world!

Who doesn't remember an embarrassing moment at school, in childhood or adolescence, when one has been overwhelmed by an uncontrollable laughter during a lesson?

And forget those teachers' eyes with her unforgiving look?

The phrase *"Risus abundat in ore stultorum!"* has persecuted generations of students!

In schools, with rare exceptions, the dominant values are: control and self-control, seriousness, rationality and logic (at the expense of divergent thinking and creativity), verbal language, the commitment to assigned tasks (like training to suffer: duty first, pleasure later).

The system pays little attention to happiness: children are often told "You must be an obedient, brave, conscientious, serious child," but rarely "Do everything to be happy".

Judging by the joy that holidays bring therefore if we asked children and young people to associate the word school with other words, we are almost certain that very few would answer fun, novelty, and curiosity. We fear the word school evokes words such as; duty, boredom, constraint etc. [36,37].

Irony, self-irony, sense of humor, and the capacity to laugh at our self, are important competences for a social life and for psychological health but it seems that the school is completely insensitive to see these things as great values and not vice versa. Many have come up against a school which sets out to sink any originality or initiative so as to passively follow program that stifle young people's curiosity. But schools still have remained unaltered over the centuries [38,39].

This resistance to change in schools is incredible and difficult to explain after thousands of pages have been written to support the fact that learning goes hand in hand with pleasure and enjoyment.

As in the book by Umberto Eco "The Name of the Rose" it seems many teachers fear that the laugh is the work of "the devil". Even if psychologists and pedagogists have stressed the importance of play and amusement in learning processes and on a good quality of life at school, few teachers are able to create a pleasant environment in the classroom.

It is paradoxical that laughter should be valued in certain catholic traditions

San Filippo Neri [40] and Don Bosco [41] encouraged the use of laughter in education.

San Filippo Neri was severely criticized and the church was hostile to his revolutionary methods in the 1500, where singing and games were fundamental elements for the children from the streets who he looked after.

Don Bosco included happiness as one of his main educational principles and in his oratory the children were encouraged to play and laugh freely.

Today we have several studies which supports the pedagogical implications of funniness and humor in teaching but they are generally qualitative evaluations of specific programs; unfortunately we have few experimental researchers who compare a traditional teaching method with a "humoristic method" even if the humor has been associated with several positive physiological and psychological effects.

The educators, who use the humor seems to establish a more positive relationships with their students and with their colleagues. The use of humor reduces the anxiety, creates a more positive atmosphere in the classroom, as well as facilitates the learning process [42-48].

Recently, Garner studied the impact of curriculum-specific humor, with the use of metaphor and analogy, on retention and recall, as well as student evaluations of the course and the instructor. Therefore, he underlines that the teacher's humor has not always been understood by all the students because the humor is a complex mixture of cultural and social components.

When using humor, we must be careful and recognize that differences in culture, age, belief, gender, and other distinctions can influence how the information is perceived [49].

These experiences regard on the whole children over the age of 11 and not infant or primary school.

However we consider it very important to help children to understand and develop a funny side and a sense of humor right from the beginning.

Apart from the cognitive and emotive implications of which we have spoken of, they are fundamental instruments of resilience in a world that "takes things too seriously".

One way of practicing the art of being funny in the school is one that is based on the techniques of clowning, even if this can seem very strange.

The figure of the clown, in fact, has often been used in the school context more of a heretic than anything else. Professors have often been heard saying, "Stop clowning, the school is a serious thing etc. " [36].

We feel it is important to render the school an environment a bit "more fun" and above all more aware of the importance of emotional intelligence. Man is not only "sapiens" but also "ludens" [50] and "ridens" [7] and it has been apparent for some time by now that the roots of creativity and freedom of thought grow in the field of game [51,52].

With all that has been said it is apparent the clowning method could make for excellent teaching methods for both the students and for teachers themselves.

The funniness of the clown appears ingénue, uninhibited, childish, but to appear so, it is necessary hard work because a clown isn't a child even if he aspires to be one. The famous clown Dimitri wrote that "a child is without doubt a wonderful master".

From a purely technical point of view, the clowning has in common principles of other disciplines. As the psychomotricity has based on listening, perception, trust, the study of proxemics and rounds of dialogue on an inseparable mind-body unity. At the same time, however, the clowning helps to develop self-mockery and not transfer on others sarcastic aggressivity.

Other ways, such as art and music education, the clowning encourages creative use of all materials and objects available in the environment, driving the students to become accustomed to careful observation of the same environment and objects.

From a psychological point of view, clowning reinforces the positive identity especially in those subjects who are shy or fear to be judged by others. The continuous emphasis on the need to experience the collapse and failure, both physically (learning to fall and pretend to fall), and metaphorically, inhibit in the students the shame related to error and severe criticism of others.

Shame is an important emotion, both negatively and positively [53,54].

In school shame often causes pathological anxiety, learning and interpersonal difficulties.

The clown's working on allows a comparison not only with one's own flaws but also with those of others, reinforcing the idea that everyone has something to be ashamed of.

Play is also the primary means of transmission of content and moreover in the field of play the creative processes are born in developmental age. Play stops the dimension of time to carry the player in the "realm of the possible".

Thus, desirable training would involve both students and teachers simultaneously.

We know that creative thinking is often confused with insubordination. The divergent scares because of its unpredictability, its lack of ability to follow established routes, for its greater ability to freely express emotions.

This fear often stems from the insecurity of teachers, who see it as a risk to surrender with the students and discover the new and unexpected.

Increased flexibility and the discovery of new forms of communication can make the classroom climate more conducive to developing the potential of individuals and help teachers to first listen then propose, in their aim to "educate" (literally pull out) rather than "inform" (as put in).

Furthermore in nursery's and primary schools it is important that adults rediscover the power of non-verbal messages.

The clown embodies the misfit adult that dwells in our unconscious, awkward and fear, which learns to laugh and cry at himself, and not being a child, in his profound wisdom, knows how to put into play his infant parts.

His ostentatious stupidity turns into emotional intelligence and becomes a very important educational tool.

André Casaca, in a recent conference in Cape Verde (Mindelo, 15-17 July 2009), explained that the clown, using the humor and apparent stupidity, solves difficult situations in the class, reversing the normal pattern of the events.

For example, if students do not listen to the teacher, he can speak and explain the lesson to the door. The surprise of such unusual and unexpected and seemingly stupid conduct enabled clarification and a recovery teacher-student interaction. Thus the stupidity of the clown, through self-mockery, turns into emotional intelligence, which can be therapeutic if it allows the viewer identifications and projections.

In a recent research, has been offered two years of clowning training to a group of preschool teachers.

Before and after the course the teachers has been tested with the Adjective Check List (A.C.L.) to relive if the Self Image changes.

The results show that the subjects perceived a significant increasing in the scales which regard the *Capability to Take Care* of the others and the *Nurturance*.

Also, the teachers have been asked to write a comic dairy, in which they tell the everyday comic events.

In a first time this was very difficult for the teachers because they are not able to laugh on their own life. The teachers wrote only comic episodes on the children at school.

Only after some focus groups they learnt to speak and to laugh on their own life too.

We think, that clowning could be an instrument which facilitates emotional intelligence (both personal and social), the awareness of self and the ability to react to failures and frustrations, increasing positive relationships with others through empathy and communication skills [55,56].

In particular, in the school the "clowning", could be used to help teachers to elicit the sense of humor of pupils, to defuse their role and to contribute to the children's wellbeing [37].

CONCLUSION

As we have seen, smile, laughter, funniness and humor are typically human social and cognitive responses. They bear a heavy responsibility in the entire development beginning at the prenatal period until the older age. Unfortunately precious few empirical investigations exist in this sector and few deal especially with questions about relational and social issues.

We only know a little about individual differences, which have a contributed to the development of the sense of humor, the irony, the self-mockery beginning from first stimulations to familial and scholastic education. What correlations exist between the parents' temperament and the child? And what kind of education allows first children, then at adolescents and at older persons, to express something in a humorous way and to use humor to confront difficulties?

The "positive psychology" becomes an important field of research, it's clear that "laugh is a serious thing" [57]. Even if the neuroscience showed that the laughter is an important resource, a natural therapy, which contrasts stress and diseases, there are only poor investigations regarding the way through how we can elicit and form the laughter from childhood up to adulthood We can only hope that more and more researchers work to explore the roots of humor and laugh and promote experimental studies. There are in fact a lot of variables; environmental, cultural, temperamental and social which cause the laughter and humor development.

REFERENCES

[1]   Brown, J. (1967). Physiology and Phylogenesis of emotional expression. *Brain Research, 5*, 1-14.
[2]   Parvizi, J., Anderson, S. W., Martin, C. O., Damasio, H. and Damasio, A. R. (2001). Pathological laughter and crying: A link to the cerebellum. *Brain, 124*, 1708-1719.
[3]   Wild, B., Rodden, F. A., Grodd, W. and Ruch, W. (2003). Neural correlates of laughter and humour. *Brain, 126*, 2121-2138.
[4]   Lockard, C. E., Fahrenbruch, J. L., Smith, J. L. and Morgan, C. J. (1977). Smiling and laughter: Different phyletic origins? *Bulletin of the Psychonomic Society, 10*, 183-186.
[5]   Kraut, R. E. and Johnston, R. E. (1979). Social and emotional messages of smiling: An ethological approach. *Journal of Personality and Social Psychology, 37*, 1539-1553.
[6]   Jones, N. B. (Ed.) (1972). *Ethological Studies of Child Behavior* (pp. 97-127). Cambridge: University Press.
[7]   Berger, P. L. (1997). *Redeeming Laughter. The Comic Dimension of Human Experience*. New York: Walter de Gruiter and Co.
[8]   Spitz, R. A. (1946). The smiling response: a contribution to the ontogenesis of social relations. *Genetic Psychology Monographs, 34*, 57-125.
[9]   Spitz, R. A. (1965). *The First Year of Life. A Psychoanalytic Study of Normal and Deviant Development of Object Relations*. New York: International Universities Press Inc.
[10]   Morton, J. and Johnson, M. H. (1991). CONSPEC and CONLERN: A two-process theory of infant face recognition. *Psychological Review*, 98, 164-181.
[11]   Sroufe, L. A. and Waters, E. (1976). The ontogenesis of Smiling and Laughter: A Perspective on Organization of Development in Infancy. *Psychological Review, 83*, 173-189.
[12]   Sroufe, L. A. and Wunsch, P. (1972). The development of laughter in the first Year of life. *Child Development, 43*, 1326-1344.

[13] Branningan, C. R. and Humphries, D. (1972). Human nonverbal Behaviour A Means Of Communication. In N. B. Jones (Ed.) *Ethological Studies In Child behavior* (37-64). Cambridge, U.K.: Cambridge University Press.

[14] Cheyne, J.A. (1976). Development of Forms and Functions of Smiling in Preschoolers. *Child Development, 47*, 820-823.

[15] Ekman, P., Friesen, W. V. and Davidson, R. J. (1990). The Duchenne Smile: Emotional Expression and Brain Physiology II. *Journal of Personality and Social Psychology, 58*, 342-353.

[16] Sarra, S. and Otta, E. (2001). Different types of smiles and laughter in children. *Psychological Reports, 89*, 547-558.

[17] Ziajka, M. L. (1981). *Changes in Early Mother Child Communication Modes.* New York: Praeger.

[18] Washburn, R. W. (1929). A study of the smiling and laughing in infants in the first year of life. *Genetic Psychology Monographs, 6*, 396-537.

[19] Justin, F. (1932). A Genetic Study of Laughter Provoking Stimuli. *Child development, 3*, 114-136.

[20] Kenderdine, M. (1931). Laughter in the preschool child. *Child Development, 2*, 228-230.

[21] Ambrose, A. (1963). The age of onset of ambivalence in early infancy: indication from the study of laughing. *Journal of Child Psychology and Psychiatry, 4*, 167-181.

[22] Humphreys, A. P. and Smith, P. K. (1987). Rough and tumble, friendship, and dominance in schoolchildren: Evidence for continuity and change with age. *Child Development, 58*, 201-212.

[23] Anzieu-Premmereur, C. (2009). The Development of a Sense of Humor in a Young Child During Psychotherapy. *Journal of Infant, Child and Adoscent Psychotherapy, 8*, 137-144.

[24] Provine, R. R. (1992). Contagious laughter: Laughter is a sufficient stimulus for laugh and smile. *Bulletin for Psychonomic Society, 30*, 1-4

[25] Provine, R. R. (2001). *Laughter: A scientific Investigation.* New York: Penguin Press.

[26] Wicki, W. (2000). Humor und Entwicklung: Eine kritische Übersicht. *Zeitschrift für Entwicklungspsychologie und Pädagogische Psychologie, 32*, 173-185.

[27] Farneti, A. (Ed.) (2001). *Psicologia in gioco: modelli ludici per la formazione degli educatori.* Bologna: CLUEB.

[28] Wolfenstein, M. (1954). *Children's Humor: A Psychological Analysis.* Glencoe, 111: Free Press.

[29] Falkenberg, I. (2010). Entwicklung von Lachen und Humor in den verschiedenen Lebensphasen. *Zeitschrift für Gerontologie und Geriatrie, 43*, 25-30.

[30] Fellini, F. (1970). *I clowns.* Bologna: Cappelli.

[31] Starobinski, J. (1984). *Ritratto dell'artista da saltimbanco.* Torino: Bollati Boringhieri.

[32] Fo, D. (1987). *Manuale minimo dell'attore.* Torino: Einuadi.

[33] Galante Garrone, A. (1980). *Alla ricerca del proprio clown.* Firenze: La Casa Usher.

[34] Farneti, A. (2004). *La maschera più piccola del mondo. Aspetti psicologici della clownerie.* Bologna: Perdisa.

[35] Carreri, C., Farneti, A. and Cadamuro, A. (2008). Il clown nella rappresentazione dei bambini. *AIP XII Convegno Nazionale – Sezione di Psicologia dello Sviluppo. Sintesi dei contributi*; Padova, Italy; 231-232.

[36] Farneti, A. (2010). Pagliacci a scuola. *Psicologia e Scuola, 30*, 50-57.

[37] Farneti, A. and Palloni, F. (2010). Clowning: the effects on Self Image and Interpersonal Relationships in Nursery Schools. *Procedia - Social and Behavioral Sciences Journal, 5*, 23-27.

[38] Papini, G. (1992). *Chiudiamo le scuole*. Viterbo: Stampa Alternativa.

[39] Parisi, D. (2000). *Scuol@. it*. Milano: Mondadori.

[40] Cerrato, E.A. (2006). *San Filippo Neri. "Chi cerca altro che Cristo...". Massime e ricordi*. Milano: San Paolo.

[41] Chiavarino, L. (1988). *Don Bosco che ride. I "fioretti" di San Giovanni Bosco*. Milano: San Paolo.

[42] Bryant, J. Comisky, P., Crane, J. and Zillman, D. (1980). Relationship between college teachers' use of humor in the classroom and students' evaluations of their teachers, *Journal of Educational Psychology, 72*, 511-519.

[43] Bryant, J. and Zillman, D. (1988). Using humor to promote learning in the classroom. *Journal of Children in Contemporary Society, 20*, 49-78.

[44] Berk, R. (1996). Student ratings of ten strategies for using humor in college teaching. *Journal on Excellence in College Teaching, 7*, 71-92.

[45] Berk, R. (1998). *Professors are from mars, students are from snickers*. Mendota Press: Madison, WI.

[46] Glenn, R. (2002). Brain research: Practical Applications for the classroom. *Teaching for Excellence, 21*, 1-2.

[47] Hill, D. (1988). *Humor in the classroom: A handbook for teachers*. Charles C. Thomas, Springfield, Il.

[48] Pollio, H. and Humphreys, W. (1996). What award-wining lecturers say about their teaching: It's all about connection. *College Teaching, 44*, 101-106.

[49] Garner, R.L. (2006). Humor in Pedagogy: How Ha-Ha Can Lead to Aha! *College Teaching, 54*, 177-180.

[50] Huizinga, J. (1946). *Homo ludens*. Torino, Einuadi.

[51] Winnicott, D. W. (2005). *Playing and reality*. New York: Routledge.

[52] Singer,D.G. and Singer J.L. (1990). *The house of make-believe. Children's Play and the Developing Imagination*. Harvard: University Press.

[53] Battacchi, M. W. and Codispoti, O. (1992). *La vergogna*. Bologna: Il Mulino.

[54] Battacchi, M. W. (2002). *Vergogna e senso di colpa. In psicologia e nella letteratura*. Bologna: Il Mulino.

[55] Gardner, H. (1983). *Frames of mind: The theory of multiple intelligence*. New York: Basic Books.

[56] Goleman, D. (1995). *Emotional intelligence. Why it can matter more than IQ*. New York: Bantam Books.

[57] Francescato, D. (2002). *Ridere è una cosa seria. L'importanza della risata nella vita di tutti i giorni*. Milano: Mondadori.

In: Humor and Health Promotion
Editor: Paola Gremigni

ISBN: 978-1-61942-657-3
© 2012 Nova Science Publishers, Inc.

Chapter 8

IS HUMOR THE BEST MEDICINE?

Paola Gremigni
Department of Psychology, University of Bologna, Italy

ABSTRACT

This chapter presents a brief and somewhat selective survey of the recent empirical studies dealing with humor and physical health. After summarizing the possible mechanisms by which humor and laughter may affect health, the results of fifty relevant articles published between 2001 and 2011 were analyzed.

Overall, findings suggest that mirthful laughter may cause muscular relaxation, beneficial effects on vascular function, reduction of pain, and have beneficial immunological and endocrine effects, whereas inconsistencies were found about the beneficial effects of laughter on asthma and COPD.

Results also suggest that people with a greater sense of humor are not objectively healthier than others and are more likely to engage in unhealthy lifestyles. However, promising findings suggest that a good sense of humor may lead to a longer life. Some support was found for the idea of humor as a stress-moderator, although the results of studies on coping humor and stress are contradictory.

Finally, results support the hypothesis that different styles of humor may facilitate or inhibit the potential to deal effectively with stressors and may promote or impede more general positive life outcomes. Indications for future research include distinguishing between different types of laughter that may have different health-promoting effects, and between objective and subjectively perceived health as determined by various humor styles.

INTRODUCTION

The title of this chapter is taken from a study from the early seventies in which Fry and Williams questioned the positive effects of laughter on health [1]. Forty years have passed since then, and a number of studies have been conducted in this field, but this issue has not found a strictly evidence-based answer yet.

When we talk about humor, we refer to a term, with positive connotations, indicating the ability to perceive, enjoy, or express what is amusing, comical, incongruous, or absurd.

Max Eastman says: *"We come into the world endowed with an instinctive tendency, to laugh and have this feeling in response to pains presented playfully"* [2: 45].

This idea that humor is a natural tendency that mitigates the impact of pain is consistent with the adage that *"laughter is the best medicine."* In the humor literature, the assumption that a greater sense of humor promotes physical health has also been very popular [3]. However, only towards the seventies did doctors and psychologists begin to show a growing interest in the influence of laughter, sense of humor, and other positive experiences on the human body. Since then, several authors have shared the belief that humor/laughter is the basis of quality mental and physical health, an effective antidote or at least a moderator in the stress-health relationship, and a valid social lubricant. In more recent years, a positive attitude toward humor has characterized part of the research, which has sought to determine the benefits of humor on physical health. Nevertheless, previous reviews of the empirical literature found controversial findings and concluded that a weak link could be established between humor or laughing and health [4–6].

This chapter presents a brief and somewhat selective survey of the recent empirical literature dealing with humor and physical health. The review is based on a search of Scopus and PubMed to locate articles published in the last 10 years (i.e., from 2001 to 2011). It reports original, empirical research relating to humor or laughter and various aspects of physical health. For articles published before 2001, I am referring to the review of the literature published by Rod Martin in 2001 [4]. Fifty relevant publications were found, the results of which are briefly reported in the following paragraphs.

First, however, I consider two preliminary issues. The first one is related to the fact that the findings presented here include research on the effect of both humor and laughter on health. Humor is a multifaceted concept, which involves cognitive, emotional, behavioral, psychophysiological, personological, and social aspects. For example, sense of humor is viewed as a personality trait or an individual-differences variable, whereas laughter is the most common behavioral expression of the humorous experience. Although laughter may also be caused by non-humorous stimuli (e.g., tickling or embarrassment) and can be triggered by imitation [7], humor is seen as both the cause for and the effect of laughter. That is why humor and laughter are so closely associated [8]. It is probably by assuming this close association that few studies analyzed whether the effects or benefits they found were due to the experience of humor, the act of laughter or the combined influence of both. Therefore, research findings are classified here based on outcomes rather than on the relative contribution of humor vs. laughter. Typical outcomes include physical health, pain and stress reduction, longevity, etc.

Second, in the next paragraph, I briefly summarize the possible mechanisms by which humor and laughter may affect health.

MECHANISMS LINKING HUMOR TO HEALTH

A dominant conceptualization in the study of humor is that it has positive effects on health. However, the health-humor relationship is more complicated than it seems. First, health is not a unitary concept; in fact, it consists of different aspects and components, such as physical, mental and social wellbeing, according to the World Health Organization. Second, even humor is a complex phenomenon that includes physiological, emotional, cognitive, social, and behavioral components. We can, therefore, assume that distinct components of humor can affect different aspects of health in a variety of ways.

Several possible mechanisms by which humor and laughter may affect physical health have been proposed [7]. The first mechanism considers the physiological changes produced by laughter the crucial element in the humor-health relationship. This approach stresses the importance of laughter, which should not be necessarily accompanied by fun and humor. In this regard, various authors suggest that laughing out loud trains and relaxes muscles, improves breathing, stimulates circulation, increases the production of endorphins that reduce pain, decreases the production of stress hormones and strengthens the immune system [9]. So this first approach suggests that laughter in itself has beneficial effects because it stimulates the entire body.

A second mechanism suggests that the benefits of humor in health are related to the positive emotional states accompanying humor and laughter. This approach, unlike the previous one, does not believe that laughter influences health directly, but rather that it is a way to generate positive emotional states. Positive emotions, for their part, can affect health, for example, increasing tolerance to pain, strengthening the immune system, or reducing the cardiovascular consequences of negative emotions [10].

The third proposed mechanism suggests that humor affects health indirectly by moderating the impact of stressful events. According to this perspective, a humorous vision and ability to see the funny side of problems mitigate the negative consequences of adversity. Referring to the transactional model of stress proposed by Lazarus and Folkman [11], humor can be considered as a form of cognitive assessment that allows an individual to identify potentially stressful situations in a more positive, less threatening way. This approach gives more importance to the perceptual-cognitive component of humor and to the ability to maintain a humorous vision during stressful situations. Humor is, therefore, seen as a coping strategy in daily life.

Humor can affect health by promoting healthy lifestyles. A great sense of humor is expected to be linked with involvement in behaviors that promote health such as taking regular physical activity, follow proper nutrition, maintaining appropriate weight, and avoid smoking or consuming too much alcohol. This mechanism is grounded on an assumed underlying link between sense of humor, self-esteem, optimism, and self-protective health behaviors [6].

All the supposed mechanisms presented above might suggest that people with a great sense of humor have a better physical condition than the others, as indicated by few symptoms (chronic pain or cardiovascular problems), improved physiological functioning (low-pressure level), and high satisfaction with their health. However, looking at the studies published before 2001, it was difficult to find a simple, direct relation between sense of humor and a good health status. For example, some studies have found negative correlations between sense of humor and symptoms of disease [12], while others have found no associations [13]. Furthermore, most studies were not driven by an explicit intention, to verify one or more of the above-mentioned possible mechanisms that link humor to health. Martin [4] provided a comprehensive review of the empirical studies investigating associations between humor/laughter and various aspects of health (i.e., immunity levels, pain tolerance, self-reported illness, stress-moderating effects, and longevity). This review concluded that there was only little evidence for the positive effect of humor and laughter on physical health-related variables. Since Martin clearly highlighted the methodological weaknesses of research in this field, my goal for this chapter is to see if the latest research offers more powerful and reliable evidence of the link between humor and health.

LAUGHTER AND PHYSICAL HEALTH

Cardiovascular Activity

A very common notion is that the physiological changes associated with laughter, such as increased cardiovascular activity, have a positive impact on physical health [3]. However, previous studies based on physiological measures found that laugher manipulation did not result in a lower heart rate or decrease blood pressure [14].

More recently, a link between laughter and the healthy function of blood vessels was reported by researchers at the University of Maryland Medical Center, indicating that laughter after watching a comic movie segment caused the dilatation of the inner lining of blood vessels, the endothelium, and increased blood flow [15].

Vlachopouloset and his colleagues [16] investigated the effect of laughter and mental stress on arterial stiffness and central hemodynamics, which are independent predictors of cardiovascular risk. The effects of viewing a 30-minute segment of two films inducing laughter or stress were assessed, using carotid-femoral pulse wave velocity as an index of arterial stiffness and augmentation index as a measure of wave reflections. Results indicated that laughter decreased pulse wave velocity, augmentation index, and cortisol levels, and increased total oxidative status, whereas stress produced opposite effects, and hence laughter seems to have a protective role against cardiovascular risk.

Another study published in 2010 [17] investigated the effects of mirthful laughter on endothelial function and central artery compliance, using a controlled crossover study and ultrasound imaging to measure the impact of watching 30 minutes of a comic movie vs. a documentary. The results were that heart rate and blood pressure, ischemia-induced brachial artery flow-mediated vasodilation, and carotid arterial compliance increased significantly, while watching the comedy, whereas no such changes were seen while watching the documentary. Comedy-induced changes in arterial compliance were significantly associated with baseline flow-mediated dilation. These results suggest that mirthful laughter elicited by comic movies has a beneficial effect on vascular function.

Miller and Fry [18], overviewing the studies on the effect of laughter on endothelial vasoreactivity, hypothesized that mirthful laughter may induce the release of beta-endorphins, which in turn activates receptors on the endothelial surface to release nitric oxide (NO).

Endothelial derived NO induces smooth muscle relaxation, vessel dilation and may reduce vascular inflammation.

Overall, empirical studies suggest that laughter may produce beneficial effects on the vasculature.

Although there is not a lot of research specifically looking at the impact of humor on heart health, the findings discussed above suggest that humor can play a role in promoting cardiac health in both healthy individuals and cardiac patients. The first study to examine purposely this issue was conducted in 2000 by Michael Miller, at the University of Maryland Medical School [19]. This correlational study found that patients who had a heart attack or had undergone a cardiac surgery, found less humor in life and were 40% less likely than the heart-healthy individuals to laugh in a variety of different situations. These findings suggest that a sense of humor may provide some protection against heart disease, but the correlational design of the study did not allow analyzing whether patients were less inclined to respond to situations with humor due to their recent cardiac event. Prospective studies are, therefore, needed to determine whether non-symptomatic people with a low sense of humor are likely to develop heart disease at a later time.

Muscular Relaxation

Reduced muscle tension is one of the physiological changes associated with laughter, which were proposed to have a positive effect on physical health [3].

The effect of laughter on muscle relaxation was recently documented [20], based on Paskind's earlier work that indicated a period of muscular relaxation follows laughter. The Overeem and co-workers' study examined how laughter and several other respiratory movements influenced spinal motor excitability, as measured by the Hoffmann reflex (H-reflex). The H-reflex is a clinical method of measurement, where the stimulus is an electric shock to sensory fibers coming from muscle spindles, and the answer is recorded using an electromyography. When looking at the H-reflex, increased twitching indicated increased spinal cord excitability. Findings from this study indicated that both laughter and simulated laughter decreased spinal motor excitability and that true laughter evoked more H-reflex depression than simulated laughter. This suggests that mirth on its own can reduce the H-reflex, leading to the post-laughter muscle relaxation response noted in Paskind's earlier work. From studies of the same authors, we can conclude that laughter produces relaxation automatically, and naturally, periods of intense laughter are followed by relaxed muscle tone, and genuinely mirthful laughter (i.e., laughter associated with the experience of humor) triggers a stronger muscle relaxation effect than laughter without mirth [20,21]. Two distinct mechanisms may cause the relaxation. Muscles not directly participating in the act of laughter tend to relax while laughing. When we stop laughing, muscles that were contracted when involved in laughing relax. As in any other physical activity, these two mechanisms, in combination, produce a general pattern of muscle relaxation throughout the whole body. This natural relaxation effect may help reduce stress, alleviate headaches, rheumatism, neuralgia, or other conditions characterized by a spasm-pain-spasm cycle.

Respiratory Function

In addition to changes in muscle tone, there is evidence that laughter leads to changes in respiratory function. Fry's work demonstrated that laughter leads to episodes of sharply sporadic deep breathing [3]. Laughing consists of repeating over and over a process where the air is pushed out of the lungs, followed by the taking of a deep breath. This process helps to get rid of the excess carbon dioxin and water vapor that is built up and to replace it with oxygen-rich air. Individuals with a respiratory disease are more likely to have a superficial breathing pattern, which leaves a larger than desired volume of residual air in the lungs. After some time, in this residual air the oxygen content decreases and water vapor and carbon dioxin increase, creating a favorable condition for pulmonary infection. Therefore, it seems safe to assume that laughter may contribute to pulmonary health in patients with respiratory illness. Unfortunately, very little research has been done on the pulmonary benefits of humor and laughter.

One pulmonary condition for which researchers have recently investigated the benefit from humor is asthma. Asthma is a chronic condition characterized by muscle spasms, mucous, and inflammation of the airways rapidly spreading. In a 2004 paper, Kimata compared watching a humorous or non-humorous film on patients with bronchial asthma and their response to triggers [22]. Watching the funny movie reduced the asthmatic reactions, by significantly reducing the level of bronchial constriction among asthmatics, enabling them to breathe more easily. Laughter appears then to be useful in controlling allergic asthma.

However, it should be noted that Kimata's work on asthma appears to contradict an earlier Australian study that indicated that hard laughter was a common trigger for asthma attacks in children [23]. Laughter was more frequently reported as a trigger than excitement. Coughing was the most prominent symptom, and symptoms typically occurred within 2 minutes of the mirthful stimulus. The same author reported a year later that 42% of the 105 patients surveyed reported mirth-triggered asthma [24]. Bronchial asthma can be triggered by allergic reactions, various pharmacological agents, the environment, occupation, infections, exercise and emotions. It was suggested that laughter, as a form of exercise and as an emotional response, is a potent stimulus that triggers bronchial asthma. Furthermore, hyperventilation might be a source of laughter-associated-asthma, in addition to stimulation of irritant receptors, in the airway epithelium.

These inconsistencies in asthma research may be reconciled by shifting the focus on the level of emotional arousal experienced. Moderately humorous events accompanied by mild laughter support healthy pulmonary function among asthmatics while extreme funniness accompanied by extended laughter interferes with it.

A very recent area of research is related to the possible value of harm of laughter for a patient with chronic obstructive pulmonary disease (COPD). COPD condition is characterized by impaired ability, to rid the lungs of air that leads to hyperinflation. In COPD patients, strong laughter could increase the amount of trapped air, because their lungs do not allow the rapid expulsion of air that occurs with a strong laugh. One recent study [25] showed that laughter can reduce hyperinflation and air-trapping through repeated expiratory efforts in patients with severe COPD, although this decrease was no longer extant two hours later. Nevertheless, it was moderate laughter that was associated with reduced lung volume while strong laughter was associated with increased hyperinflation. A more recent study also found that laughing aloud may cause acute deterioration in pulmonary function, secondary to worsened hyperinflation, in COPD patients [26].

These studies on COPD lead to the same conclusion reached for asthma: in people with respiratory diseases extended hearty laughter leads to lung health detriments whereas mild laughter supports healthy pulmonary function.

Physical Symptoms

Past research attempting to determine if an association exists between an increased sense of humor and a reduced number of physical symptoms has been inconclusive. Several investigators have reported findings supporting the link between greater humor and fewer physical symptoms, including colds, upper respiratory infections, nausea, diarrhea, pounding heart, dyspnea, musculoskeletal pain, and blood pressure, whereas some others have found no evidence for such a relationship. In his review, Martin [4] concluded that very little evidence supports a simple relationship between measures of humor and disease symptoms.

A more recent study [27] explored the extent to which different humor styles and negative affect predict physical health. Results showed that an increased number of physical symptoms was associated with higher levels of negative affect, but were unrelated to the humor styles. Neither adaptive humor was associated with a decrease in physical symptoms nor was maladaptive humor associated with an increase in symptoms. As such, these findings were consistent with previous work demonstrating that sense of humor is not linked to physical symptoms.

A study by Svebak, Martin and Holmen [28], conducted in Norway on a sample of more than 65,000 subjects, also offers few confirmations for a direct relationship between humor and physical symptoms. This large study included health-related measures such as common bodily symptoms (e.g., nausea, diarrhea, pounding heart, dyspnea, musculoskeletal pain, and blood pressure), subjective health satisfaction, and measures of sense of humor and laughter expressiveness. There was no significant correlation between sense of humor and symptoms of illness, or between humor and objective indicators of health, although the study found a weak correlation between sense of humor and the satisfaction of participants with their health status.

Overall, these results suggest that people with a great sense of humor are not objectively healthier than others. Nevertheless, they seem to be subjectively more satisfied with their health. This could be because people with more sense of humor, having a more positive outlook on life, tend to underestimate their physical symptoms.

HUMOR AND PAIN REDUCTION

A major impetus for the increased popularity of humor and health was the publication, in 1976, of Norman Cousins' article "Anatomy of an Illness" in the *New England Journal of Medicine,* expanded into a best-selling book in 1979. Cousins claimed that 10 minutes of hearty laughter a day had a reliable analgesic effect, providing pain-free sleep, and contributed to his recovery from ankylosing spondylitis, a progressive and painful rheumatoid disease involving inflammation of the spine. Although it is unknown whether Cousins' recovery can be attributed to the laughter or to other factors (e.g., the massive use of Vitamin C, personality traits such as optimism, a misdiagnosis in the first place, etc.), his experience has given rise, in particular, to the idea that laughter reduces pain.

In the recent literature, several studies have addressed the study of humor and/or laughter and their effects on pain perception and tolerance.

Pain threshold and tolerance are usually measured using procedures that were developed in traditional, experimental studies of pain, in which participants are exposed to painful stimuli. The most common is the cold pressor test, in which participants are asked to immerse their arm in a tub of frozen water for up to a few minutes. Pain threshold is defined as the amount of time elapsed before the participant reports the stimulus to be painful, while pain tolerance is the extent of time before the individual cannot tolerate the stimulus any longer and wishes to terminate it.

In past research, although there was considerable experimental evidence of increased tolerance to pain stimuli after exposure to humor [29], contradictory results were also presented [30].

Of great interest are more recent studies on the impact of humor and laughter on pain perception and tolerance, as they investigated issues rarely examined before. An experiment by Karen Zweyer and her colleagues [31] was designed to clarify whether the effects of humor on pain reduction are due to laughing, in particular, to the positive emotion of mirth, or to other factors such as the cognitions involved in humor. In this study, participants watched a comedy film that contained sound effects but no dialogue, and they were instructed to enjoy the film but inhibit all smiling and laughing, or smile and laugh as much as possible during the film, or produce a humorous narrative while watching the movie. Using the cold pressor procedure pain tolerance was measured before, immediately after and 20 minutes after the film. The researchers also videotaped the participants during the procedure, and subsequently coded their facial expressions for genuine (Duchenne) and forced (non-Duchenne) smiling and laughing. The three conditions yielded similar, significant increases in pain threshold and tolerance. Results indicated that exposure to a humorous stimulus *per se* had a lowering effect on pain, probably due to feelings of amusement; while neither laughter nor humor productions were required. Moreover, the observed increases in pain tolerance were found to be positively associated with genuine enjoyment smiles (Duchenne display), but not with the frequency or intensity of laughter.

A study by Diana Mahony and her colleagues [32] investigated the role of expectancies in humor-related increases, in pain tolerance. In this study, before being shown a humorous videotape, the participants were told that humor is known to increase pain tolerance (positive expectancy condition), or that humor has been shown to reduce pain tolerance (negative expectancy condition), or they were told nothing about the effects of humor on pain (no expectancy condition). Following exposure to the comedy, the positive and no expectancy groups both showed significantly greater increases in pain thresholds than the negative expectancy group. These results suggest that humor-related increases in pain tolerance are mediated by expectancies.

Some explanations of the effect of humor on pain tolerance suggest that laughter may stimulate the production of endogenous opioids such as beta-endorphins, thereby increasing pain tolerance in the face of physical illness or disease. Recently, Dunbar and colleagues

[33] recalled the notion that laughter plays a crucial role in increasing pain tolerance through an endorphin-mediated opiate effect. Endorphins are endogenous opioid peptides produced in the central nervous system that function as neurotransmitters, but also play a crucial role in the management of pain through their analgesic properties. A series of six experimental studies in both the laboratory (watching videos) and naturalistic contexts (watching stage performances), using change in the pain threshold as an assay for endorphin release, showed that pain threshold was significantly higher after the laughter than in the control condition. This pain-tolerance effect was due to laughing itself and not merely to a change in positive affect.

The biological hypothesis of an endorphin-mediated opiate effect is not contradicted by the results of the studies mentioned above. Even in the case of placebo analgesic effects of humor [32], this does not negate the possibility that they are mediated by physiological processes, including endorphin production in the brain.

Despite the consistent results of studies linking pain tolerance to humor or laughter, a recent study showed that the effectiveness of humor in enhancing pain tolerance is the same as that of other distracters such as music, arithmetic and horror [34]. The authors concluded that compelling distraction increases pain tolerance in adults, regardless of whether or not the distraction is humorous.

Relatively little research has been done on the relationship between humor or laughing and pain in children. Studies focusing on procedural pain, a distressing problem for children, parents and healthcare providers, have not specifically looked at laughing as a mechanism for mitigating pain. A preliminary study was recently conducted, the findings of which may be extended to healthy children going through painful procedures, such as diagnostic tests or preventative interventions [35]. This study involved 18 healthy children watching comic video-tapes before, during and after the cold-pressor test. Pain appraisal and pain tolerance were examined in relation to humor indicators (number of laughs during each video and child ratings of how funny the video was). Although humor indicators were not significantly associated with pain appraisal or tolerance, children showed significantly greater pain tolerance while viewing funny videos than when viewing the videos immediately before or after the cold-water task. The results suggest that humorous distraction is useful to help children tolerate painful procedures.

Another study [36] examined the humor-pain interface in hospitalized preadolescent children who had undergone a medical intervention. It was a non-experimental study using a correlational design. Use of pain-specific humor-coping was positively associated with an adaptive problem-focused coping style and was also more strongly (and inversely) associated to ratings of pain unpleasantness rather than sensory intensity. The results were opposite to those of Stuber's research [35] in that humor was here associated with more subjective aspects of pain (i.e., appraisal or unpleasantness), rather than objective aspects (i.e., pain tolerance and intensity).

Chronic pain is another area that has received little attention in recent studies on humor. Chronic pain is regarded as pain that persists past the normal time of healing, which is usually three months for nonmalignant pain [37]. It is associated with negative mood states and poor life satisfaction and is very common in later life. Among older people chronic pain has important consequences, including loneliness, social isolation, depression, impaired physical functionality, and increased healthcare utilization and costs [38]. Since the use of medication for pain relief has proven inadequate, especially in older people, researchers have tried to see if humor could be an alternative. Recently, a study involved a group of older people with chronic musculoskeletal pain in a randomly controlled study where an 8-week humor therapy intervention, based on reading funny jokes and stories, was administered to the experimental group but not to the control group [39]. In the post-intervention, there was a significant reduction in pain intensity and loneliness and an increase in happiness and life satisfaction in the experimental group that was not found in the control group. Unfortunately, the design of the study does not allow the effects of the humor therapy to be disentangled from those of the therapeutic relation. Nevertheless, it seems to provide some support to the link between humor and chronic pain management.

Rod Martin [6] suggests that experiments in the field of humor and pain tolerance have been more methodologically rigorous than in other fields such as the immunity research. Most studies have, in fact, control groups and controlling for confounding variables. Nevertheless, the mechanisms involved in pain control and threshold are still not completely clear. According to the gate control theory, distraction is essential in the relief and control of pain [40]. According to the neurotransmitters theory, the release of endorphins in the brain is another mechanism of pain management [41]. Humor is an effective distractor, but there is also evidence that it triggers activation of the endorphin system. Furthermore, it is not clear which stimulus generates positive effects, and whether the effect is due to laughter *per se* or to the amusement-related positive emotion of mirth, or to the effect of a distractive stimulus.

In summary, in the current experimental literature, there is some empirical support for Norman Cousins' observation that laughter reduces pain, although further studies are needed to explain the exact mechanisms through which this reduction occurs.

HUMOR AND STRESS

Humor as a Stress Moderator

In addition to the direct physiological effects of humor and laughter on health, it has also been suggested that there may be some indirect links. Humor might improve health through cognitive mechanisms that moderate the negative effects of stress on health. In this hypothesized stress-moderator mechanism, particularly relevant are the cognitive-perceptual aspects of humor, which would be more important than laughter.

Kuiper and Nicholl [42] proposed that two mechanisms, cognitive appraisals and distancing, may play a critical role in the perceptions that more humorous individuals have about various facets of their physical health. Those with greater senses of humor may have a more positive orientation toward life, which is congruent with a more positive cognitive appraisal regarding the threats they face. A second mechanism, which may assist people with a greater sense of humor to develop fewer negative perceptions, involves the use of cognitive distancing from potential stressors as a way of protecting the self. This change in perspective was suggested to minimize the potential consequences of unfavorable events, allowing those with greater senses of humor to more effectively cope with life's adversities and frustrations [43].

Previous research found that a great sense of humor promoted a positive appraisal of potentially stressful events [44]. In turn, it was suggested that these indirect effects contributed to lower stress levels, having a beneficial impact on physical health. Results of studies suggested that a humorous outlook on life helps one to see the funny side of problems that in turn enables individuals to cope more effectively with stress by allowing them to gain a different perspective and distance themselves from stressful situations, ultimately enhancing their feelings of mastery and wellbeing in the face of adversity. However, Martin, in his 2001 review [4], concluded that empirical evidence in support of this capacity for humor to mediate the effects of stress on health was insufficient.

Two more recent studies offered some support to this idea of humor as a stress-moderator. A study confirmed that a higher sense of humor positively influenced the perception of stress in a sample of community adults and undergraduates [45]. Abel [46] found that, when dealing with the same number and types of daily hassles, individuals characterized by a high sense of humor reported having perceived less stress, in the last month, than individuals with a lower sense of humor. More positive appraisals of stressful situations mitigated the level of negative affective arousal. They also favored the use of positive coping strategies, aimed at redefining a direct action on the source of stress. This study seems to confirm what Lefcourt and colleagues [47] suggested, namely that humor can perform its role as a coping strategy. Specifically, as a coping strategy, humor may allow individuals to find something funny in the stressful situation, thereby reducing the negative emotional reaction associated with it, or it may stimulate actions aimed at changing the situation itself.

Humor as a Coping Strategy

Research on stress was followed by a major development after the redefinition of the concept of a stressful event by Lazarus and Folkman [11]. According to the transactional model, no event can be defined as stressful in itself, but only when the individual perceives a discrepancy between the demands of the situation and their ability to cope with it. This emphasizes the role of the subject as an active agent able to influence the impact of stressful events by adopting specific coping strategies. Coping is defined as the variety of cognitive, emotional and behavioral efforts that the person does to process requests, over-rated as surplus, and available resources. Humor has been identified as one of the healthiest coping strategies, which make those who use them psychologically and physically healthier. Research on coping humor has focused primarily on populations with special needs and clinical populations, since coping humor was seen as a mechanism for managing the inevitable stresses of aging or being chronically ill.

A study exploring the relationship between stress and coping strategies in middle-aged women found that a higher coping humor was associated with lower perceived stress and higher self-esteem (Park, 2010). Another study [48] examined the associations among coping humor, other personal/social factors and the health status of community-dwelling older adults. Results showed that coping humor and self-efficacy contributed to mental health status in older adults. Moreover, correlations among coping humor, self-efficacy and social support suggested that a sense of humor may play an important role in reinforcing self-efficacious approaches to the management of health issues.

Other recent studies contradicted these findings. Celso and colleagues [49] investigated the relationships between humor coping, health status and life satisfaction, among older residents of assisted-living facilities. It was hypothesized a direct association of humor coping on life satisfaction and a role of humor coping as a mediator in the relation between health status and life satisfaction. Both the direct association of humor coping on life satisfaction and the intervening role between health status and life satisfaction were not supported. Another study [50] assessed the relationship between humor and physical/mental health variables in a longitudinal study of individuals with systemic sclerosis, a progressive rheumatic disease that can be fatal in severe cases. Humor coping did not significantly predict any of the disease-related outcomes (i.e., severity, pain, disability, and distress), either cross-sectionally or longitudinally. These studies contribute to a growing body of evidence that humor coping may not be directly beneficial to quality of life in those suffering from chronic disease.

To summarize, the basic idea, emerging from recent studies, is that humor as a coping strategy may allow, through a humorous outlook, individuals to achieve more positive interpretations of demanding and difficult situations. This process weakens the negative relationship between stressful life events and well-being. However, this mechanism does not work in the case of chronic disease.

Humor Styles and Stress

The contradictory results of studies on coping humor and stress reinforce the importance of considering sense of humor as a multidimensional variable, with components that can be either positive or negative in influencing experiences. Martin [51] proposed the presence of individual differences in four styles of humor, reflecting an adaptive or a maladaptive use of humor. Specifically, affiliative humor characterized by efforts to build relationships through humor and self-enhancing humor characterized by use of humor to maintain a positive outlook on life might positively influence how the individual copes with stress. The other two styles, aggressive humor involving humor that attacks or demeans others and self-defeating humor characterized by humor that demeans the self in efforts to build relationships might, by contrast, exacerbate stress rather than reduce it.

Self-enhancing humor was found to be negatively related to evaluations of past stressors and anticipated future stressors, while self-defeating humor was positively related to them [52] . This study also provided preliminary evidence to support a mediator model in which the role of humor styles in explaining perceptions of stress was mediated through a composite of positive personality styles (i.e., optimism, hope, and happiness). This new mediator model is based on recent studies, showing that positive personality qualities are more reliable predictors of health and effective coping than sense of humor. Research supports health benefits of great optimism [53], high hope as a stable trait [54], and stable happiness [55,56].

In a subsequent study, Arnie Cann and his colleagues [57] used a longitudinal model, to capture the mediation role of positive personality traits on the relation between humor styles and perceived stress. They assessed humor styles and personality at baseline and perceived stress 8 weeks later, in a sample of college students. Results indicated that the positive personality qualities fully mediated the relationship between self-enhancing humor and perceived stress. These personality traits also partially mediated the relationship between self-defeating and perceived stress. Thus, a self-enhancing humor style appeared to buffer the effects of stressors, while other styles, such as self-defeating humor, had negative effects, through the mediation of positive personality qualities. These results also support the hypothesis that person's style of using humor facilitates (or inhibits) the potential to deal effectively with stressors through promoting (or restraining) a more general positive personality style. Consequently, people who stably manifest high levels of optimism, hope, and happiness, supported by a good sense of humor tend to perceive their lives as little stressful, thus report positive levels of both physical and mental health. Cann's recent study [57] also showed that self-directed humor styles are much more important than humor styles that focus on others, in understanding how people respond to potential stressors. In fact, self-enhancing humor style appears to buffer the effects of stressors, self-directed humor that demeans the self is positively related to the levels of stress experienced, and, therefore, negatively related to self-reported health, whereas the other-directed humor styles are of little importance in understanding the relationship between sense of humor and health outcomes, as confirmed by previous studies [52].

Taken together, findings to date suggest that a more complex approach to the relation between humor and stress is needed to more clearly identify the role that sense of humor might play, in relation to stress and coping [57].

HUMOR AND THE IMMUNE SYSTEM

Almost thirty years ago, Dillon and colleagues [58] hypothesized that humor, as a positive emotional state, may be a possible immune system enhancer. This idea was based on research indicating that stressful events and their associated negative affect may cause immunosuppression. According to psychoneuroimmunology theory, it has been postulated that laughter or sense of humor may affect health through moderation of stress chemicals and/ or immune-enhancement.

The greatest amount of research in this area has focused on immunoglobulin A. Secretory IgA, a part of the immune system, is an antibody found in mucosal areas, including saliva, which represents the first defense against antigens in these areas. Research carried out on relatively small samples showed significant, positive correlations between scores on humor and the values measured by saliva (spit) IgA immunoglobulin [58]. However, other studies with larger samples failed to find any correlation between these variables [59]. Rod Martin [4] especially criticized methodological weaknesses in research on humor and the immune system.

More recent experiments have reported humor-related changes in various components of immunity measured in blood samples. In one of the most comprehensive reports, Berk

[60] reported the results of a series of five separate studies involving a total of 52 healthy males, who viewed a comedy video for one hour. Blood samples (taken before, during, and after the intervention) showed increased immunoglobulins A, G and M, with immunoglobulin effects lasting at least 12 hours. IgM and IgG are other immunoglobulins that, in addiction to IgA, form part of the immune response. These findings seem to support the modulation of neuroimmunologic parameters by laughter.

Along with IgA, some other cells offer a different immune protection; the most studied among these are natural killer (NK) cells. NK cells take the role of seeking out and destroying tumor cells, viruses, and other foreign organisms in the body. Berk [60], in the cited series of five studies, reported that exposure to a humorous stimulus also significantly increased NK activity.

Results of another study [61] involving 33 adult women indicated that the effect of humor was mediated by humor response, as the amount of mirthful laughter correlated with the decreased stress in subjects who viewed a humor video. Humor response also played a role in change, in NK cell activity, following the video. This finding indicated that although sense of humor was not directly related to a change in NK activity, a significant relationship exists between the amount of laughter and reduced stress and improved NK activity.

Laughter's impact on NK cells was also seen in studies with diabetic patients. Hayashi and colleagues [62] reported changes in gene expression, in patients with type 2 diabetes who had been induced to laugh. They analyzed the changes in 18,716 genes, finding that 23 were significantly changed after listening to a comic story compared with a boring lecture. Of the genes changed, 4 were involved in an immune response, and 5 were related to the cell cycle, apoptosis, and cell adhesion. In a second study [63] on diabetic patients, 41,000 genes were analyzed, and the laughter experience up-regulated 39 genes, 14 of which were related to NK cell activity. Laughter improved postprandial blood-glucose levels by modulating NK cell activity. A more recent study [64] showed that laughter again lowered 2-hour postprandial blood sugar levels in type 2 diabetics by decreasing the levels of prorenin in blood (prorenin is involved in the onset of diabetic complications). Laughter also normalized the expression of the prorenin receptor gene on peripheral blood leukocytes, which is reduced in diabetic patients. Another study also found a decrease in plasma prorenin concentrations, together with an increase in plasma angiotensinogen, in type 2 diabetics over a 6-month period in which they engaged in laughter therapy [65]. Overall, these findings suggest that laughter may inhibit the onset or progress of diabetic complications starting at the level of gene-expression. They again showed that laughter affected those genes that mediate NK cell activity and this produced improvement in glucose levels.

A strong interest in the potential health benefits of humor appears to be present among researchers in Japan. In a Japanese study, after watching a comedy videotape, healthy participants showed in their saliva increased levels of certain molecules that are involved in the elimination of free radicals from the mouth [66]. Free radicals are molecules implicated in inflammation, aging, and the development of some types of cancer. Another study investigated the effect of laughter on salivary endocrinological stress marker chromogranin A (CgA) in a small sample of 11 healthy men [67]. Saliva samples taken after watching a comic film showed increased levels of CgA, while the control samples showed no significant change in CgA levels. This preliminary study also showed a stress relief effect of laughter after watching the comic film.

Hajime Kimata recently reported research on the role of humor and laughter in reducing allergic reactions in individuals with allergies. Individuals with dermatitis showed a less severe allergic reaction to skin prick tests after watching a humorous movie than after watching a documentary [68]. Viewing a humorous film was found to reduce IgE production by seminal B cells cultured with sperms from 24 male patients with atopic eczema, suggesting that it may be helpful for the treatment of allergy in the reproductive tract [69]. Viewing a humorous film markedly elevated salivary, testosterone levels and reduced trans-epidermal water loss values, in elderly patients with atopic dermatitis. On the contrary, viewing a control non-humorous film failed to do so [70]. Decreased salivary testosterone levels and increased trans-epidermal water loss characterized elderly patients with atopic dermatitis. Laughter increased levels of breast-milk melatonin in both mothers with atopic eczema and healthy mothers, and feeding infants with increased levels of melatonin-containing milk reduced allergic responses to latex and house dust mite in infants with atopic eczema [71]. Patients with an allergy-related bronchial asthma showed reduced asthmatic reactions to allergens after watching a comedy videotape, whereas no such effect was found with a non-humorous film [22]. Finally, a reduction in allergy-related immunoglobulins in the tears of patients with allergic conjunctivitis was found after watching a comedy film, but not a non-humorous control film [72]. Taken together, these experiments suggest that humor may suppress the excessive immune responses that occur in certain allergic reactions by reducing the secretion of immunoglobulins such as IgE and IgG.

Several studies have investigated the effects of mirthful laughter on the neuroendocrine-immune system in patients with rheumatoid arthritis (RA). The most recent is also a Japanese study focusing on the growth hormone (GH). GA plays an auxiliary role in the regulation of immune function and is increased in patients with RA, compared with healthy people [73]. After experiencing mirthful laughter, induced by a comical story, the level of serum GH in the rheumatoid arthritis group significantly decreased, approaching that in the control group.

These Japanese investigations suggest beneficial immunological and endocrine effects of laughter. The criticism directed at previous studies, including the use of small numbers of participants or inadequate controls [4], is less applicable to more recent studies, since they have used more rigorous methodologies. However, the evidence is not yet conclusive, and further research is needed to investigate the mechanisms of these effects in greater detail, using larger samples.

HUMOR AND LIFESTYLES

Lifestyle is the summary of the ways people relate to themselves, with others, with their problems, besides the diet, luxury habits (smoking, alcohol, coffee, and drugs), physical activity, and leisure management. Lifestyle models provide an explanation for poor health where the factors considered as determinants of disease are perceived as modifiable [74].

A lifestyle that is not healthy (e.g. sedentary lifestyle, smoking, unhealthy diet and excess weight, excessive stress, etc.) accelerates the aging process and then exposes individuals to a significantly elevated risk of developing disabling medical conditions by reducing life expectancy and quality of life. Low-risk lifestyle factors, on the contrary, exert a powerful and beneficial effect on mortality [75]. The relationship between humor and life styles was investigated in the general effects of humor on health. Previous studies do not support the hypothesis that a greater sense of humor is associated with healthier lifestyles; instead, they seem to emphasize the opposite effect [4]. At present, two main studies reach the same conclusion.

A research, conducted by Kerkkanen, Kuiper, and Martin [76], aimed to capture the effects of humor on health during three years involving 34 leaders of the Finnish police. The measures of health indices included blood pressure, cholesterol level, alcohol consumption, body mass index, and smoking. Results did not support the hypothesis that humor positively influences health. In fact, further analysis found some conflicting associations, such as that high scores in some aspects of humor were associated with increased obesity, smoking and cardiovascular risk. These results suggest that people with a great sense of humor tend to adopt a healthy lifestyle.

The Terman life-cycle study, which followed a large sample of intellectually gifted individuals over several decades [77], found that those who had a greater sense of humor and optimism as children were more likely to smoke and drink as adults. This study used a composite cheerfulness measure that included a sense of humor as a component. Findings indicated that more cheerful people grow up to be more careless about their health, drink more alcohol, smoke more cigarettes, and engage in riskier activities and hobbies than less cheerful people. These detrimental effects were equally evident when only the sense of humor component was used to predict outcomes. Overall, these longitudinal findings suggest that a greater sense of humor may contribute to a riskier lifestyle and to poorer health habits, resulting in premature mortality rates. This association between humor and unhealthy lifestyles could be partly because people with a greater sense of humor have extrovert personality traits [78]. Previous research has shown that extroverts more likely than introverts consume alcohol, smoke, and are obese [79,80]. Although research supports an association between humor and unhealthy lifestyles, the mechanisms that underlie this association should be studied in more detail. Findings suggest that humor may have different health consequences, some of them positive, while others are potentially harmful. Future research should consider the role humor styles might play in the processes connecting stable differences in the self and the world view to health outcomes.

HUMOR AND LONGEVITY

Up to this point, we have seen that humor and laughter, albeit with some uncertainty, make contributions to good health by strengthening the immune system, as well as reducing cardiovascular reactivity, damaging effects of stress, and pain. If humor has some beneficial effects on physical health, then we can reasonably assume that people who more frequently engage in humor and laughter tend to live longer than their less humorous counterparts. Nevertheless, Martin [4], reviewing the literature, concluded that the research evidence in this regard is not very encouraging. A paradigmatic example is Rotton's study [81] on longevity and humor, reporting that famous comedians, comedy writers, and humorous authors did not live longer than serious authors and entertainers. Consistent with these results are those from a long-term longitudinal study (the Terman Life Cycle Study, begun in 1921).

Individuals found to be more cheerful at age 12 had higher death rates than their less cheerful peers [82]. Cheerfulness is a personality trait that tends to be associated with a greater sense of humor. An explanation offered for this finding was that a more cheerful person engages more often in behaviors known to have health risks. More recently, studies from Norway documented evidence showing that humor predicts survival rates among both healthy and seriously ill individuals. One study [83] explored the role of sense of humor in survival status, measured two years later, in patients diagnosed with end-stage renal failure, a life-threatening condition that requires regular dialysis.

A highly significant increase in survival was essentially accounted for by sense of humor. Those who scored above the median in the sense of humor increased their odds for survival by on average 31%. The HUNT-2 study [84] tracked the health status of an adult county population over a seven-year period. Among persons who developed cancer during this period, individuals with a high sense of humor had a 70% higher survival rate than those with a low sense of humor.

A more recent report of the HUNT-2 study [85] showed that while hazard ratios increased with traditional risk factors such as cardiovascular disease, diabetes, and cancer, they decreased with sense of humor. Sense of humor appeared to increase the likelihood of survival in both individuals with poor and good subjective health. However, above the age of 65 this effect became less evident. Even though the causal mechanism behind the better survival rates of individuals with a high sense of humor is not clear in these Norwegian studies, humor seems to protect against damaging effects of stressors and disease-related stressors upon survival. Svebak hypothesized that the link between humor and survival is mediated by better coping skills shared by those with a higher sense of humor. A recent, original study [86] indirectly confirmed the positive effect of humor on longevity. Researchers rated for smiling photographs of 196 professional baseball players that had been taken in 1952. Smile intensity in photographs predicts mortality occurring by 2009, accounting for 35% of the explained variability in survival, after controlling for other variables (i.e., college attendance, marital status, birth year, career length, age at entrance year, and BMI). Chida and Steptoe [87] conducted a meta-analysis of the prospective studies examining the association between positive well-being and mortality in both healthy and diseased populations. Positive characteristics associated with reduced risk of mortality in healthy populations included a sense of humor, besides other variables such as life satisfaction, hopefulness, optimism and positive personality qualities.

To conclude, while in studies prior to 2000 there was no evidence of a positive effect of humor on longevity, recent studies are promising in their suggestion that humor may lead to a longer life. Nevertheless, the mechanisms that underlie this association are still unknown, thus requiring further investigation.

CONCLUSION

Results of the recent (2001-2011) studies discussed in this chapter show a promising, positive trend regarding the relationship between humor/laughter and physical health outcomes. Overall, empirical studies suggest that mirthful laughter may cause muscular relaxation, have beneficial effects on vascular function, reduce pain, and provide favorable immunological and endocrine effects, whereas inconsistencies were found in asthma and COPD research about the effects of laughter.

With regards to the study of sense of humor and health, results suggest that people with a greater sense of humor are not objectively healthier than others and are more likely to engage in unhealthy lifestyles. However, recent studies are promising in their suggestion that humor may lead to a longer life. Some support was also found for the idea of humor as a stress-moderator, although results of studies on coping humor and stress are contradictory. Finally, results of recent studies support the hypothesis that different styles of humor may facilitate or inhibit the potential to deal effectively with stressors and may promote or impede more general positive life outcomes.

Mahoney and colleagues [88] have proposed that different types of laughter, ranging from chuckles and giggles to belly laughs, may have quite different health-promoting effects. They also pointed out that only laughter that is associated with positive emotions and the lack of malice may be critical for physical health benefits. Given the purported theoretical mechanisms linking laughter and health [3], it may prove valuable for future research to continue to explore the potential relationships between laughter and health with more refined constructs of laughter. In considering the possible effects of sense of humor on health, Kuiper and Nicholl [42] have introduced an important distinction between physical health objectively measured and subjectively perceived, and speculated that a greater sense of humor contributes to a more positive perception of health than shown by objective indices. Using a sample of undergraduate students, they found that individuals with higher scores on sense of humor measures reported more positive health-related perceptions, such as less fear of serious illness or death, less negative somatic preoccupation, and fewer concerns about pain, although they did not have healthy lifestyles. These results confirmed the hypothesis and were consistent with findings from studies of Svebak, Martin and Holmen [28], showing that a higher sense of humor was related to greater subjective satisfaction with health but not with more objective indicators of health status. People with a greater sense of humor seem to perceive themselves to be healthier, showing fewer concerns and preoccupation with symptoms of illness, even though they are not objectively healthier. It may be useful for future research to continue to explore the possible relationships between humor and health, considering the distinction between objectively and subjectively perceived physical health.

REFERENCES

[1]   Fry, W. F., and Stoft, P. E. (1971). Mirth and Oxygen Saturation Levels of Peripheral Blood. *Psychotherapy and Psychosomatics, 19,* 76-84.
[2]   Eastman, M. (1936). *Enjoyment of Laughter.* New York, Halcyon House.
[3]   Fry, W. (1994). The biology of humor. *Humor, International Journal of Humor Research, 7(2),* 111–126.
[4]   Martin R. (2001). Humor, laughter, and physical health, methodological issues and research findings. *Psychological Bulletin, 127,* 504–519.

[5] Martin, R. A. (2004). Sense of Humor and Physical Health, Theoretical Issues, Recent Findings, and Future Directions. *Humor, International Journal of Humor Research, 17*, 1-20.

[6] Martin, R. A. (2007). Approaches to the Sense of Humor. A Historical Review. In W. Ruch (Ed.), *The Sense of Humor. Explorations of a Personality Characteristic* (pp. 15-62). Berlin: Mouton de Gruyter.

[7] Attardo, S. (1994). *Linguistic Theories of Humor*. New York, Mouton.

[8] Chapman, A. J., Foot, H. C. (1977). It's a Funny Thing, Humour. Oxford, England: Pergamon Press.

[9] Dionigi, A., and Gremigni, P. (2010). *Psicologia dell'umorismo*. Roma, Carocci.

[10] Fredrickson, B. L., and Levenson, R. W. (1998). Positive emotions speed recovery from the cardiovascular sequelae of negative emotions. Cognition and Emotion, 12(2), 191-220.

[11] Lazarus, R. S., and Folkman, S. (1984). *Stress, Appraisal, and Coping*. New York, Springer.

[12] Ruch, W. (1996). Measurement approaches to the sense of humor, Introduction and overview. *Humor, International Journal of Humor Research, 9*, 239-250.

[13] Porterfield, A. L. (1987). Does sense of humor moderate the impact of life stress on psychological and physical well-being? *Journal of Research in Personality, 21(3)*, 306-317.

[14] White, S., and Camarena, P. (1989). Laughter as a stress reducer in small groups. Humor, *International Journal of Humor Research*, 2(1), 73–80.

[15] Miller, M., Mangano, C., Park. Y., Goel, R., Plotnick, G.D., and Vogel, R. A. (2006). Impact of cinematic viewing on endothelial function. *Heart, 92(2)*, 261-262.

[16] Vlachopoulos, C., and Panagiotis, X. (2009). Divergent effects of laughter and mental stress on arterial stiffness and central hemodynamics. *Psychosomatic Medicine, 71(4)*, 446-453.

[17] Sugawara, J., Takashi, T., and Hirofumi, T., (2010). Effect of Mirthful Laughter on Vascular Function. *The American Journal of Cardiology, 106(6)*, 856-859.

[18] Miller, M., and Fry, W. F. (2009). The effect of mirthful laughter on the human cardiovascular system. *Medical Hypotheses, 73(5)*, 636-639.

[19] Clark, A., Seidler, A., and Miller, M. (2001). Inverse association between sense of humor and coronary heart disease. *International Journal of Cardiology, 80(1)*, 87–88.

[20] Overeem, S., Taal, W., Ocal Gezici, E., Lammers, G., and Van Dijk, J. (2004). Is motor inhibition during laughter due to emotional or respiratory influences? *Psychophysiology, 41*, 254–258.

[21] Overeem, S., et al. (1999). Weak with laughter. *The Lancet, 354*, 838.

[22] Kimata, H. (2004). Effect of viewing a humorous vs. non-humorous film on bronchial responsiveness in patients with bronchial asthma. *Physiological Behavior, 81*, 681–684.

[23] Liangas, G., Morton, J.R., and Henry, R. L. (2003). Mirth-triggered asthma, is laughter really the best medicine? *Pediatric Pulmonology, 36(2)*, 107-112.

[24] Liangas, G., Yates, D. H., Wu, D., Henry, R. L., and Thomas, P. S. (2004). Laughter-associated asthma. *Journal of Asthma, 41(2)*, 217-221.

[25] Brutsche, M. H., Grossman, P., Müller, R. E., Wiegand, J., Pello, B. F., and Ruch, W. (2008). Impact of laughter on air trapping in severe chronic obstructive lung disease. International *Journal of Chronic Obstructive Pulmonary Diseases, 3(1)*, 185–192.

[26]   Lebowitz, K. R., Sooyeon, S., Diaz, P. T., and Emery, C. F. (2011). Effects of humor and laughter on psychological functioning, quality of life, health status, and pulmonary functioning among patients with chronic obstructive pulmonary disease, A preliminary investigation. *Heart and Lung, The Journal of Acute and Critical Care, 40(4)*, 310-319.

[27]   Kuiper, N. A., and Harris, A. L. (2009). Humor styles and negative affect as predictors of different components of physical health. *Europe's Journal of Psychology, 1*, 1-18.

[28]   Svebak, S., Martin, R. A., and Holmen J. (2004). The prevalence of sense of humor in a large, unselected country population in Norway, Relations with age, sex, and some health indicators. *Humor, International Journal of Humor Research, 17(1-2)*, 121-134.

[29]   Weisenberg, M., Raz, T., and Hener, T. (1998). The influence of film-induced mood on pain perception. *Pain, 76*, 365–375.

[30]   Zilmann, D., Rockwell, S., Schweitzer, K., and Sundar, S. S. (1993). Does humor facilitate coping with physical discomfort? *Motivation and Emotion, 17(1)*, 1-21

[31]   Zweyer, K., Velker, B., and Ruch, W. (2004). Do cheerfulness, exhilaration, and humor production moderate pain tolerance? A FACS study. Humor, *International Journal of Humor Research*, 17(1-2), 85–119.

[32]   Mahony, D. L., Burroughs, W. J., and Hieatt, A.C. (2001). The effects of laughter on discomfort thresholds, does expectation become reality? *Journal of General Psychology, 128*, 217–226.

[33]   Dunbar, R. I. M., et al. (2011). Social laughter is correlated with an elevated pain threshold. *Proceeding of the Royal Society B (Biological Science)*, doi, 10.1098/rspb.2011.1373.

[34]   Mitchell. L. A., MacDonald, R. A. R., and Brodie, E. E. (2006). A comparison of the effect of preferred music, arithmetic and humour on cold pressor pain. *European Journal of Pain, 10*, 343–351.

[35]   Stuber, M., Dunay Hilber, S., Libman Mintzer, L., Castaneda, M., Glover, D., and Zeltzer, L. (2009). Laughter, humor and pain perception in children, a pilot study. *eCAM, 6(2)*, 271–276.

[36]   Goodenough, B., and Ford, J.(2005). Self-reported use of humor by hospitalized pre-adolescent children to cope with pain-related distress from a medical intervention. Humor, I*nternational Journal of Humor Research*, 18(3), 279–298.

[37]   Merskey, H., and Bogduk, N. (1994). *Classification of Chronic Pain. Descriptions of Chronic Pain Syndromes and Definitions of Pain Terms* (2nd edition). Seattle, WA, IASP Press.

[38]   Yonan, C. A., and Wegener, S. T. (2003). Assessment and management of pain in the older adult. *Rehabilitation Psychology, 48(1)*, 4-13.

[39]   Tse, M. M. Y., et al. (2010). Humor therapy, relieving chronic pain and enhancing happiness for older adults. *Journal of Aging Research*, doi: 10.4061/2010/343574.

[40]   Melzach, R., and Wall, P. D. (1965). Pain mechanisms, A new theory. *Science, New Series, 150(3699)*, 971-979.

[41]   Haig, R. A. (1988). The Anatomy of Humor, Biopsychosocial and Therapeutic Perspectives. Springfield, Ill: Charles C. Thomas Publisher.

[42]   Kuiper, N. A., and Sorrel, N. (2004). Thoughts of feeling better? Sense of humor and physical health. *Humor, International Journal of Humor Research, 17(1-2)*, 37-66.

[43]   Kuiper, N. A., and Martin R. A. (1993). Humor and self-concept. *Humor, International Journal of Humor Research, 6*, 251-270.

[44] Kuiper, N. A., and Olinger, L. J. (1998). Humor and mental health. In H. S. Freedman (Ed.), *Encyclopedia of Mental Health* (vol. 2, pp.445-457). San Diego, CA, Academic Press.

[45] Mauriello, M., and McConatha, J. T. (2007). Relations of humor with perceptions of stress *Psychological Reports 101(3II),* 1057-1066.

[46] Abel, M. H. (2002). Humor, stress, and coping strategies. *Humor: International Journal of Humor Research, 15,* 365-381.

[47] Lefcourt, H. M., Davidson K., Prkachin, K. M., and Mills D. E. (1997). Humor as a stress moderator in the prediction of blood pressure obtained during five stressful tasks. *Journal of Research in Personality, 31,* 523-542.

[48] Marziali, E., McDonald, L., and Donahue, P. (2008). The role of coping humor in the physical and mental health of older adults. *Aging and Mental Health, 12(6),* 713-718.

[49] Celso, B. G., Ebener, D. J., and Burkhead, E. J. (2003). Humor coping, health status, and life satisfaction among older adults residing in assisted living facilities. *Aging and Mental Health, 7(6),* 438-445.

[50] Merz, E. L., Malcarne, V. L., Hansdottir, I., Furst, D. E., Clements, P. J., and Weisman, M. H. (2009). A longitudinal analysis of humor coping and quality of life in systemic sclerosis *Psychology, Health and Medicine, 14(5),* 553-566.

[51] Martin, R. A., Puhlik-Doris, P., Larsen, G., Gray, J., and Weir, K. (2003) Individual differences in the uses of humor and their relation to psychological well-being, Development of the Humor Styles Questionnaire. *Journal of Research in Personality, 37,* 48-75.

[52] Cann, A., and Etzel, K.C., (2008). Remembering and anticipating stressors: Positive personality mediates the relationship with sense of humor. *Humor: International Journal of Humor Research,* 21, 157-178.

[53] Carver, C. S., Scheier, M. F., Miller, C. J., and Fulford, D. (2009). Optimism. In C. R. Snyder, and S. J. Lopez (Eds.), *Oxford Handbook of Positive Psychology* (2nd edition, pp. 303–11). New York: Oxford Univ. Press.

[54] Richman, L. S., Kubzansky, L., Maselko, J., Kawachi, I., Choo, P., and Bauer, M. (2005). Positive emotion and health: Going beyond the negative. *Health Psychology, 24(4),* 422-429.

[55] Siahpush, M., Spittal, M., Singh, G. K., (2008). Happiness and life satisfaction prospectively predict self-rated health, physical health, and the presence of limiting, long-term health conditions. *American Journal of Health Promotion, 23(1),* 18-26.

[56] Veenhoven, R. (2008). Healthy happiness. Effects of happiness on physical health and the consequences for preventive health care. *Journal of Happiness Studies, 9,* 449-469.

[57] Cann, A., Stilwell. K., and Taku, K. (2010). Humor Styles, Positive Personality and Health. *Europe's Journal of Psychology, 6(3),* 213-235.

[58] Dillon, K., Minchoff, B., Baker, K. (1985). Positive emotional states and enhancement of the immune system. *International Journal of Psychiatric Medicine, 15,* 13–18.

[59] Lefcourt, H, M., Davidson-Katz, K., and Kueneman K. (1990). Humor and Immune System Functioning. *Humor: International Journal of Humor Research, 3,* 305-321.

[60] Berk, L. S., Felten, D. L., Tan, S. A., Bittman, B. B., and Westengard, J. (2001). Modulation of neuroimmune parameters during the eustress of humor-associated mirthful laughter. *Alternative Therapy and Health Medicine, 7(2),* 62-76.

[61] Bennett, M. and Lengacher, P. C. (2007). Humor and laughter may influence health: III. Laughter and health outcomes. *Evidence-based Complementary and Alternative Medicine, 5(1),* 37-40.

[62] Hayashi, T., et al. (2006). Laughter regulates gene expression in patients with type 2 diabetes. *Psychotherapy and Psychosomatics, 75(1),* 62-65.

[63] Hayashi T., et al. (2007). Laughter up-regulates the genes related to NK cell activity in diabetes. *Biomedical Research, 28(6),* 281-285.

[64] Hayashi, T., and Murakami, K. (2009). The effects of laughter on post-prandial glucose levels and gene expression in type 2 diabetic patients. *Life Science, 85(5-6),* 185-187.

[65] Nasir, U. M., et al. (2005). Laughter therapy modulates the parameters of renin-angiotensin system in patients with type 2 diabetes. *International Journal Molecular Medicine, 16(6),* 1077-1081.

[66] Atsumi, T., et al. (2004). Pleasant feeling from watching a comical video enhances free radical scavenging capacity in human whole saliva. *Journal of Psychosomatic Research 56,* 377–379.

[67] Toda, M., Kusakabe, S., Nagasawa, S., Kitamura, K., Morimoto, K. (2007). Effect of laughter on salivary endocrinological stress marker chromogranin A. *Biomedical Research, 28(2),* 115-118.

[68] Kimata, H. (2001). Effect of humor on allergen-induced wheal reactions. *JAMA, 285(6),* 738.

[69] Kimata, H. (2009). Viewing a humorous film decreases IgE production by seminal B cells from patients with atopic eczema. *Journal of Psychosomatic Research., 66(2),* 173-175.

[70] Kimata, H. (2007). Elevation of testosterone and reduction of trans epidermal water loss by viewing a humorous film in elderly patients with atopic dermatitis. *Acta Medica (Hradec Kralove), 50(2),* 135-137.

[71] Kimata, H. (2007). Laughter elevates the levels of breast-milk melatonin *Journal of Psychosomatic Research, 62(6),* 699-702.

[72] Kimata, H. (2004). Differential effects of laughter on allergen-specific immunoglobulin and neurotrophin levels in tears. *Perception and Motor Skills, 3,* 901–908.

[73] Ishigami, S., Nakajima, A., Tanno, M., Matsuzaki, T., Suzuki, H., and Yoshino, S. (2005). Effects of mirthful laughter on growth hormone, IGF-1 and substance P in patients with rheumatoid arthritis. *Clinical Experimental Rheumatology, 23,* 651–657.

[74] Hansen, E., and Easthope G. (2006). *Lifestyle in Medicine.* London: Routledge.

[75] Ford, E. S., Zhao, G., Tsai, J., Li, C. (2011). Low-Risk Lifestyle Behaviors and All-Cause Mortality, Findings From the National Health and Nutrition Examination Survey III Mortality Study. *American Journal of Public Health, 101(10),* 1922-1929.

[76] Kerkkanen, P., Kuiper N. A., and Martin R. A. (2004). Sense-of-Humor, Physical Health and Well-Being at Work, A Three-Year Longitudinal Study of Finnish Police Officers. *Humor: International Journal of Humor Research,17(1-2),* 21-35.

[77] Martin, L. R., et al. (2002). A life course perspective on childhood cheerfulness and its relation to mortality risk. *Personality and Social Psychology Bulletin, 28,* 221-231.

[78] Ruch W. (1994). Temperament, Eysenck´s PEN system, and humor-related traits. *Humor: International Journal of Humor Research, 7,* 209-244.

[79] Patton, D., Barnes, G. E., Murray, R. P. (1993). Personality characteristics of smokers and ex-smokers. *Personality and Individual Differences,* 15(6), 653-664.

[80] Haellstroem, T., and Noppa, H. (1981) Obesity in women in relation to mental illness, social factors and personality traits. *Journal of Psychosomatic Research, 25,* 75-82.

[81] Rotton, J. (1992). Trait humor and longevity. Does comics have the last laugh? *Health Psychology, 11,* 262-6

[82] Friedman, H. S., et al. (1993). Does childhood personality predict longevity? *Journal of Personality and Social Psychology, 65,* 176-85.

[83] Svebak S., Kristoffersen B., Aasarød K. (2006). Sense of humor and survival among a county cohort of patients with end-stage renal failure. A two-year prospective study. *International Journal of Psychiatric Medicine, 36,* 269-81.

[84] Svebak S., Romundstad S., Holmen J. (2007). Sense of humor and mortality, A seven-year prospective study of an unselected county population and a sub-population diagnosed with cancer. The Hunt Study. American Psychosomatic Society 65th Annual Meeting, March 7-10, 2007. *Psychosomatic Medicine, 69,* A-64.

[85] Svebak, S., Romundstad, S., and Holmen, J. (2010). A 7-year prospective study of sense of humor and mortality in an adult county population. The HUNT-2 study. *International Journal of Psychiatry in Medicine, 40,* 125-146.

[86] Abel, E. L., and Kruger, M. L. (2010). Smile intensity in photographs predicts longevity. *Psychological Science, 21,* 542–544.

[87] Chida Y., and Steptoe A. (2008). Positive Psychological Well-Being and Mortality. A Quantitative Review of Prospective Observational Studies. *Psychosomatic Medicine, 70,* 741-756.

[88] Mahony, D. L., Burroughs, W. J., and Lippman, L, G. (2002). Perceived Attributes of Health-Promoting Laughter, A Cross-Generational Comparison. *The Journal of Psychology, 136(2),* 171–81.

In: Humor and Health Promotion
Editor: Paola Gremigni

Chapter 9

HUMOR AND MENTAL HEALTH

Paola Gremigni
Department of Psychology, University of Bologna, Italy

ABSTRACT

The idea that humor can be associated with mental well-being has been spreading in recent years; therefore, a discrete body of research has investigated the potential benefits of humor for mental health and psychological well-being. Some evidence has emerged that humor produces positive short-term emotional changes and may attenuate negative emotions as a result of cognitive distraction. Nevertheless, cross-sectional studies have found no single correlations between sense of humor and the ability to regulate negative emotions. Different humor styles have been found to mediate the relationship between positive personality qualities and well-being, although the mediator models used to explain this relationship are still far from producing conclusive results. Research findings make clear that humor is a multidimensional construct, consisting of components that can affect mental health and well-being either positively or negatively. Consequently, various humor styles may have different effects on social interactions as well as mental health.

Therefore, in examining the potential role of humor in improving mental health processes and psychological well-being we should take into consideration various humor styles, contexts and circumstances.

INTRODUCTION

In contemporary Western culture, a sense of humor is widely viewed as a highly desirable personality characteristic. Individuals with a greater sense of humor are thought to cope better with stress, to get along well with others and enjoy better mental and even physical health [1] . The idea that humor is associated with mental well-being has spread in recent years. In this regard, we can recall a work of Carol Ryff [2], which was intended to verify whether the six criteria of psychological well-being she proposed were similar to those shown by ordinary people. This study found that the best indicators associated with positive functioning identified by middle-aged and older adults also included a sense of humor.

During the late 1990s, humor was included in the list of the core strengths of character or enduring positive human traits identified by Positive Psychology [3]. The Values in Action (VIA) Classification of Strengths identifies 24 components of good character that contribute to optimal human development and organizes them under six broad virtues. Virtues are the core characteristics valued by moral philosophers and religious thinkers: wisdom, courage, humanity, justice, temperance, and transcendence. The last one (i.e. transcendence) includes strengths that build connections to the larger universe and provide meanings: appreciation of beauty and excellence, gratitude, hope, humor, and spirituality. Humor in the VIA is conceptualized as a unipolar and unidimensional strength, which scope is restricted to those forms that serve some moral good. However, humor is a multidimensional concept and the VIA classification does not cover all of the virtues-related humorous behaviors; hence, further research is required to investigate the role of virtue in humor [4]. Unfortunately, the strength of humor has not received much attention from Positive Psychology researchers, although it has much to offer for the promotion of well-being.

Components of humor have been seen as effects of psychological and physical states of a person. Such psychological conditions include depression, autism, borderline personality disorder, hysteria, schizophrenia, mood disturbance, psychological repression, aggression, and anxiety [5]. A recent review reported scientific evidence of the influence of depression on the ability to laugh [6]. It suggests that reduction of laughter frequency is a symptom of depression, and its increase may be used as a marker of clinical improvement.

On the other hand, aspects of humor could also be determinants of physical and mental conditions. I tried to summarize the research on humor's effects on physical health in the previous chapter. The aim of this chapter is to review the relevant, recent research on the effects of humor on psychological conditions.

First to address this issue, I briefly describe the mechanisms that have been hypothesized to explain the influence of humor and laughter on mental health and well-being.

An important mechanism through which a sense of humor may be beneficial to mental health is by contributing to one's ability to regulate emotions, which is an essential aspect of mental health [7]. Sense of humor might produce "habitual amusement-related positive emotions or moods" [8]; in other words, it might directly affect psychological well-being by making people feel better emotionally. This conceptualization of sense of humor asserts that it should be positively related to measures of positive affect (including happiness) and negatively related to measures of negative affect (including depression).

An indirect contribution of sense of humor to mental health is to enhance the performance on tasks that demand directed attention by inclining a person toward positive affect. This indirect contribution was demonstrated experimentally in the late eighties by Isen and her colleagues [9]. The positive mood and flexible thinking induced by several methods, including exposure to humorous material, was found to contribute to the effective functioning in attention-demanding situations.

Another mechanism states that humor might indirectly benefit health and mental well-being through an interpersonal mechanism, by increasing one's level of social support. Individuals who use humor in an affiliative and non-hostile manner are able to reduce effectively interpersonal conflicts and tensions and enhance positive feelings in others. As a result, they may enjoy more numerous and satisfying social relationships [10]. In fact, it may be easier for individuals with a great sense of humor to establish and maintain friendships, to develop a rich network and thus, to get the mental and physical health benefits that derive from social support. This hypothesized mechanism focuses on interpersonal aspects of humor and the social competence with which individuals express humor in their relationships, rather than the frequency with which they engage in laughter. This model emphasizes the distinction between styles of humor that facilitate relationships and enhance social support, and other forms that are potentially maladaptive.

Finally, Can and colleagues [11] provided a model to understand the actual processes through which effective and ineffective styles of humor may be relevant to psychological well-being. The proposed model assumes that humor promotes well-being through positive personality qualities that serve as mediators in the relationship between humor styles and perceptions of stress. Using humor effectively, through higher levels of self-enhancing humor and lower levels of self-demeaning humor, can help to maintain a more positive personal style, characterized by higher positive affectivity and positive qualities like optimism, happiness, and hope.

In conclusion, implications of humor for positive mental health were proposed to be related to the abilities to regulate negative emotions and enjoy positive emotions, to establish meaningful relationships with others, and possess a set of positive personality characteristics and resources.

A review published in 1999 [5] indicated that, in general, humor as a response (e.g. laughter) may contribute to a reduction of existing mental health problems, whereas a great sense of humor can beneficially influence mental health by moderating the perceived intensity of negative life events. A more recent review [10] described research investigating the potential benefits of humor in regulating negative emotions, coping with stressful events, and establishing meaningful social relationships. Crucial points emerge from this review. Experimental laboratory research confirmed a short-term beneficial effect of humor and laughter but provided little evidence for longer-term psychological benefits. Correlational studies found weak or inconsistent evidence for mental benefits of a sense of humor. Research on humor styles found that positive and negative styles of humor are differentially correlated with the individuals' experiences of close relationships, emotional well-being and healthy functioning.

DOES HUMOR PREDICT POSITIVE AFFECT?

Positive affect can be defined as a state of pleasurable engagement with the environment eliciting feelings, such as happiness, joy, excitement, enthusiasm, and contentment [12]. Positive affect is part of the concept of subjective well-being that includes life satisfaction, absence of negative emotions, optimism, and positive emotions [13]. It is also part of the concept of psychological well-being that encompasses trait-like dispositions, such as optimism and cheerfulness [14]. The literature on the relationship between affectivity and health is consistent. The strongest link with health was found with trait affective styles, which reflects a person's typical emotional experience, rather than state affect. The presence of positive affect as a dispositional state was found to be associated with positive health experiences (i.e., strong immune response, few illness symptoms and pain reported, good health, and longevity) [13,15–17]. Positive affect was also associated with protective psychosocial and behavioral factors (i.e., strong social connectedness, perceived social support, preference for adaptive coping responses, and performing health behaviors) [13]. To the extent that humor produces a positive emotional state [18], we can safely say that it has a direct effect on psychological well-being of individuals.

Investigations of humor and emotions have demonstrated, in a number of laboratory experiments, the effects of humor on mood. In particular, smiling and laughing are expressions of the positive emotion of mirth that is induced by the perception of humor. The act of smiling and laughing by itself, even when done artificially, may induce feelings of amusement and mirth, at least temporarily [19–22]. These experiments provided fairly consistent evidence of short-term effects of humor on positive mood and feelings of well-being in the laboratory.

A more recent cross-sectional study [23] confirmed that a good sense of humor predicted well-being of the people who use it. Results indicated that only humor appreciation was an effective predictor of emotional well-being and personal development, whereas another dimension evaluated in this study (i.e., contact with nature) was a predictor of psychological functioning.

However, in the literature there are also studies that did not confirm the hypothesis that humor has positive effects on mental well-being. Among them, we recall the study of Kuiper and Martin [24] indicating that individuals with a greater tendency to laugh at everyday life did not show higher levels of positive affect. In conclusion, findings for the role of laughter and sense of humor as predictors of psychological well-being are to date consistent, although less than those on the relationship between stable differences in affectivity and health.

CAN HUMOR ATTENUATE NEGATIVE EMOTIONS?

Chronic negative affect has been shown to be related to poorer health experiences [25], and recent levels of negative affect have proven to be a reliable predictor of physical health [26]. For example, negative emotions can intensify a variety of health threats and contribute to prolonged infection and delayed wound healing. Accordingly, Kiecolt-Glaser and colleagues [27] argued that distress-related immune deregulation may be one core mechanism behind the health risks associated with negative emotions.

Besides increasing positive moods, there is experimental evidence that humor can reduce negative moods, thus bringing benefits to health. Laboratory experiments found that exposure to a humorous video led to a significant reduction in reported levels of anxiety [28,29]. There is also some evidence that humor can reduce the effects of experimentally induced depressed moods [30]. A recent study of medical education explored the effectiveness of humor, when used as intervention in a large group teaching over negative emotions amongst students [31]. Humor was found to be truly effective in relieving students on their negative emotions of depression, anxiety and stress. Taken together, these findings suggest that humor produces positive short-term emotional changes. Cross-sectional studies have found the presence of at least moderate negative correlations between some humorous aspects and measures of neuroticism, anxiety, and depression [32]. Nevertheless, other studies did not confirm the relationship between humor, anxiety and depression [10,33].

A recent study aimed to demonstrate that the cognitive demands involved in humor processing can attenuate negative emotions [34]. The authors hypothesized that humorous stimuli attenuate negative emotion to a greater extent than do equally positive non-humorous stimuli. Participants reported less negative feelings in both mild and strongly negative trials with humorous, positive stimuli than with non-humorous positive stimuli, whereas humor did not differentially affect emotions in the neutral trials. Cognitive demanding stimuli were more effective in regulating negative emotions than those that were less demanding. These findings supported the idea that humor may attenuate negative emotions as a result of cognitive distraction.

HUMOR STYLES AND PSYCHOLOGICAL WELLBEING

Martin and colleagues [35] have recently proposed a new approach to the study of individual differences in the use of humor that takes into account the multidimensionality of this construct. They identified four different styles of humor, or ways in which people use humor in their daily lives: two potentially detrimental styles (aggressive and self-defeating humor) and two potentially beneficial styles (affiliative and self-enhancing humor). Benevolent humor is used to be accepted socially (affiliative) or to deal with stressful situations (self-reinforcement), whereas non-benevolent humor is used to tease others (aggressive) or self-mock (worthlessness). Different humor styles were associated with health and psychological well-being in different ways [35]. The self-reinforcing and affiliative styles correlated negatively with anxiety and depression, and positively with self-esteem and psychological well-being. On the other hand, higher scores on the worthlessness humor style were associated with increased anxiety, depression, psychiatric symptoms, and lower self-esteem and well-being. The aggressive style was related to hostility and aggression. These results were confirmed by other studies. In one of them [36], the benevolent humor styles were associated with higher self-esteem, lower levels of depression and anxiety, and multiple self-competencies associated with better coping. The non-benevolent humor styles were instead associated with a lower self-esteem, higher levels of anxiety and depression, and lower perceptions of empowerment and self-competencies. In another study [37], self-enhancing humor was negatively related, and self-defeating was positively related to both evaluations of past stressors and anticipated future stressors. The two self-directed styles of humor were reliably related to well-being outcomes, although they were not shown to be both adaptive: self-defeating humor style was associated with poorer adjustment and lower well-being than self-enhancing humor style [37,38].

In a cross-cultural study, Kazarian and Martin [39] investigated the differences in the use of humor styles, by gender and culture, among Lebanese, Canadian and Belgian students. Lebanese students showed a lower use of adaptive humor, compared to the Canadians and less use of affiliative and aggressive humor styles than the Belgians. Canadian and Belgian males used aggressive humor more than the female of their own country. In this study, the association between humor styles and mental health was only partly supported by empirical evidence. These results confirm the hypothesis that only some types of humor are associated with mental well-being, while others may even have a harmful effect [35].

Taken together, these studies support the idea that sense of humor is a multidimensional construct, consisting of components that can affect mental health and well-being either positively or negatively.

HUMOR AND OTHER PERSONAL RESOURCES

People who are high on positive personality qualities, such as optimism, autonomy, and personal growth tend to report a higher level of positive functioning, including experiencing higher levels of positive affect, greater life satisfaction, increased level of self-esteem, in addition, to the absence of negative affect. These positive personality qualities are also associated with more positive approaches to coping with stressful situations and to a better overall health. Research supports the health benefits of greater optimism [40], higher levels of hope as a stable trait [41], and stable differences in happiness [42]. Effective use of humor may be one way that people with more positive personality qualities use to maintain their positive outlooks. Indirect support to this idea came from research indicating that a good sense of humor was associated with higher levels of cheerfulness [35]. Another positive quality that was associated with humor was hopefulness. In fact, a study found that participants who watched a comedy video, as compared to those who viewed a non-humorous video, reported a greater increase in feelings of hopefulness [43]. Some research has also shown that people with a greater sense of humor have a better vision of themselves. For example, employees engaged in a guided program of non-humor dependent laughter demonstrated a significant increase in several different aspects of self-efficacy in the workplace, including self-regulation, optimism, positive emotions, and social identification, and they maintained these gains at follow-up [44].

Several studies on humor styles explored the relation between adaptive and maladaptive humor and positive personality characteristics. Affiliative and self-enhancing humor styles positively correlated with indicators of positive mental health (i.e., psychological well-being, self-esteem, and optimism) [35,45], while they negatively correlated with depression [46,47], anxiety [48], loneliness [49], and global distress [38]. On the other hand, aggressive and self-defeating humor showed negative associations with indicators of positive mental health, and positive correlations with various negative emotions and impaired psychosocial functioning (for a review see Martin [10]). In a recent study [37], initial evidence was found to support a mediator model in which the role of humor styles in explaining perceptions of stress was mediated through a composite of positive personality styles, including optimism, hope, and happiness (i.e., humor styles → positive personality → perception of stress). A different mediator model was tested in another recent study [50] involving a sample of Serbian young adults. A mediating role of humor styles in the relationship between personality traits and psychological well-being was partially shown. Self-enhancing humor style mediated the relationship between extraversion, neuroticism and satisfaction with life, whereas affiliative humor style partially mediated the relationship between neuroticism and affective well-being (i.e., personality → humor styles → affective well-being).

A recent study [51] investigated humor styles in the context of explicit (i.e., conscious, deliberate) and implicit (i.e., automatic, habitual) self-esteem. Results showed that participants with a self-defeating humor style had damaged self-esteem, defined as a combination of low explicit and high implicit self-esteem. A possible mechanism behind these results could be that the frequent use of self-defeating humor might result in a downward spiral of social rejection, resulting in low explicit social self-esteem. Nevertheless, the correlational design of this study did not allow making causal inferences. Other recent studies found that humor styles mediated the relationships between positive and negative self-evaluation standards and psychological well-being. For example, Dozois and colleagues [52] found that self-enhancing and self-defeating humor styles mediated the relationship between early maladaptive schemas and depressed mood. Early maladaptive schemas influenced information processing, emotional reactions to life situations, self-control, and interpersonal relationships. Furthermore, the relationship between the primary evaluative component of the self-schema and psychological well-being (rated in terms of social self-esteem and lower depression) was mediated by a more affiliative humor, whereas a more self-defeating humor, induced by negative self-evaluative standards, led to a decrease in social self-esteem [53].

Taken together, these findings show that a good sense of humor or humor styles might be reliable predictors of a better mental health, even if their predictive power is less than that of other positive personality qualities. Nevertheless, the mechanisms linking these variables and the mediator models used to explain them are still far from exhaustive and conclusive.

DOES HUMOR IMPROVE INTERPERSONAL PROCESSES?

Research has only recently been directed to investigate the potential effect of humor on interpersonal relationships, since humor was supposed to improve interpersonal processes and facilitate social relationships [1].

Studies of dating and married couples have shown that a great satisfaction with the relationship is associated with a good sense of humor of the partner and the amount of laughter shared between the spouses [10]. A more recent study [54] found that partners tended to resemble each other with regard to the sense of humor. However, couple similarity on sense of humor was unrelated to the relationship quality, in contrast with what was expected. On the contrary, another recent study found little similarity within couples on humor styles, but it found that the best predictors of satisfaction were perceptions of a partner's humor style [55].

In a qualitative study of dating relationships, Amy Bippus [56] drew a distinction between humor that serves a bonding function and more negative types, such as cruel, inappropriate, and overbearing humor that may be injurious to the relationship. Humor styles, together with conflict styles, were found to serve as a mediator between the attachment style and relationship satisfaction in the context of romantic relationships [57]. Specifically, humor styles reflecting attitudes about others were related to the avoidance attachment style, while those reflecting attitudes about the self were related to the anxiety attachment dimension.

Another study on humor in close relationships underlined the necessity to evaluate separately positive, negative, and instrumental uses of humor by each partner, since they were differentially associated with marriage satisfaction [58].

A few recent studies have examined associations between potentially healthy and unhealthy humor styles and variables having to do with close relationships. The distinction between positive and negative uses of humor appeared to be critical, since affiliative and aggressive styles had opposed relationships with the couples' satisfaction [59]. Moreover, a recent study showed that the two other-directed humor styles explained much more variance of the relationship satisfaction than the self-directed styles. Thus, they were crucial to consider as personal qualities, but their relevance likely was greater when the uses of humor were directed toward interpersonal, rather than intrapersonal, goals [55].

Overall, correlational studies examining associations between trait humor and several variables relevant to personal relationships found a positive correlation of humor with intimacy, empathy, social assertiveness, and interpersonal trust [10].

Studies on general social relationships confirmed the role of humor styles in facilitating social interactions. A recent study [60] found that labeling social comments as humorous had positive effects on recipients' reactions to these comments. Furthermore, when the acquaintance was described as feeling depressed, affiliative comments made in a humorous fashion led to more positive reactions than did non-humorous affiliative comments. A correlational study on the relation between shyness and humor styles found a significant negative correlation between shyness and affiliative humor and a positive correlation between shyness and self-defeating humor, indicating that shy people, who have difficulties in social situations, tend to use less adaptive humor styles [61]. Finally, coping humor was found to be positively associated with pleasure and self-confidence people attributed to their interactions and with time they spent with others although the strength of this relation was moderated by depression [62].

Studies on peer-relations in childhood and adolescence also seem to provide initial empirical support to the relationship between humor styles and peer acceptance. One of these studies investigated how different humor styles may bear on peer relationships and bullying during middle childhood. Results indicated that adaptive humor styles helped the child's status within the peer group, whereas maladaptive humor styles hindered it [63]. Another study showed that positive humor styles and trait cheerfulness were positively correlated with various domains of social competence in undergraduate students, whereas negative humor styles and trait lousy mood were negatively correlated with social competence [64].

However, there is also some evidence that humor may play a negative role in interpersonal relationship. For example, one study on close relationships found that for men higher coping humor was associated with lower marital satisfaction and greater negative affect and verbal negativity during marital discussions [65]. Another study indicated that greater humor expression by husbands, during a problem discussion, predicted a greater likelihood of separation in newly married couples, in the context of serious life stress [66].

A qualitative study found that violent humor was used by Finnish school boys as a strategy to construct masculinity and gain social status [67]. The effect of such a negative humor strategy might have serious consequences on students' lives.

This emerging body of research makes clear that humor styles, as expressions of a sense of humor, cannot be regarded as uniformly positive in relation with social interaction. Findings demonstrate the usefulness of treating humor as a multidimensional variable to understand the roles it might play across relationships. Therefore, in examining the potential role of humor in improving interpersonal processes we should take into consideration various humor styles, gender differences, and specific interpersonal contexts and circumstances.

THE USE OF HUMOR IN MENTAL ILLNESS

Probably due to what seems to be the potential benefit of humor and laughter, in the last 30 years we have seen an increase in the use of humor with individuals with mental illness. A recent review [6] reported some evidence supporting the hypothesis of the therapeutic action of laughter on depression. Empirical findings seem to demonstrate that laughter may improve mood directly, moderate negative consequences of stressful events on psychological well-being and mediate the normalization of the hypothalamic, pituitary, adrenocortical system dysfunctions involved in the depression pathogenesis. Through these mechanisms, laughter can counteract depressive symptoms. Furthermore, the favorable effects of laughter on social relationships and physical health may have a role in influencing the ability of depressed patients to face the disease. Results of empirical studies on the therapeutic use of humor in depressed patients showed that humor proved to be helpful. This was the case with the use of humor in the group therapy of geriatric patients with depression and Alzheimer's [68]. A recent pilot study found significant short-term mood improvement after training addressing humor skills in patients with major depression, although there was no significant long-term improvement of depressive symptoms [69]. In a study of hospitalized adolescent psychiatric patients, higher coping humor was associated with lower levels of depression and higher self-esteem, although it was unrelated to feelings of hopelessness [70]. A study of hospitalized, adult psychiatric patients found that higher sense of humor tended to be associated with lower depression and higher self-esteem and positive moods, among clinically depressed patients [71]. Overall, these findings give some support to a general protective role of humor in mood disturbance. Studies on the effect of humor styles on mental health specify that only the benevolent styles of humor have a protective role. Recently, Düşünceli [72] investigated the effect of humor styles on psychopathology among university students in Turkey. Results of a structural equation model indicated that the self-enhancing humor style decreased symptoms of a variety of psychological disturbances, such as somatization, obsessive compulsive disorder, anxiety and phobic anxiety, interpersonal sensitivity, depression, anger-hostility, and psychotic disorder. The affiliative humor style also decreased the symptoms of mood disorders. The self-defeating humor style, in contrast, increased the symptoms of mood and anxiety disorders. These findings support the result of previous studies [35] showing that self-enhancing humor style predicted anxiety disorders negatively, whereas self-defeating humor style predicted anxiety disorders positively. Despite the presence of studies that have not confirmed an inverse relationship between humor and levels of anxiety and depression [73], other studies supported this view. For example, in a study on personality-vulnerability dimensions and positive and negative styles of humor, undergraduates with higher levels of depressed mood reported less use of self-reinforcing and affiliative humor, and an increased use of self-depreciating humor [74]. This study took into account two personality traits, autonomy and social dependency (i.e., tendency to base their self-esteem on the opinions of others). It suggested that self-reinforcing style, being inversely correlated with social dependency, could protect people from depression in response to situations of social rejection. Olson and colleagues [75] found that among individuals with high rumination, those with higher adaptive humor styles (especially self-reinforcing humor style) had significantly lower levels of dysphoria than individuals with high rumination and lower adaptive humor. Rumination is a negative, anxious repetitive thought that is highly correlated with depression.

Based on these results, humor was hypothesized to act as a distracter from ruminative thoughts, also to mitigate the negative effects of rumination, thus indirectly helping prevent depressive episodes [76]. However, an experimental study did not confirm that humor effectively distracted for rumination or reduced the amount of rumination [76].

In a community sample of Israeli adults, affiliative and self-enhancing humor styles, on one hand, and aggressive and self-defeating humor styles, on the other, mediated the relationship between self-criticism (a trait that confers vulnerability to depression) and neediness (which is related to levels of depressive symptoms) [77]. Pietrantoni and Dionigi found that Italian people who experienced negative events, and used aggressive and worthlessness styles of humor were more prone to develop anxiety and depression, than those using adaptive humor styles [78].

Hugelshofer and colleagues found that high levels of affiliative and self-enhancing humor, and low levels of self-defeating humor were associated with few depressive symptoms, in a large sample of students [79]. Additionally, higher levels of affiliative humor provided a buffer against the deleterious effects of a negative attributional style, even though this relation varied between women and men. Chen and Martin [38] reported a similar pattern of relationships when looking at mental health based on self-reported symptoms. Although a greater sense of humor seems to be related to lower severity of disturbance in clinically depressed individuals and to fewer depressive symptoms in healthy people, this does not seem to be the case among patients with schizophrenia.

In one study, hospitalized patients with chronic schizophrenia were shown 70 comedy movies over a three-month period, while those in a control group were shown an equal number of non-humorous dramatic movies [80]. After these interventions, patients who had watched the comedy movies were rated by the staff as having significantly lower levels of verbal hostility, anxiety/depression and tension than those in the control group. The patients themselves reported greater perceived social support from the staff. The authors of the study acknowledged that these findings may have had more to do with the effects of the movies on the perceptions of the hospital staff than on the actual functioning of the patients. Another study of humor in hospitalized schizophrenic patients similarly found no relation between coping humor and self-report and psychiatrist-rated hostility, aggression, and anger [81]. Overall, the rather limited research on this topic provides little evidence that schizophrenic patients with high humor have a better psychological adjustment than are those with less of a sense of humor.

In a recent review of the literature, Marc Gelkopf [82] stated that empirical studies on the use of humor and laughter in people with serious mental illness have not produced consistent results, because of serious methodological shortcomings. In particular, most studies lack control groups, use non-standardized assessment tools, involve extremely small samples, and do not administer an adequate control stimulus for distinguishing between the effects of humor and those of positive emotions in general. Therefore, this field needs further investigation.

CONCLUSION

A discrete body of research has investigated the potential benefits of humor for mental health and psychological well-being. Findings for the role of laughter and sense of humor as predictors of psychological well-being are consistent, although less than those on the relationship between stable differences in affectivity and health. Some evidence has emerged that humor produces positive short-term emotional changes and may attenuate negative emotions as a result of cognitive distraction. Nevertheless, cross-sectional studies have found no clear correlations between sense of humor and the ability to regulate negative emotions. A good sense of humor or humor styles might mediate the relationship between positive personality qualities and well-being, although the mediator models used to explain this relationship are still far from exhaustive and conclusive. Research findings make clear that humor is a multidimensional construct, consisting of components that can affect mental health and well-being either positively or negatively. Consequently, humor styles cannot be regarded as uniformly positive in relation with social interaction or with severity of disturbance in clinically depressed individuals and other mentally ill patients. Therefore, in examining the potential role of humor in improving mental health processes and psychological well-being we should take into consideration various humor styles, contexts and circumstances. An area of research that has been understudied is related to the connection between humor and quality of life (QoL) outcomes in chronic disease. The few studies in the literature show conflicting results. In patients with head and neck squamous cell carcinoma, sense of humor, but not depression or anxiety levels, at diagnosis predicted QoL and depression level at 6 years follow-up [83]. In patients with systemic sclerosis, a progressive rheumatic disease that can be fatal in severe cases, humor coping did not significantly predict any of the disease-related outcomes, either cross-sectionally or longitudinally [84]. More recently, a sense of humor among patients with chronic obstructive pulmonary disease has proven to be associated with positive psychological functioning and enhanced quality of life, but laughing aloud was shown to cause acute deterioration in pulmonary function secondary to worsen hyperinflation [85]. Overall, these results indicate that humor may not be directly beneficial to QoL in chronic disease. We can speculate that conflicting results in research on humor and mental health may be related to difficulties in conceptualization and measurement of the sense of humor. The various pieces of this process have been identified, as much progress has been made in defining the key aspects of humor; however, what is still missing is the full view of the complex connection between them.

REFERENCES

[1]   Lefcourt, H. M. (2001). *Humor: The psychology of living buoyantly.* New York: Kluwer Academic.

[2]   Ryff, C. D. (1989). Happiness is everything, or is it? Explorations on the meaning of psychological well-being. *Journal of Personality and Social Psychology, 57,* 1069-1081.

[3]   Peterson, C., and Seligman, M. E. (2004). *Character strengths and virtues: A handbook and classification.* Washington: American Psychological Association.

[4]   Müller, L., and Ruch, W. (2011). Humor and strengths of character. *The Journal of Positive Psychology*, *6*, 368-376.

[5]   Galloway, G., and Cropley, A. (1999). Benefits of humor for mental health: Empirical findings and directions for further research. *Humor: International Journal for Humor Research*, *72*, 301-314.

[6]   Fonzi, L., Matteucci, G., Bersani, G. (2010). Laughter and depression: Hypothesis of pathogenic and therapeutic correlation. *Rivista di Psichiatria*, *45*, 1-6.

[7]   Gross, J. J., Muñoz, R. F. (1995). *Emotion regulation and Mental Health Clinical Psychology: Science and practice*, *2*, 151-164.

[8]   Martin, R. A. (2001). Humor, laughter, and physical health: Methodological issues and research findings. *Psychological Bulletin*, *127*, 504-519.

[9]   Isen, A. M., Daubman, K. A., Nowicki, G. P. (1987). Positive affect facilitates creative problem solving. *Journal of Personality and Social Psychology*, *52*, 1122-1131.

[10] Martin, R. A. (2007). *The psychology of humor: An integrative approach*. New York: Academic Press.

[11] Cann, A., Stilwell, K., and Taku, K. (2010). Humor styles, positive personality and health. *Europe's Journal of Psychology*, *3*, 213-235.

[12] Watson, D., Clark, L. A., and Tellgen, A. (1988). Development and validation of brief measures of positive and negative affect: the PANAS Scale. *Journal of Personality and Social Psychology, 54*, 1063–1070.

[13] Diener, E., Chan, M. Y. (2011). Happy people live longer: Subjective well-being contributes to health and longevity. Applied Psychology. *Health and Well-Being*, *3*, 1–43.

[14] Ryan, R. M., Deci, E. L. (2001). On happiness and human potentials: A review of research on hedonic and eudaimonic well-being. *Annual Review of Psychology*, *52*, 141–166.

[15] Cohen, S., and Pressman, S. D. (2006). Positive affect and health. *Current Directions in Psychological Science*, *15*, 122-125.

[16] Segerstrom, S. C., and Sephton, S. E. (2010). Optimistic expectancies and cell-mediated immunity: The role of positive affect. *Psychological Science*, *21*, 448–455.

[17] Berges, I., Seale, G., and Ostir, G. V. (2011). Positive affect and pain ratings in persons with stroke. *Rehabilitation Psychology*, *56*, 52-57.

[18] Celso, B. G., Ebener, D. J., and Brkhead, E. J. (2003). Humor, coping, health status, and life satisfaction among older adults residing in assisted living facilities. *Aging and Mental Health*, *7*, 438-445.

[19] Ruch, W., Köhler, G., and van Thriel, C. (1997). To be in good or bad humour: Construction of the state form of the State-Trait-Cheerfulness-inventory—STCI. *Personality and Individual Differences*, *22*, 477-491.

[20] Ruch, W. (1997) State and trait cheerfulness and the induction of exhilaration: A FACS study. *European Psychologist*, *2*, 328-341.

[21] Foley, E., Matheis, R., and Schaefer, C. (2002). Effect of forced laughter on mood. *Psychological Reports*, *90*, 184.

[22] Neuhoff, C. C., and Schaefer, C. (2002). Effects of laughing, smiling, and howling on mood. *Psychological Reports*, *91*, 1079-80.

[23] Herzog, T. R., and Strevey S: J. (2008). Contact with nature, sense of humor, and psychological well-being. *Environment and Behavior*, *40*, 747-776.

[24] Kuiper, N. A., and Martin, R. A (1998b). Laughter and stress in daily life: Relation to positive and negative affect. *Motivation and Emotion, 22,* 133-153.

[25] Friedman, H. S., and Booth-Kewley, S. (1987). The "disease-prone personality": A meta-analytic view of the construct. *American Psychologist, 42,* 539-555.

[26] Kuiper, N. A., and Harris, A. L. (2009). Humor styles and negative affect as predictors of different components of physical health. *Europe's Journal of Psychology,* February. Retrieved from http://www.ejop.org/ archives/2009/02/humor-styles-and-negative-affect-as-predictors-of-different-components-of-physical-health.html

[27] Kiecolt-Glaser, J. K., McGuire, L., Robles, T. F., and Glaser, R. (2002). Emotions, morbidity, and mortality: New perspectives from psychoneuroimmunology. *Annual Review of Psychology, 53,* 83-107.

[28] Szabo, A. (2003). The acute effects of humor and exercise on mood and anxiety. *Journal of Leisure Research, 35,* 152-162.

[29] Szabo, A., Ainsworth, S. E., and Danks, P. K (2005). Experimental comparison of the psychological benefits of aerobic exercise, humor, and music. *Humor: International Journal of Humor Research, 18,* 235–246.

[30] Danzer, A., Dale, J. A., and Klions, H. L. (1990). Effect of exposure to humorous stimuli on induced depression. *Psychological Reports, 66,* 1027-1036.

[31] Narula, R., Chaudhary, V., Narula, K., and Narayan, R. (2011). Depression, anxiety and stress eduction in Medical Education: Humor as an intervention. *Online Journal of Health and Allied Sciences, 10,* 7. Retrieved online June 2011, http://www.ojhas. org/issue37/2011-1-7.htm

[32] Kuiper, N.A., and Borowicz-Sibenik, M. (2005). A good sense of humor doesn't always help: Agency and communion as moderators of psychological well-being. *Personality and Individual Differences, 38,* 365-377.

[33] Nezu, A. M., Nezu, C. M., and Blissett, S. E. (1988). Sense of humor as a moderator of the relationship between stressful events and psychological distress: A prospective analysis. *Journal of Personality and Social Psychology, 54,* 520-525.

[34] Strick, M., Holland, R. W., van Baaren, R. B., and van Knippenberg, A. (2009). Finding comfort in a joke: Consolatory effects of humor through cognitive distraction. *Emotion, 9,* 574-578.

[35] Martin, R. A., Puhlik-Doris, P., Larsen, G., Gray, J., and Weir, K. (2003) Individual differences in the uses of humor and their relation to psychological well-being: Development of the Humor Styles Questionnaire. *Journal of Research in Personality, 37,* 48-75.

[36] Kuiper, N. A., Grimshaw, M., Leite, C., and Kirsh, G. A. (2004). Humor is not always the best medicine: Specific components of sense of humor and psychological well-being. *Humor: International Journal of Humor Research, 17,* 135-168.

[37] Cann, A., and Etzel, K. C. (2008). Remembering and anticipating stressors: Positive personality mediates the relationship with sense of humor. *Humor: International Journal of Humor Research, 21,* 157-178.

[38] Chen, G., and Martin, R. A. (2007). A comparison of humor styles, coping humor, and mental health between Chinese and Canadian university students. *Humor: International Journal of Humor Research, 20,* 215-234.

[39] Kazarian S. S., and Martin, R. A. (2004). Humour styles, personality, and well-being among Lebanese university students. *European Journal of Personality, 18,* 209-219.

[40] Carver, C. S., Scheier, M. F., and Miller, C. J. (2009). Optimism. In S. J. Lopez, and C. R. Snyder (Eds.), *Oxford handbook of positive psychology* (pp. 303-312). New York: Oxford University Press.

[41] Richman, L. S., Kubzansky, L., Maselko, J., Kawachi, I., Choo, P., and Bauer, M. (2005). Positive emotion and health: Going beyond the negative. *Health Psychology, 24*, 422-429.

[42] Siahpush, M., Spittal, M., and Singh, G. K. (2008). Happiness and life satisfaction prospectively predict self-rated health, physical health, and the presence of limiting, long-term health conditions. *American Journal of Health Promotion, 23*, 18-26.

[43] Vilaythong, A. P., Arnau, R. C., Rosen, D. H., Mascaro, N. (2003). Humor and hope: Can humor increase hope? *Humor: International Journal of Humor Research, 16*, 79–89.

[44] Beckman, H., Regier, N., and Young, J. (2007). Effect of workplace Laughter groups on personal efficacy beliefs. *Journal of Primary Prevention, 28*, 167-182.

[45] Kazarian, S. S., and Martin, R. A. (2006). Humor styles, culture-related personality, well-being, and family adjustment among Armenians in Lebanon. *Humor: International Journal of Humor Research, 19*, 405-423.

[46] Erickson, S. J., Feldstein, S. W. (2007). Adolescent humor and its relationship to coping, defense strategies, psychological distress, and well-being. *Child Psychiatry AND Human Development, 37*, 255-271.

[47] Hugelshofer, D. S., Kwon, P., Reff, R. C., and Olson, M. L (2006). Humour's role in the relation between attributional style and dysphoria. *European Journal of Personality, 20*, 325–336.

[48] Bilge, F., and Saltuk, S. (2007). Humor styles, subjective well-being, trait anger and anxiety among university students in Turkey. *World Applied Sciences Journal, 2*, 464-469.

[49] Fitts, S. D., Sebby, R. A., and Zlokovich, M. S. (2009). Humor styles as mediators of the shyness-loneliness relationship. *North American Journal of Psychology, 11*, 257-272.

[50] Jovanovic, V. (2011). Do humor styles matter in the relationship between personality and subjective well-being? *Scandinavian Journal of Psychology 52*, 502–507.

[51] Stieger, S., Formann, A. K., and Burger, C. (2011). Humor styles and their relationship to explicit and implicit self-esteem. *Personality and Individual Differences, 50*, 747–750.

[52] Dozois, D. J., Martin, R. A., and Bieling, P. J. (2008). Early maladaptive schemas and adaptive/maladaptive styles of humor. *Cognitive Therapy and Research, 33*, 585-596.

[53] Kuiper, N. A., and McHale, N. (2009). Humor styles as mediators between self-evaluative standards and psychological well-being. *The Journal of Psychology, 143*, 359–376.

[54] Barelds, D. P., and Barelds-Dijkstra, P. (2010). Humor in intimate relationships: Ties among sense of humor, similarity in humor and relationship quality. *Humor: International Journal of Humor Research, 23*, 447–465.

[55] Cann, A., Davis, H. B., and Zapata C. L. (2011). Humor styles and relationship satisfaction in dating couples: Perceived versus self-reported humor styles as predictors of satisfaction *Humor: International Journal of Humor Research, 24*, 1–20.

[56] Bippus, A. M. (2000). Making sense of humor in young romantic relationships: Understanding partners' perceptions. *Humor: International Journal of Humor Research, 13*, 395–418.

[57] Cann, A., Norman M. A., Welbourne, J. L., and. Calhoun L. G. (2008). Attachment styles, conflict styles and humour styles: Interrelationships and associations with relationship satisfaction. *European Journal of Personality, 22*, 131–146.

[58] De Koning, E., and Weiss, R. L. (2002). The Relational Humor Inventory: Functions of humor in close relationships. *American Journal of Family Therapy, 30*, 1-18.

[59] Cann, A., Zapata, C. L., and Davis, H. B. (2009). Positive and negative styles of humor in communication: Evidence for the importance of considering both styles. *Communication Quarterly, 57*, 452-468.

[60] Ibarra-Rovillard, M. S., and Kuiper, N. A. (2011). The effects of humor and depression labels on reactions to social comments. *Scandinavian Journal of Psychology 52*, 448–456.

[61] Hampes, W. P. (2006) Humor and shyness: The relation between humor styles and shyness *Humor: International Journal of Humor Research, 19*, 179–187.

[62] Nezlek, J. B., and Derks, P. (2001). Use of humor as a coping mechanism, psychological adjustment, and social interaction. *Humor: International Journal of Humor Research, 14*, 395–413.

[63] Klein, D. N., and Kuiper, N. A (2006). Humor styles, peer relationships, and bullying in middle childhood. *Humor: International Journal of Humor Research, 19*, 383–404.

[64] Yip J. A., and Martin, R. A. (2006). Sense of humor, emotional intelligence, and social competence. *Journal of Research in Personality, 40*, 1202–1208.

[65] Lefcourt, H. M., and Martin, R. A. (1986). *Humor and life stress: Antidote to adversity.* New York: Springer.

[66] Cohan, C. L, Bradbury, T. N. (1997). Negative life events, marital interaction, and the longitudinal course of newlywed marriage. *Journal of Personality and Social Psychology, 73*, 114-128.

[67] Huuki, T., Manninen, S., and Sunnari, V. (2010). Humour as a resource and strategy for boys to gain status in the field of informal school. *Gender and Education, 22*, 369-383.

[68] Walter, M., Hänni, B., Haug, M., Amrhein, I., Krebs-Roubicek, E., Müller-Spahn, F., and Savaskan, E. (2007). Humour therapy in patients with late-life depression or Alzheimer's disease: A pilot study. *International Journal of Geriatric Psychiatry, 22*, 77–83.

[69] Falkenberg, I, Buchkremer, G., Bartels, M., and Wild, B. (2011). Implementation of a manual-based training of humor abilities in patients with depression: A pilot study. *Psychiatry Research, 186*, 454–457.

[70] Freiheit, S. R., Overholser, J. C., and Lehnert, K. L. (1998). The association between humor and depression in adolescent psychiatric inpatients and high school students. *Journal of Adolescent Research, 13*, 32-48.

[71] Kuiper, N. A., and Martin, R. A (1998). Is sense of humor a positive personality characteristic? In W. Ruch (Ed.), *The sense of humor: Explorations of a personality characteristic* (pp. 159-178). Berlin: Walter de Gruyter.

[72] Düşünceli, B. (2011). The effect of humor styles on psychopathology: examination with structural equation mode. *International Journal of Academic Research, 3*, 224-231.

[73] Porterfield, A. L. (1987). Does sense of humor moderate the impact of life stress on psychological and physical well-being? *Journal of Research in Personality*, *21*, 306-317.

[74] Frewen, P. A., Brinker, J., Martin, R. A., and Dozios, D. J. (2008). Humor styles and personality-vulnerability to depression. *Humor: International Journal of Humor Research*, *21*, 179-195.

[75] Olson, M. L., Hugelshofer, D. S., Kwon, P., and Reff, R. C. (2005). Rumination and dysphoria: The buffering role of adaptive forms of humor. *Personality and Individual Differences*, *39*, 1419-1428.

[76] Ferrin, T., King, B., Morelock, N., Olson, J., and O'Neil, R. (2008). Rumination: A laughing matter? The effects of humor on depressive moods. *Intuition*, *4*, 12-18.

[77] Besser, A., Luyten, P., Blatt, S. J. (2011). Do humor styles mediate or moderate the relationship between self-criticism and neediness and depressive symptoms? *Journal of Nervous and Mental Disease*, 199, 757-764.

[78] Pietrantoni, L., Dionigi, A., (2006). Quando ridere fa male: La relazione tra eventi di vita, stili umoristici e disagio psicologico. *Psicoterapia Cognitiva e Comportamentale*, *12*, 301–316.

[79] Hugelshofer, D. S., Kwon, P., Reff, R. C., and Olson, M. L. (2006). Humour's role in the relation between attributional style and dysphoria. *European Journal of Psychology*, *20*, 325-336.

[80] Gelkopf, M., Kreitler, S., and Sigal, M. (1993). Laughter in a psychiatric ward: Somatic, emotional, social, and clinical influences on schizophrenic patients. *Journal of Nervous and Mental Disease*, *181*, 283-289.

[81] Gelkopf, M., and Sigal, M. (1995). It is not enough to have them laugh: Hostility, anger, and humor-coping in schizophrenic patients. *Humor: International Journal of Humor Research*, *8*, 273–284.

[82] Gelkopf, M. (2011). The use of humor in serious mental illness: A review. *Evidence-Based Complementary and Alternative Medicine*, 1-8.

[83] Aarstad, H. J., Aarstad, A. K., Heimdal, J. H., Olofsson, J. (2005). Mood, anxiety and sense of humor in head and neck cancer patients in relation to disease stage, prognosis and quality of life. *Acta Oto-Laryngologica*, *125*, 557-565.

[84] Merz, E. L., Malcarne, V. L., Hansdottir, I., Furst, D. E., Clements, P. J., and Weisman, M. H. A longitudinal analysis of humor coping and quality of life in systemic sclerosis. *Psychology, Health and Medicine*, *14*, 553-566.

[85] Lebowitz, K. R., Suh, S., Diaz, P. T., and Emery, C. F. (2011). Effects of humor and laughter on psychological functioning, quality of life, health status, and pulmonary functioning among patients with chronic obstructive pulmonary disease: A preliminary investigation. *Heart and Lung: The Journal of Acute and Critical Care*, *40*, 310-319.

In: Humor and Health Promotion
Editor: Paola Gremigni

ISBN: 978-1-61942-657-3
© 2012 Nova Science Publishers, Inc.

Chapter 10

HUMOR IN PSYCHOTHERAPY

Alberto Dionigi

Department of Education, University of Macerata, Italy

ABSTRACT

Humor is a healing matter. The benefits of it are nowadays well known. Even if its healing potential is evident, there is a shortage of interest in studying humor in psychotherapy.

The use of humor in psychotherapy is a controversial topic, but in recent years many therapists and researchers have put their attention on this field. For a long period of time, the interest of humor in psychotherapy has been addressed by psychoanalytic or psychodynamic clinicians, but in the last years interest has been shown by therapists of a variety of orientations. Some clinicians show great interest and emphasis in the use of humor in psychotherapy while others see it only as a negative or non-serious matter.

The purpose of this chapter is to explore the research on the beneficial potential and on maladaptive role of humor in therapy and to encourage skilled, practicing psychotherapists, as well as students, to think about humor as a valuable intervention in psychotherapy.

With this chapter I will take the reader through the use of humor in the psychotherapeutic process and address some specific areas such as the use of humor as an assessment tool and as a facilitator element in building therapeutic alliance. A section will be dedicated to the different orientations that include humor as a technique and a particular attention will be given to the role of humor in group therapy.

A review of humor in therapy would not be complete without mentioning some problems that have been voiced in regard to the therapeutic use of humor and for this reason the last section is dedicated to deepen this aspect.

INTRODUCTION

In the past three decades, the medical and the psychological world has begun to take more seriously the healing power of humor and the positive emotions associated with it. A great deal of evidence establishes a relationship between humor and increased levels of personal well-being and there has been a continuous movement amongst therapists around the world to use humor in psychotherapy [1].

This change has happened in the last few years, while for a very long time humor and psychotherapy appeared as a strange juxtaposition. It could seem strange if we think about the fact that humor has been connected to a number of important human functions such as social acceptance, coping, and physical and mental health, among others [2, 3, 4]. It sounds reasonable to ask why for such a long time little about humor in psychotherapy has been investigated. Researchers of this field suppose that therapists hardly ever agree to incorporate humor into their session because of the idea that a serious person does not use humor and because of the fact that psychotherapy is a serious matter, humor cannot take place, at least in voluntary way.

According with the notion of seriousness of mental disorders, psychotherapists usually tend to take themselves too seriously [5]. Moreover, not only do they see their professional work as important and serious, they see themselves as very important and serious too [6].

Franzini [6] states, "the call for the use of humor in therapy has been longstanding and is growing stronger, even though most of the salubrious claims remain essentially untested empirically" (p. 171). Nevertheless, it must be said that in every relationship, including one where humor is used or appears in the therapeutic process, the use of humor may have positive therapeutic effect if used properly but, if it is used inappropriately or is misinterpreted, humor can have a detrimental effect on the therapeutic relationship. This could be a reason that explains why psychotherapists have been resistant to incorporating humor into their repertoire.

Another possible explanation for the lack of research in this field is the fact that although some psychotherapists use humor in their sessions, they do not make it known. The scarcity of literature about humor in psychotherapy may be seen as a sign of the therapists' tendency to keep their use of humor private in order to avoid criticism [7]. Moreover, psychodynamic therapists who support humor in sessions almost never report their own humor [8].

The way in which humor is employed is an important variable for clinicians to carefully consider in any decision to use humor in clinical practice.

As we have seen in this volume, humor has a high potential in enhancing healing, and if it is used in a positive way can be very useful in strengthening and enhancing therapeutic outcome.

One of the first therapists who expressed interest in the presence of humor in psychotherapy was Sigmund Freud [9], even if he focused on the role of humor as a coping strategy used by the client rather than a useful tool that can be used by therapists to improve personal well-being. Over the years many therapists came into this subject and some of them have had the intuition to give their attention to it and to integrate it as therapeutic skills (e.g. Albert Ellis).

In this regard, has been noted that, even if there is a great deal of research around social functions of humor, much of what is written about humor in therapy is largely opinion-based with little investigated empirically [10].

The study of humor can be quite difficult, and to study humor in psychotherapy can be more difficult due to the fact that when we refer to humor we must keep in mind that its perception is very individual and what can be appreciated as humorous by one person might not be so for another. Humor is a very complex subject, consisting of several constructs and an individual reaction to a humorous stimulus can include the individual's emotional and or cognitive changes as a result of stimulus. With reference to these aspects, the *experience* of humor is a complex interaction that engages an individual's psychological response (laughter), emotional response (mirth) and/or cognitive response (wit) to a humorous stimulus [11].

For some clinicians there is a close relationship between personality and different types of humor that a person finds most amusing. For this reason, some clinicians have proposed that asking psychotherapy patients to tell their favorite jokes might be an useful type of projective test that could be analyzed to diagnose their problem and identify their unresolved needs and conflicts [12].

Furthermore, perception of humor can differ from situation to situation and during the same psychotherapeutic process, due to changes happening during it and to the mental state of the patient: humor is often "situation specific". This last topic states that there is not a "recipe" which explains how to use humor in psychotherapy: to really be completely effective, humor requires a spontaneity, and even an element of surprise. However, it could be useful to have some guidelines in order to help therapists on the way to utilize humor in psychotherapy.

Humor can, in fact, cover several functions: it can represent a way to "break the ice" or begin a counseling relationship while still formative. Furthermore, another very important aspect is the ability to laugh at oneself that is one of the main characteristics of man.

Longitudinal studies found that mature defenses, including the sense of humor, predict greater levels of mental and physical health, life satisfaction, job success, and marital stability, as well as less mood disturbance in stressful times, and the ability to see obstacles, such as exams, as challenges rather than threats [2, 13].

Bennet [14], stated that clients enjoyed humor in therapy and those that did not experience humor in therapy reported terminating therapy due to the lack of humor.

We have seen how many topics are linked to the use of humor in psychotherapy, and to be exhaustive an entire book on it could be written. Unfortunately, most of the literature on humor is based on clinical and other observational and professional experience, rather than findings based on experimental data: not a large number of empirical investigations exist to explore this interesting field.

The aim of this chapter is to provide an updated review of the literature on the use of humor in psychotherapy. The reader is encouraged to explore further the topics which, for a lack of space, could not be presented in this chapter. In this contribution, the terms *psychotherapy* and *counseling,* as well as *patient* and *client,* are used interchangeably.

HUMOR POTENTIAL IN PSYCHOTHERAPY

The use of humor in psychotherapy has been strongly defended and brutally criticized [15]. Humor can be a useful treatment technique in the hands of some psychotherapists or can have destructive effects. In this chapter I intend to analyze the potential, positive and negative, of using humor in a specific setting such as psychotherapy. With the term psychotherapy, we refer to an intentional process by trained psychotherapists to create intervention strategies that are designed to help patients in problems of living with the aim to increase the individual's sense of their own well-being and to decrease psychopathology.

Psychotherapy may be performed by practitioners with a number of different qualifications, including several specialties (e.g. psychotherapists, psychiatrists, psychoanalysts) and they employ a wide range of techniques. The techniques used are based on experiential relationship building, coming from their specific framework as communication, dialogue, homework and so on which are designed to improve the mental health of patients or to improve group relationships (such as in a family).

The goal of psychotherapy is to promote change in clients' emotions, behavior, cognitions, and/or physiology [11]. These four areas interact with each other and one change in one aspect (e.g. cognition) can modulate a change in another (e.g. emotion).

Even if the beneficial effects of humor are widespread, the use of humor in psychotherapy still has a lot of limitations. Freud defined it as the "the most prominent defense mechanism" and very often humor is used to release high levels of anxiety. Starting from him, many theorists and psychologists began to be interested in practicing humor during clinical sessions to test its healing effect. Recently, Corey [16] stated that humor can be effective in counteracting painful effects. He refers to the ability of the therapist in demonstrating the ironic aspects of a situation in order to lead clients to experience some lightheartedness, and help them to overlap their sadness.

Humorous interventions have therapeutic power because of the capacity to produce changes in all the four areas above [17]. Gelkop and Kreitler [18] agree with this vision; for the two researchers, emotional and cognitive aspects of humor are closely interwoven: optimism, for example, may be considered as a direct effect of cognitive aspects of humor. In a similar way, a decreased hostility may reflect a directional emotional change or a mediate cognitive effect due to the increase in positive attitudes towards people.

Moreover, humor can serve several functions: it represents a very effective means of communication and for this reason it is often claimed to be a "social lubricant" and it represents an opportunity for the therapists and the patients alike to share in a meaningful experience which can have therapeutic possibilities [19].

Humor can provide some emotional self-control assistance. Humor can condense a message and say something worth learning. The basic assumption is that if you can laugh at a problem, you imply that you will prevail against it [20]. Another salient aspect is that humor humanizes: it can take you from being a part time professional to the realm of being a full time human. Borcherdt, [20] states that humor ignites 37 different functions in the service of mental health. Far from being exhaustive and complete I will now underline some subjects that can be, in my opinion, the most interesting for psychotherapy.

First of all, humor may *prevent emotional confusion and dizziness* providing relief for the stresses and strains that are a part of resolving permanent individual differences. Second, humor may *increase tolerance*. Ellis [5] points out that when you laugh at yourself, you increase your tolerance levels. Not taking yourself too seriously in this way will facilitate this same tolerance in relating to others and improve your social relationship.

In Borcherdt analyses humor may serve to *discourage self-proving conduct* because those who have the capacity to laugh at themselves can be less inclined to try to prove themselves to one another.

Another important function of humor is that it can *separate your faults from yourself*. According to Ellis [5], humor allows you to take your faults seriously, but yourself lightly. Humor can teach to overreact less and to accept yourself more by taking yourself and others less seriously. This function is strictly related to the fact that humor may be helpful in combating fear of relationships. Moreover, thanks to humor it is possible to expose personality flaws and shortcomings in a non-threatening way.

The last two functions I will focus on refer to the ability that humor has to become a mechanism of self and other discovery and to maintain attention and retention. Laughter can reveal character because humor lowers your guard while exposing thoughts, feelings, and behaviors that you may have never known existed in you.

With regard to the beneficial functions of humor in psychotherapy, humor may function as affiliative behavior [21]. Through humor it is possible to establish and maintain a positive therapeutic relationship and facilitate the therapeutic alliance [22]. Moreover, in general conversation, feelings that might normally be blocked by the lack of a socially acceptable outlet may be communicated safely through the use of humor and it is possible to express emotions and feelings that otherwise would be silent because of the embarrassment they cause to the patient [23].

Very often, we hear the phrase: "Someday, we'll look back at this and laugh". This statement points out that there is a humorous side of stressful events, but our negative emotions deny us any real experience of humor connected with it [24]. With the passage of time, the negative emotions decrease, and we can appreciate the light side of the experience. Some therapists focus on this notion to introduce to their clients incongruous or bizarre aspects that can be viewed in incidents and trauma.

Humor may have several functions and one of them is represented by the role of the psychotherapist in identifying the painful emotions and responding empathetically to the client.

Progress in therapy may be made for the first time after humorously introducing a painful topic which the patient initially laughs about, but then cries about [25].

Sultanoff [17] investigated the role of humor in crisis and found that experiencing a crisis situation is likely to integrate the crisis into the internal emotional being. In this way, people are unable to separate their emotional self from the emotional experience of the crisis.

The reason for reporting these findings is twofold: first, patients may require the help of a psychotherapist after having lived through a crisis event. Second, there is a similarity in emotive response between living a crisis event and an event lived as a crisis. For these reasons, I found it useful to report Sultanoff's ideas in order to lead therapists to bear in their mind that humor can be used across the psychotherapeutic process.

One factor influencing an individual's receptivity to humor about a crisis situation is distance. Distance from the crisis experience may be proximal, emotional, or temporal [11].

With *proximal distance* Sultanoff refers to the experience of being on the outer edges of the crisis but not immersed in it. Individuals who are not in the "proximity" of the crisis are more likely to be receptive to crisis humor.

Emotional distance may be rooted in how individuals view or place meaning on the crisis situation. It is important to take into account that people react differently depending on the meaning each one places on the emotional experience of the crisis. Identical humor about the crisis might be helpful to one individual and harmful to another.

Temporal distance is illustrated by the passage of time. The expression: "Time heals all wounds" illustrates this point. Humor helps to place crisis in perspective and helps to make the crisis more manageable.

Psychotherapists should choose carefully if using humor in crisis situations: sometimes humor may be received negatively and it is clinicians' responsibility to "repair" the interpersonal damage that may result. One way to repair it is to listen carefully to the upsets and pain of the person [11].

Very often clients use humor to transform negative emotions and feelings. Wolfstein [26], investigating the role of humor in loss, believed that patients required an emotional transition from pain and anxiety to more pleasant emotion. "This retaining of contact with a disappointing reality combined with the urgent demand to continue to feel, but to feel something pleasant, is decisive for joking" (p. 25). In this way, humor can help a client transition from negative to coping emotional strategies and to accept their emotional experience [26].

The experience of humor offers a client alternative ways to perceive the events. Humor provides new perspectives [18,15] and increases problem-solving abilities [27]

Meyer [28] argues that thanks to the relaxing elements of humor, people can lower defenses and be more open to seeing the new perspectives required to appreciate humor. Viewing new perspectives and laughing together at them can enhance communication with each other.

Facilitating clients in alternative thoughts, humor invites the client to change distorting thinking patterns. In these ways humor can be used as a useful tool to take apart resistance within the session and makes it possible to create a flexible conversation compared to the rigidity of the previous one [22].

HUMOR IN ASSESSMENT

The use of humor in an early session is generally not recommended because the relationship has still not developed [11]. However, evidence shows how there are a lot of occasions when humor can be effective.

In the first session, patients may initiate humor to serve several purposes, one of most common is to reduce emotional distress and is usually associated with nervous laughter. According to Freud, Vaillant [29] points out that the use of humor is an adaptive and mature defense mechanism which helps clients to gain distance from painful events and memories. Paying attention to nervous laughter and being able to diagnose the reasons may indicate the importance for the therapist to focus on the issues stimulating the laughter.

Moreover, in the first sessions, where client and psychologist are still not confident, there could be a high rate of embarrassment due to the fact that one has to open up and talk about his own problems to a stranger. In this part of the clinical interview it is very common to observe nervous laughter the aim of which is to defuse anxiety and "save face".

Humor, at this time, can be useful to break the ice and put the client at ease, in order to empathize with him and make the clinical session less scary.

Adler [30], endorsed the comment of Dostoyevsky "one can recognize a person's character much better by his or her laughter than by a boring psychological examination" (p.199). Moreover, the lack of joking ability could be associated with disturbances in other emotional areas [31].

Assessing the client's readiness to receive a humorous intervention is not simple, but Sultanoff [11] suggests some guidelines. Psychotherapists could directly ask the clients what they find humorous in order to share the experiences of it, which can reveal styles of humor with which they are most connected. If the therapist knows which type of humor a client enjoys, he/she can adapt humorous interventions to match the client's styles. A client could use humour in a number of ways to mask critical issues, for example by using sarcasm or self-deprecating comments [32].

In agreement with the findings of Martin et al. [33] people who used self defeating humor generally scored lower in self-esteem and this could have led to avoiding positive comments. The self defeating humor would be a deflection of the real issues and an avoidance tactic. It is important to shed light on this exaggerated humor in order to present to the client a more positive reality. Once the client noticed that humor utilized in this way represents an avoidance tactic, the client would begin to focus on the issue at hand [32].

It is important to note that discussing with the client about why something that they produce (in language or in behavior) was funny can provide clues about their intellectual development [34]. Moreover, if the therapist pays attention to humorous behavior (e.g., asking why the client is laughing when talking about some aspects) he can help the client raising self-awareness [16].

Another way to use humor as an assessment tool is to use it as a projective text, just like Rorschach Test. In an early study it was explored the use of cartoons with images open to client interpretation as a tool for establishing the frame and the goal of psychotherapy [35]. Open-ended cartoons were used to provide diagnostic insight and in order to explore thoughts and feelings in a way that minimizes the power-differential. In this study, it is reported the case of a client who, at the end of therapy, thought about the cartoons which related to his own problems because they were truthful: "It made me realize that if I can laugh about that, why couldn't I laugh about my own problems and do something about it" (p. 195). The authors state that using cartoons in this way can help make daunting problems seem manageable [35].

Schnarch [36] discusses clients' use of humor and joke telling within therapy as a demonstration of the changes that were occurring in the clients' lives and the decrease in symptomatology.

Furthermore, the ability to engage in humor can be an assessment of cognitive functioning, [34, 37] and sharing with the therapist a client's favorite joke from his/her own family can be a gateway into other critical incidents or disputes in the client's life [9, 37].

Knowledge of what a client or group laughs at or finds humorous can provide a good deal of information into what they feel and what they are experiencing, and such insight would seem a helpful addition to the interpretive skills of the therapist [38].

Another way to test how a person is humorously gifted is to ask him/her to produce a humorous story in three minutes. If he/she is not able to do it, you can ask him/her to describe an object such as a clock, a pen or a photograph. This method allows us to assess if they are able to produce humor in a situation that, in appearance, is not humorous at all [39].

On the other hand, the lack of humor in a client represents an interesting factor: people who don't use humor could be experiencing a great trauma in their lives [40]. Several studies [1] show how stress, trauma and depression could make an individual humorless and unable to deal with many aspects of daily life. In this way, a lack of humor may represent an indicator of depression or personality disorders [41]. A careful therapist would note the lack of humor as a potential area of concern: the inability to find happiness, joy and humor in life would be an indicator of a client's therapeutic need level [40].

Obviously, humor isn't the only assessment tool used to assist a client: we must keep in mind that the individual response to humor and interpretation of what is humorous would vary for every patient. Moreover, not everybody considers humor as an appropriate strategy to cope with trauma or stress and it could be a great error if a counselor considered a lack of humor response as a pure indicator without considering the communication and appreciation link.

Humor may be used by patients in three major areas: they can use humor to understand incongruity in their lives, to find relief from stress and to express a feeling of superiority [43].

It must be noted that humor as an expression of superiority can be either a mechanism of control or a form of resistance. Patients may use it in order to dissolve their negative feelings of inferiority. With reference to the use of humor as stress relief, clients who utilized it in this way would offer insight into the issues of their lives. The third area is represented by the incongruous use of humor which lets a client recognize the inconsistencies in their environment. The client would reframe the situation with incongruent information. This new focus would allow clients to discover the flaw in fatalistic or dichotomous thinking [42].

Finally, Allport [43], notes that the use of humor (especially sarcasm) by patients may convey rebellion and dissatisfaction with life.

HUMOR AND THERAPEUTIC ALLIANCE

A great deal of research has indicated that one of the most important factors for client change in psychotherapy is the nature of the therapeutic alliance [16, 44].

In establishing a proper alliance between psychotherapist and client, empathy is identified as essential for the development of therapeutic alliance.

Rogers [45], has hypothesized that, in order to be therapeutic and effective and to lead to a change in the client, six specific conditions are necessary. These conditions can be applied to all psychotherapy, not just to client-centered therapy.

These conditions require genuineness in the therapeutic relationship between therapist and client, the ability of the therapist to empathize with the client in this relationship, to have an unconditional positive regard for the client (warmth), and to be able to communicate empathy. Out of these conditions, empathy is the construct that has evoked the most attention from psychotherapists and researchers.

Meyers and Hayes [46] found that therapists who self-disclose general information in relation to client content were found to be more expert than those who did not self-disclose, even if the therapeutic alliance is positive. On the other hand, therapist self-disclosures were related with low expertness by patients if therapeutic alliance was weak.

Humor may have an important role in constructing empathy and in the building of the relationship, because of its property as a social lubricant. Use of humor in relationships of all kinds is related to relationship satisfaction, closeness, and effective resolution of conflict [13].

Moreover, humor may be used by the client to measure the terapist's empathy. When there is a positive alliance, it is easier for humor to appear and in this way clients would open up and feel more relaxed during psychotherapy [47].

It must be said that humor should be genuine, and so should be its use. A therapist who tries in every way to be humorous to his client makes a big mistake, because non-genuine humor is likely to be perceived by the client as manipulative and insincere. Honest humor is more likely to be trusted and can increase the probability of therapeutic alliance.

However, while the potential association between the use of humor in therapy and therapeutic alliance is mentioned consistently, there are currently no published empirical studies dedicated to exploring this relationship specifically [47].

Evidence which investigates the role of humor in building therapeutic alliance is ambivalent: some researchers such as Ackerman and Hilsenroth [48] encourage the open expression of affects and the use of humor in order to develop positive therapeutic alliance. Humor will help foster a degree of mutuality between the clinician and the patient, increasing the alliance [47]. Buckman [49], studying the role of humor in couple therapy, found that humor may be useful in helping to reduce the tension and to offer the clients an acceptable means of expressing strong emotions and that humor can be exposed as the strongest defense mechanism that exists within a couple's relationship. In Buckman's thought an "overuse" of humor by partners is a sign that their emotional intimacy has been disabled, and they are avoiding true connection with one another.

On the other hand, Saper, who has stated that research on humor's use in therapy would be "formidable, if not impossible" [50: 366], cites the results of Golub [51] who in his dissertation tried to investigate the relationship between humor and the therapeutic alliance. In this study significant results were found and no difference was displayed in the clients' preference for either a humorous or non-humorous counselor.

O'Brien [52], conducted a study in which he attempted to control the presence of humor in therapy sessions. He instructed ten therapists, asking them to increase the number of humorous comments made in their sessions to one client.

Results showed no relationship between the use of humor and the therapeutic relationship: alliance was found in both cases. Meyer, who reported this study in his dissertation [47] claims that the main problem with this study may lie with how O'Brien attempted to "control" humor in his study. According to Franzini [6], this methodological issue, where humor is not spontaneous, is an obstacle for the study and new researchers of humor will need to overcome this.

Not only humor, but laughter may have an important role in influencing an attachment relationship between client and therapist: psychoanalytically oriented researchers focus their attention on this theme [52]. Nelson [21] states that the emergence of laughter, and specially of sharing laughter, in a therapy session can be related to an attachment behavior that can give great information about the degree of alliance between client and therapist.

HUMOR AS A THERAPEUTIC TECHNIQUE

The therapeutic potential of humor is nowadays well known and its widespread utility is made known thanks to the Association for Applied and Therapeutic Humor (AATH) founded in 1987 by Alison Crane. AATH is a non-profit professional organization that advances the understanding and application of humor and laughter for their positive benefits. According to this association therapeutic humor is:

> Any intervention that promotes health and wellness by stimulating a playful discovery, expression or appreciation of the absurdity or incongruity of life's situations.

> This intervention may enhance health or be used as a complementary treatment of illness
> to facilitate healing or coping, whether physical, emotional, cognitive, social or spiritual [54].

Another interesting definition of therapeutic humor was given by the editors of the Handbook of Humor and Psychotherapy. Fry and Salameh [55] define therapeutic humor as "constructive, empathic humor, which is totally unrelated to sarcasm, racist or sexist humor, deformations, put-downs and other abuses of humor" (p. xix).

Due to the complexity of the construct, to help the classification, some specific interventions have been categorized as therapeutic humor techniques. Some example of humor techniques employed in psychotherapy are jokes, riddle telling, spontaneous punning, recognizing the absurd, extreme exaggerations, repetition of amusing punch lines, illustrations of illogical reasoning, therapist self-depreciation, demonstration of common human weakness, humorous observations of social interactions, critical humor to promote change, teasing, being provocative, using nicknames, and imagery [6, 14, 56]. Clinicians have different ways to use and to apply it, and the purpose of the next pages is to shed light onto the different techniques.

Due to the fact that there are several ways to use humor in therapy, psychotherapists must take care to use that which is most appropriate for the moment, for the client and for the presented problem [57].

Buttny [58], analyzing a transcript of couple therapy, suggested that humor is useful in therapy activity because it disarms client resistance and creates a space in which to explore contrasting explanations. In his study, the majority of instances were initiated by the therapist in order to design various therapeutic purposes. Humorous interventions may included hyperbole, hypothetical, metaphors, non-lingual vocalizations, repetition, quotes and irony.

In his study, a humorous approach was mainly adopted when disagreement arose, and one of the main conclusions he came up with was that one of the main functions of humor is as a lubricant to decrease potential conflict rather than as a break from therapeutic activity.

Here below, I will focus on some humorous interventions used both alone and in specific therapeutic techniques.

Provocative Therapy

In Freud thought, jokes enable individuals to defend against fear, anxiety, anger, and other disturbing emotions. For the famous psychoanalyst, who used humor in his own sessions when illustrating points or clarifying an insight, humor has a liberating effect on people, providing comfort and help in relieving the pains of misfortunes.

Freud's ideas have been brought into "Provocative Therapy" developed by Farrelly, where humor plays a central role [59]. Provocative therapy assumes the client is not as psychologically fragile as usually considered and that challenging the pathology that the client shows will cause significant change.

Saper [50] notes that among the techniques used by the therapists such as ridicule, exaggeration, distortion, jokes, sarcasm and irony, humor is one of the best ways to highlight clients' maladaptive behaviors while revealing their worst thoughts and fears about themselves. These tactics deprive clients of their usual defensive strategies and therapists are encouraged to ridicule the maladaptive behavior the client displays, rather than the client. Thus humor is employed in a benign and friendly manner [59].

Paradoxical Intention

Frankl, [60] employed a technique called "Paradoxical Intention" in which clients are encouraged to exaggerate their symptoms to the point of absurdity. He claimed that this develops their ability to laugh at their neurotic behaviors, which in turn permits divestment and extinction of symptoms. In paradoxical intention's technique clients are encouraged to try to increase the frequency and exaggerate the severity of their symptoms. This technique has been used to treat several problems such as anxiety disorder, obsessive-compulsive disorder, agoraphobia and depression.

Frankl [60] reports the case of a young physician who consulted him because of his fear of perspiring. In order to cut this circle formation, he advised the patient, in the event that sweating should recur, to resolve deliberately to show people how much he could sweat. This indication had the paradoxical effect of stopping him from sweating and, after suffering from his phobia for four years, he was able, after a single session, to free himself permanently from it within one week. Frankl utilized this technique for several symptoms. Martin [1] stated that the efficacy of this technique is due to the potential of putting the client into a sort of "double bind" that can only be resolved by recognizing the absurdity of their symptoms, enabling them to develop the ability to laugh at their neurotic behavior and to take a feeling of detachment from them.

Rational Emotive Therapy (RET)

Albert Ellis, the founder of Rational Emotive Therapy (RET), believed that people disturb themselves cognitively, emotively, and behaviorally. Ellis [5] stated that "human disturbance largely consists of exaggerating the significance or the seriousness of things, and the ripping up of such exaggerations by humorous counter-exaggeration may well prove one of the main methods of therapeutic attack" (p. 4).

He had the idea to propose humor in therapy, arguing its benefits in an article [5] and video [61] in which he demonstrated some of his own therapeutic strategies through humor. Humor and absurdity are used in RET as "disputing interventions" to challenge clients' false and irrational belief systems. Thanks to the nature of humor, it is possible to lead to change in cognition, emotions and behavior.

Cognitively, humor may be used to present new ideas to the absolutistic and rigid client's thought. Cognitive restructuring can be promoted by puns, witty remarks, shocking language, and sarcasm. Emotively, humor brings enjoyment, leading life to be more worthwhile. Behaviorally, humor may encourage acting differently because it constitutes an anti-anxiety activity and it serves as a diverting relaxant.

Ellis [5] showed that humor may help a person to take a more tolerant view of themselves and what they see as their imperfections, but also of the world when it falls short of their expectations or generates feelings of uncertainty. Humor is also applicable in cognitive-behavioral therapy, as a way to raise awareness of a client's irrational cognitive processing [15].

McGhee in his book reported a piece of a session which a colleague told him about [24: 127]:

"A woman whose husband had died spent a couple of years in therapy, with no real progress. She felt guilty about her husband's death, and could not get past this. She had insisted that her husband do some outside yard work when he preferred to putter around inside. He died of a heart attack while working in the yard. She constantly said to herself, 'If I hadn't insisted on him working outside, he'd be alive today'. She went from therapist to therapist, but no one seemed to be able to help her. Finally, one therapist who had several sessions with her said to her one day, "You know, I've been thinking about it, and I've decided you are right. You killed him. I think you should march right down to the police station and turn yourself in".

The shocked patient suddenly sat up straight and stared at him. After a brief puzzled look, a smile came across her face, and then a short laugh. That was the turning point in her therapy. From that point on, she continued to improve".

This is an interesting example of how a therapist can use exaggeration to help a patient achieve a fundamental insight, specifically that she was not responsible for the conditions inside her husband's body that actually triggered the heart attack.

In cognitive psychotherapy the focus is on changing clients' thoughts, behavior or emotions (or all three). In the example above the targets were emotions and thoughts. The intellectual insight regarding the absurdity of turning herself in for murder generated the positive emotion of joy and exhilaration via the laughter, which in turn helped her begin to unload her guilt [15].

Cognitive Therapy

Humor consists of cognitive processes and contents such as distancing, shifting and optimism. Kreitler and Kreitler [62] show that cognitive acts correspond to specific patterns of meaning variables that characterize the contents (e.g., sensory qualities, function), the structure and the processes (e.g., superordination, modification) of meaning and meaning assignment. The cognitive approach emphasizes, for example, the effects of humor on increasing optimism, and self-efficacy beliefs [63].

Kreitler, Drechsler, and Kreitler [64] discovered that each humorous event is based on two closely interwoven cognitive shifts: a small shift that enables the evocation of a feeling of superiority and helps in bolstering self-esteem and coping with fear and a large shift which fulfills primarily a cognitive role (e.g. evokes surprise and poses a kind of riddle whose solution is intellectually gratifying).

These two modes of humor may have different impacts on physical and psychological well-being: the smaller shifts create an immediate emotional gratification, which might lead to abreaction and catharsis, while the larger shifts enable one to take a new and different view of things.

The two shifts may make life more interesting and intellectually satisfying and may enhance the ability to face conflict with less emotional stress.

Because of its functions, humor seems to be a broad-spectrum tool of cognitive therapy particularly adequate for integration into a variety of therapeutic systems.

Psychodynamic Therapy

Grotjahn [65], according to Freud suggested that the use of humor by a client would allow for tension release. He believed in the potential role of humor to help clients in distressing emotionally harmful situations: he believed this fosters and, as a form of interpretation, enables the bypassing of client resistance.

Thanks to humor the client is able to see both the tragic and humorous simultaneously. Grotjahn stated: "The situation needs not be a comic one. Laughter and tears may be interchanged and may appear in the same person simultaneously" [65: 198].

Grotjahn believed that humor would be an expression often following danger or perceived danger for the client. The dangerous situation creates emotional energy that the client releases as humor or laughter. The response of crying and laughing is the emotional release to understanding the perceived danger has past. A psychotherapist who could identify the seriousness of the joy and tears response would have an empathetic understanding of the perceived danger and the impact on the client.

Behavior Therapy

In an early case study, Ventis [66] compared the efficacy of muscle relaxation and the use of humorous imagery during a session of systematic desensitization in the treatment of a woman who suffered from social anxiety. In that study, Ventis demonstrated that desensitization with humor was effective in only a single session. In the same year, [67] he found that humorous desensitization worked when traditional desensitization failed. Smith found that introducing humor in nine sessions with a young woman, helped her in reducing strong, maladaptive anger.

More recently, Ventis and his colleagues [68] carried on a more carefully controlled study to investigate the use of humor in systematic desensitization in the treatment of spider phobia. Forty students with spider phobia were randomly assigned to either four individual treatment sessions using traditional systematic desensitization with muscle relaxation, four sessions of desensitization using humor, or a third group which did not receive treatment.

In the humor conditions, participants were given homework assignments in which they were asked to generate humorous statements and images relating to spiders.

The results reported that participants in both the humor group and in the standard treatment group showed significant and equally large reductions in their fear of spiders while those in no-treatment did not show any significant improvement.

PROMOTING THE USE OF HUMOR IN THE CLIENT

Humor can directly change a client's emotional state and for this reason it can be used as a treatment modality to relieve negative emotions. Not only can psychotherapists be engaged in producing humor, but they can teach clients to use humor to relieve, for example, anxiety and depression. Using humor in a therapeutic manner can be useful to clients for learning that they can both relieve their emotional distress and be empowered to manage their emotional reactions.

A client suffering from depression can derive benefit when he/she experiences humor, even for a short time. In this way, clients can be taught to seek out humorous experiences outside the therapy sessions as modality of managing their emotional distress.

There are many ways to use humor in counseling without needing to be a comedian. One of the most important factors for humor is the ability to be childlike [69]. Specifically, a counselor, a psychotherapist or other healing professional could give some homework to patients.

The most simple humor "homework" is to prescribe the client to increase his or her opportunities to experience humor [70]. In the mean time it is particularly important to design the homework as well as possible. This means to assess the client's specific humorous appreciation (e.g. comedians, types, etc.) and to focus on it.

To improve a client's sense of humor in face of adversity a therapist could, for example, ask the client, "How would an 8 year old see this situation?" Another technique is to give the client a cartoon that touches on the problem in a more playful way: in this way the client is helped to reframe the issue into a less troublesome perspective.

The therapist could also encourage the client to keep a humor journal every week recalling things that made them laugh or an amusing incident that happened that day or encourage clients to watch funny films, read joke books and attend comedy shows.

To test humorous ability the clinician can ask the clients to share an amusing anecdote or observation during the session or ask him/her to develop a *"Humor First Aid Kit"* including things that make her laugh or bring a smile to her face.

To not take themselves too seriously, psychotherapists could also write a "laughter prescription" asking the client to read their favorite comic strip every morning with coffee.

These are only some of the recommendations suggested by Godfrey [69] and they can be viewed as an interesting way to insert humor in psychotherapeutic process. It must be said, that as medical prescriptions, the laughter prescriptions must be appropriate to the patients and their problems.

TRAINING HUMOR IN THE THERAPISTS' COURSES

Humor is not yet considered a serious matter which can be learned and practiced in academic or specialist courses for psychotherapists.

Psychotherapy is an interpersonal process, in which the relationship between the therapist and the client is arguably the main vehicle for therapeutic change [71]. Clinicians and clients know how often humor and laughter occur during their interactions. For this reason, I believe that clinicians should know both the adaptive and maladaptive function of humor and the way in which it can be useful.

An interesting recent study of individual psychodynamic psychotherapy sessions found that laughter in either the therapist or the client occurred on average every three minutes, with clients laughing more than twice as often as therapists [72].

One possible explanation for the large differences between patient and therapist laugh responses can be the natural reserve of therapists during a psychotherapy session. As we have seen, this supports the idea psychotherapists tend to suppress their expressions of affect in a therapeutic setting. This suppression of affective communication by the therapist is probably due to the desire to focus on the patient.

In the same research, it emerges that therapists were much more likely to laugh in response to comments from the patients than in response to their own comments [72].

In accordance with Sultanoff [73] I believe that integrating humorous interventions into clinical practice follows a process similar to the integration of any therapeutic skill. Psychotherapists need to practice it, just as they do with other communication (e.g. active listening, empathic understanding and so forth).

As the capacity to be empathetic can be trained, the same can be done to improve the sense of humor of a clinician: therapists who have a core capacity to express humor can be trained to improve their sense of humor and to integrate humor into therapy.

In the meantime, we must keep in mind that humor is not always "the best medicine": it is therapeutic if used by clinicians in a genuine manner, in order to communicate empathy and concern for the client. Sharing humorous comments and laughing together may promote feelings of intimacy and friendliness and facilitate the client's trust in the therapist. On the other hand, humor can be harmful if it is used to denigrate clients feelings and perceptions [1]. However, humor can be used in a positive way, teaching the client how to use it in a functional mood [74].

These above are only some examples of how humor can take place in the psychotherapeutic process and recent findings state how it is possible to improve one's personal sense of humor [24].

To learn and practice humor skills, a therapist can begin sharing humorous material such as cartoons and jokes with friends and family. This is on the assumption that the more clinicians practice humor in nonclinical settings, the more humor becomes integrated into their clinical work [73]. Even if it could be a good way to start improving sense of humor, in view of the increasing interest in using humor in therapy, Franzini [75] proposes that effort be directed to developing a formal course in humor training to offer to all psychological therapists, regardless of their specific orientation.

With reference to the improving of the sense of humor there are several models already realized. Although they have not been set up specifically for therapists, I assume that they can be a good beginning that must be integrated with more specific components referring to clinical intervention. Here below, I focus the attention on a couple of programs that I have personally found interesting. The first program I introduce is the one realized by Nevo, Aharohson and Klingman [76]. This program for the improvement of the sense of humor consists of 14 sessions, in which it is possible to work with the different aspects of humor (cognitive, social, motivational, emotional and behavioral). After a primary explanation of what humor and sense of humor consist of, the program focuses on the benefits of humor with reference to the research and the applications of humor in several fields (school, work, etc).

Participants are asked to train themselves in several tasks whose aim is to improve their sense of humor. Tasks consist of telling jokes, using cognitive ABC's method of confronting barriers to the use of sense of humor (especially in therapy), and identifying the limits of humor. Finally, a consistent part of the program consists of participants laughing at themselves to improve their ability not to take themselves too seriously. At the beginning and at the end of the course a questionnaire is given to test changes in their perception of sense of humor.

Another program I would mention is the one realized by Dr. Paul McGhee, who developed this program both to improve the sense of humor and to get the health and coping benefits of it. In his book, Mc Ghee [24] explains his "humor skills training program" and reports evidence from multiple countries documenting its effectiveness in boosting sense of humor.

The basic idea which the program led to is to build key foundation humor skills to have good days when you're in a good mood. Timing is very important for Mc Ghee, and in fact, in his opinion, strengthening one habit/skill at a time avoids extending this habit/skill to daily stressors until the habits are well developed (otherwise, the sense of humor can abandon you when you are under stress). The book provides specific exercises and activities in order to develop each skill over a 1- to 2-week period.

The aim of this program is to first build the habit of becoming a more playful person in general and then it focuses on verbal humor skills, finding humor in everyday life, laughing at yourself and other key humor skills.

As previously written, even if this program has not been specifically designed for clinicians, it can be very useful as part of a more consistent training, which could be integrated with specific notions on humor and mental disorders.

HUMOR IN GROUP THERAPY

Until now I have reported the studies and the findings about humor used in a therapeutic dyad, where a psychotherapist and a patient are involved. Now, I will focus my attention on the use of humor in group therapy, due to the fact that it is a particular setting in which more people are involved.

Within group therapy, humor has been found to have many positive effects on the group process and the work of a group. The use of humor in group therapy shares some of the effects reviewed in individual therapy but also has its own advantages. Humor has been found to help group members bond, relieve tension and hostility, encourage creativity, and add to a successful working phase [1]. Lynch [42], identified two types of humor which he called identification and differentiation. Identification humor is used to create an internal perception that increases in-group cohesiveness and validates commonly held perceptions. Fry [77] found that humor acts to relieve fear, especially social fear: individuals who laugh together become more integrated resulting in strengthened group cohesiveness. McGhee [78] found that laughter helps establish group membership. Differentiation humor separates individuals through differences such as religion, sex, race, beliefs, and so on. Differentiation humor could be interpreted as a power play in communication.

Scogin and Pollio [79] found that long-lasting groups use humor more frequently and for longer amounts of time than short-lasting groups. Peterson and Pollio [38] found that 75% of the humor of group members was negatively targeted toward others and only 7% of the humor was positively targeted. Humor in groups can serve both therapeutically enhancing and distracting functions.

Negative humor directed at someone not in the group was found to be enhancing the therapeutic work of the group, as a method of support to promote group well-being [38].

When aggressive or negative humor was directed at a group member, it has been valued as a means of diverting the conversation and the therapeutic effectiveness of the group was rated as lower.

According to Goldstein [80], humor used in this way is a manipulation tool to stay distant from the work of therapy, a way of psychologically closing oneself off from the ongoing proceedings. These findings endorse the idea that humor increases connections with others and can unite groups in a common purpose.

Specific interventions in group therapy may invite members to share a funny experience around some insight. Using humor in a group should have the function to take advantage of paradoxes within the group, to build cohesiveness, and to tolerate the absurd, the unpredictable and the unanticipated [81].

Gelkopf and Kreitler [18] exploring the studies conducted on the use of humor in group therapy found that the use of humor in group therapy may be presented in terms of the three potential beneficiaries: therapist, patient and group. The authors note that there are some aspects that must be considered such as the stage of the therapy, the type of therapy, and the selection of specific goals and means depend on the needs of the patients. In this way, it is likely that group-related aspects may predominate in the initial phases of the therapy while patient-related and-therapist-related aspects may predominate in the more advanced stages.

Therapist-related aspects: using humor in group therapy may be seen as an aspect related to therapists which can be applied in several ways.

Humor is a very important skill for the therapist: by manifesting humor the therapist shows his or her humaneness. Moreover, the use of incongruity and surprise by means of humor may stimulate the group, evoke curiosity, overcome defenses, and provide a cue for remembering the insight more readily than the verbal interpretations. Because of their role, they can display humorous behavior which the patient may imitate [82].

Patient-related aspects: people involved in group therapy may benefit from humor because it enables the development of a sense of proportion and serves as a communication tool. Humor helps interpersonal relations by strengthening the skill of telling jokes and enhancing a "lighter" view of the world. Introducing oneself in a humorous way may be useful in helping the process of self-disclosure. Humor facilitates overcoming exaggerated seriousness which often serves as a defense against ambiguity.

Group-related aspects: the last aspect refers to the group. As we have seen earlier, to share laughter together can promote a sense of intimacy, belonging, and friendliness in the group [83]. Even in the group, humor and laughter can be used for reducing tension and to introduce topics that otherwise would be difficult to discuss. Humor, may be used to understand a certain dynamic group process, just by paying attention to the timing of humor or laughter.

THE HARMFUL ROLE OF HUMOR IN PSYCHOTHERAPY

A review of humor in therapy would not be complete without mentioning some reservations that have been voiced in regard to the therapeutic use of humor [50].

So far, we have seen how beneficial the use of humor can be in healing mental health, thanks to the active role in defusing tension, approaching intolerable topics and so on. However, we must keep in mind that humor is not only positive: humor may be used for many different purposes and some of them are not positive (e.g. disparagement and ridicule).

One of the most important psychological theories focuses on superiority. Although humor may appear harmless to lay-people, the negative potential of humor has been largely considered since ancient philosophers such as Plato and Aristotle, who centuries ago warned against the dark side of laughter. Humor can have a highly destructive potential and can have opposite results to what is expected. When a therapist decides to use humor with a patient he should keep in mind several factors such as his/her age, sex, culture, mental constructs in order to avoid misunderstandings and not being clear.

Kubie [8], who is a psychoanalytically oriented therapist, highlights the risk in using humor in psychotherapy. He is the most frequently cited author for the article he wrote, entitled The destructive potential of humor in psychotherapy. Specifically, he points out that humor may mask hostility, both for the therapist and the client, may hurt or offend the patient, confuse the patient about the therapist's intent, intensify resistance and seduce the patient sexually or emotionally [21].

Kubie pointed out that the first risk a therapist can run into is that patients might not be taken seriously: whether therapists should emphasize that what was just said is just a joke, this indicates that humor has been used inappropriately and in an insensitive way, as the patient's failure to recognize the stimulus indicates a lack of interest for the feelings and needs of the patient.

Another risk related to its use in therapy occurs when the therapist touches on important topics in a humorous way and this can be perceived in a distorted manner: the patient may believe that certain topics are taboo and should not be discussed seriously. Humor can therefore have the potential to lessen the therapists' credibility in the eyes of the client by humanization of the expert.

Kubie's vision is particularly critical and Pierce [84] similarly, has suggested that although treatment can often involve laughing to be healthy and beneficial, the use of humor in therapy becomes negative when it is used to belittle, laugh at, or mimic the patient. Humor may also be negative when used in a defensive shift of attention from an highly emotional topic and when it is irrelevant to the therapeutic purpose, gratifying only the needs of the therapist and wasting valuable therapy time and energy.

Pierce [84] identified three different kinds of maladaptive humor in therapy. The first one refers to the use of humor by the therapist to aggress against the client. As we have seen earlier, in this kind of humor the therapist belittles, laughs at or mimics the client. Pierce states that this kind of humor is conveyed by feelings of anger both conscious and unconscious with reference to the client. He also suggests, in this case, to refrain from using humor or to use it very sparingly because of the harmfulness of it.

The other two types of humor are less harmful than the first one. One of them refers to the use of humor in a defensive manner, which directs attention away from emerging feelings to transfer to safer territory.

The third non-useful kind involves humorous comments produced by therapists or clients that are not pertinent to the therapeutic purpose. In this type of humor not only can defensive strategies be entered, but comments that drain attention away from the main thrust of the work. One explanation of these kind of comments by therapists could be connected to it being a way to garner a few seconds of narcissistic gratification.

Saper [50] suggested that improper humor is any humor that "humiliates, deprecates, or undermines the self-esteem, intelligence or well-being of a client" (p. 366). Moreover, the misuse of humor creates a negative counseling environment affecting counseling progress [32].

In addition, patients may feel the need to laugh with the therapist to show that they possess a good sense of humor, especially when joviality covers hidden feelings of resentment and stress.

The use of humor by the therapist may make it difficult for patients to express their negative feelings or disapproval. Moreover, even when humor is at the patient's expense he usually feels constrained to join in, if only to prove to the therapist that he has sense of humor. The humorous intervention by the therapist may be viewed in this case as a narcissist behavior, explained in order to be gratified by the patient.

Salameh [85], in an effort to increase research on the use of humor's effect in the therapeutic process, developed the Humor Rating Scale as a tool that could be used to rate live or videotaped psychotherapy sessions. Level 1 refers to destructive use of humor, such as vindictive and degrading humor towards the client, often used in a moment of anger and/or frustration by the therapist. Level 2 refers to harmful humor, which does not focus on the client's needs and is often followed by redemptive comments. Level 3 refers to minimally helpful humor, which attempts to create a warm, inviting therapeutic atmosphere, but remains mostly a response to the client's own humor. Level 4 refers to the very helpful humor, initiated by the therapist which focuses on the problem specifically, assisting the client to view their problems from an objective perspective. Level 5 refers to outstandingly helpful humor that involves an interplay between client and therapist, focusing not only on the problem at hand but also leading to new insights and solutions. As Martin [1] notes, even if the reliability and the validity of this rating scale still needs to be evaluated, it might be a useful instrument for researchers and clinicians wishing to evaluate therapeutic humor.

Using humor too early in a counseling relationship could actually cause a client such discomfort they may choose to terminate counseling. It is important that counselors understand the motivation, implication and effects of humor use with diverse populations. Counselors must also remember to be cautious of over-generalizing and stereotyping individuals during counseling.

CONCLUSION

Humor in psychotherapy is one of the most difficult areas to describe. Therapists may be tendentially divided into two groups: one of them advocates the use of humor in therapy, because they consider it useful both as a skill and technique. The other group prefers not using humor because of the destructive potential. Whether you believe humor should or shouldn't be involved in your therapy session is up to you. There are, however, some recommendations that must be made. As a basic rule, humor always should be benign and pleasant: in this way it contributes to the creation of a non-threatening therapeutic relationship and can elicit and facilitate communication and foster a favorable working relationship between therapist and client. Therapists who decide to use humor should be careful in order to avoid possible misunderstanding in comprehension by patients. For these reasons it is important to use humor therapeutically and it is important that therapists consider it as a skill that must be learned and trained, in the same way as a variety of other clinical skills.

Most of the claims that have been made about potential benefits and damages of humor in psychotherapy are based on personal experience and anecdotal evidence. In the last year an ever increasing number of studies have been emerging, and part of them are based on Conversational Analysis [22, 47, 58], in order to give a more clear example of what happens during therapy sessions and what kind of humor is involved. Further research is necessary to shed light onto this exciting theme that covers a large part of our life.

REFERENCES

[1]   Martin, R. (2007). *The Psychology of Humor. An Integrative Approach*. New York: Academic Press.
[2]   Cann, A., & Calhoun, L. (2001). Perceived personality associations with differences in sense of humor: Stereotypes of hypothetical others with high or low senses of humor. *Humor, 14*, 117-130.
[3]   Casado-Kehoe, M., Vanderbleek, L., & Thanasiu, P. (2007). Play in couples counseling. *The Family Journal: Counseling and Therapy for Couples and Families, 15*, 133-136.
[4]   Martin, R. (2001). Humor, laughter and physical health: Methodological issues and research findings. *Psychological Bulletin, 127(4)*, 504-519.
[5]   Ellis, A. (1977). Fun as psychotherapy. *Rational Living, 12*, 2-6.
[6]   Franzini, L. (2001). Humor in Therapy: The Case for Training Therapists in its Uses and Risks. *Journal of General Psychology, 128(2)*, 170-193.
[7]   Baker, R. (1993). Some reflections on humour in psychoanalysis. *International Journal of Psycho- Analysis, 74(5)*, 951-960.
[8]   Kubie, L. (1971). The destructive potential of humour in psychotherapy. *American Journal of Psychiatry, 127(7)*, 861-866.
[9]   Freud, S. (1960). *Jokes and their Relation to the Unconscious* (original edition 1928). New York, NY: Norton & Co.
[10] Golan, G. & Jaffe, E. (2007). Humour in psychotherapy. British Journal of Psychotherapy, 4(4), 393-400.

[11] Sultanoff, S. M. (1994). Choosing to be amusing: Assessing an individual's receptivity to therapeutic humor. *Journal of Nursing Jocularity, 4*, 34-35.

[12] Zwerling, I. (1955). The favorite joke in diagnostic and therapeutic interviewing. *Psychoanalytic Quarterly, 24*, 104-114.

[13] Cann, A., Norman, M., Welbourne, J., & Calhoun, L. (2008). Attachment styles, conflict styles and humour styles: Interrelationships and associations with relationship satisfaction. *European Journal of Personality, 22*, 131-146.

[14] Bennett, C. (1996). *An investigation of clients' perception of humor and its use in therapy* (Unpublished Dissertation). Denton, TX: Texas Women's University.

[15] Richman, J. (1996). Points of correspondence between humor and psychotherapy. *Psychotherapy, 33*, 560-566.

[16] Corey, G. (2005). Gestalt theory. In L. Gebo & S. Gesicki (Eds.), *Theory and Practice of Counseling and Psychotherapy* (7th edition, pp. 192-223). Belmont, CA: Brooks/Cole.

[17] Sultanoff, S. (1992). *The Impact of Humor in the Counseling Relationship. Laugh It Up*, Publication of the American Association for Therapeutic Humor, 1

[18] Gelkopf, M. & Kreitler, S. (1996). Is humour only fun, an alternative cure or magic: The cognitive therapeutic potential of humour. *Journal of Cognitive Psychotherapy, 10(4)*, 235-254.

[19] Pearson, D. F. (1980). Clinical Humor: A Positive Approach Toward Health. *AMCAP Journal*, 19-23.

[20] Borcherdt, B. (2002). Humor and its contributions to mental health. *Journal of Rational-Emotive & Cognitive-Behavior Therapy, 20, Nos. ¾*

[21] Nelson, J. (2008). Laugh and the world laughs with you: An attachment perspective on the meaning of laughter in psychotherapy. *Clinical Social Work Journal, 36*, 41-49.

[22] Jeffrey, S. (2009). *Questioning the importance of being earnest: A conversation analysis of the use and function of humour in the serious business of therapy* (Unpublished Dissertation). Hatfield, UK: University of Hertfordshire.

[23] Winick, C. (1976). The social contexts of humor. *Journal of Communication, 26(3)*, 124-128.

[24] McGhee, P. E. (2010). *Humor. The Lighter Path to Resilience and Health.* Bloomington, IN: Authorhuse.

[25] Haig, R. (1988). *The Anatomy of Humor: Biopsychosocial and Therapeutic Perspectives.* Springfield, IL: Charles C. Thomas.

[26] Wolfstein, M. (1978). *Children's Humor: A Psychological Analysis.* Bloomington, IL: Indiana University Press.

[27] Rosenheim, E., & Golan, G. (1986). Patients' reactions to humorous interventions in psychotherapy. *American Journal of Psychotherapy, 40*, 110-124.

[28] Meyer, J. (2000). Humour as a double-edged sword: Four functions of humour in communication. *Communication Theory, 10(3)*, 310-331.

[29] Vaillant, G. E. (2000). Adaptive mental mechanism: Their role in a positive psychology, *American Psychologist, 55(1)*, 89-98.

[30] Adler, A. (1956). The individual psychology of Alfred Adler. New York: Basic Books.

[31] Smith, E. E. & White, H. L. (1965). Wit, creativity, and sarcasm. *Journal of Applied Psychology, 49*, 131-134.

[32] Gladding, S. (1995). Humor in counseling: Using a natural resource, *Journal of Humanistic Education and Development, 34(1)*, 3-12.

[33] Martin, R., Puhlik-Doris, P., Larsen, G., Gray, J., & Weir, K. (2003). Individual differences in uses of humor and their relation to psychological well-being: Development of the Humor Styles Questionnaire. *Journal of Research in Personality, 37*, 48-75.

[34] Bergen, D. (1998). Development of the Sense of Humor. In W. Ruch (Ed.), *The Sense of Humor: Explorations of a Personality Characteristic* (pp. 329-360). Berlin, Germany: Mouton de Gruyter.

[35] Simon, K. (1995). Leunig cartoons as therapeutic letters: Crafting a viable therapeutic focus for change. *Australian and New Zealand Journal of Family Therapy, 16*, 190-200.

[36] Schnarch, D. (1990). Department of redundancy department: Humor in psychotherapy: Therapeutic uses of humor in psychotherapy. *Journal of Family Psychotherapy, 1*, 75-86.

[37] Lemma, A. (2000). *Humour on the Couch: Exploring Humour in Psychotherapy and Everyday Life*. Philadelphia, PA: Whurr.

[38] Peterson, J. & Pollio, H. (1982). Therapeutic effectiveness of differentially targeted humorous remarks in group psychotherapy. *Group, 6(4)*, 39-50.

[39] Turner, R. G. (1980). Self-Monitoring and Humor Production. *Journal of Personality 48(2)*, 163-172.

[40] Bordan, T., & Goldin, E. (1999). The use of humor in counseling: The laughing cure. *Journal of Counseling and Development, 77(4)*, 405-410.

[41] Forabosco, G. (1998). The ill side of humor. In W. Ruch (Ed.), *The Sense of Humor: Explorations of a Personality Characteristic* (pp. 271-292). Berlin, Germany: Mouton de Gruyter.

[42] Lynch, O. (2002). Humorous communication: Finding a place for humor in communication research. *Communication Theory*, 423-445.

[43] Allport, G. (1955). *Becoming: Basic Considerations for a Psychology of Personality*. New Haven, CT: Yale University Press.

[44] Rogers, C. (1961). *Client-centred Therapy: Its Current Practice, Implications and Theory*. London: Constable.

[45] Rogers, C. (1961). *On Becoming a Person: A Therapist's View of Psychotherapy*. London: Constable.

[46] Meyers, D., & Hayes, J. (2006). Effects of therapist general self-disclosure and countertransference disclosure on ratings of the therapist and session. *Psychotherapy: Theory, Research, Practice, Training, 43*, 173-185.

[47] Meyer, K. J. (2007). *The relationship between therapists' use of humor and therapeutic alliance*. (unpublished dissertation). Ohio, USA: School of The Ohio State University.

[48] Ackerman, S. J., & Hilsenroth, M. J. (2003). A review of the therapist characteristics and techniques positively impacting the therapeutic alliance. *Clinical Psychology Review, 23*, 1-33.

[49] Buckman, E. S. (1994). Humor as a communication facilitator in couples' therapy. In E. S. Buckman (Ed.), *The Handbook of Humor: Clinical Applications in Psychotherapy* (pp. 75-90). Malabar, FL: Krieger.

[50] Saper, B. (1987). Humor in Psychotherapy: Is It Good or Bad for the Client? *Professional Psychology: Research and Practice, 4*, 360-367.

[51] Golub, R. R. (1979). *An investigation of the effect of humor in counseling.* Unpublished doctoral dissertation, Purdue University.

[52] O'Brien, E. E. (2001). *Humor, the therapeutic relationship, and outcome.* Unpublished doctoral dissertation, Indiana University Pennsylvania.

[53] Siebold, C. (2006). Female sexual agency: Evolving psychoanalytic ideas. *NMCOP Newsletter*, Winter, 3-13.

[54] AATH - Association for Applied and Therapeutic Humor. (n.d.). Retrieved May 25, 2011, from http://www.aath.org/

[55] Fry, W. F., & Salameh, W. A. (Eds.). (1987). *Handbook of Humor and Psychotherapy: Advances in the Clinical Use of Humor.* Sarasota, FL: Professional Resources Press.

[56] Kuhlman, T. L. (1984). *Humor and Psychotherapy.* Homewood, IL: Dow Jones-Irwin.

[57] Blevins, T. L. (2010). *Humor in Therapy: Expectations, Sense of Humor, and Perceived Effectiveness* (Unpublished Dissertation). Auburn, Alabama: Auburn University.

[58] Buttny, R. (2001). Therapeutic humour in retelling the clients' tellings. *Text, 21(3)*, 303-326.

[59] Farrelly, F., & Brandsma, J. (1974). Provocative therapy. Millbrae, California: Celestial Arts.

[60] Frankl, V. E. (1960). Paradoxical intention: A logotherapeutic technique. *American Journal of Psychotherapy, 14*, 520-535.

[61] Ellis, A. (1977). Fun as psychotherapy. New York: Albert Ellis Institute.

[62] Kreitler S., & Kreitler H. (1990). *The Cognitive Foundations of Personality Traits.* New York: Plenum.

[63] O'Leary, A. (1992). Self-efficacy and health: behavioral and stress-physiological mediation. *Cognitive Therapy and Research, 16*, 229-245.

[64] Kreitler, S., Drechsler, I., & Kreitler, H. (1988). How to kill jokes cognitively? The meaning structures of jokes. *Semiotica, 68*, 297-319.

[65] Grotjahn, M. *Beyond Laughter: Humor and the Subconscious.* New York: McGraw-Hill, 1957.

[66] Ventis, W. L. (1973). Case history: The use of laughter as an alternative response in systematic desensitization. *Behavior Therapy, 4(1)*, 120-122.

[67] Smith, R. E. (1973). The use of humor in the counterconditioning of anger responses: A case study. *Behavior Therapy, 4*, 576-580.

[68] Ventis, W. L., Higbee, G., & Murdock, S. A. (2001). Using humor in systematic desensitization to reduce fear. *Journal of Genaral Psychology, 128(2)*, 241-253.

[69] Godfrey, J. (2004). Toward optimal health: The experts discuss therapeutic humor. *Journal of Women's Health, 13*, 474-479.

[70] Sultanoff, S. (1998). Humor and Wellness-Melding the Present and the Future: Humor and Heart Disease. *Therapeutic Humor, 12(5)*, 1-2.

[71] Teyber, E. (1988). *Interpersonal Process in Psychotherapy: A Guide for Clinical Training.* Chicago: Dorsey Press.

[72] Marci C. D., Moran, E. K. & Orr, S. P. Physiologic Evidence for the Interpersonal Role of Laughter During Psychotherapy. *Journal of nervous & Mental disease, 192(10)*, 689-695.

[73]   Sultanoff, S. (2002). Integrating humor into psychotherapy. In C. E. Schaefer (Ed.). *Play Therapy with Adults* (pp. 107-143). Hoboken, NJ: John Wiley & Sons.

[74]   Olson, H. A. (1994). The use of humor in psychotherapy. In H.S. Strean (Ed.), *The Use of Humor in Psychotherapy* (pp. 195-198). Northvale, NJ: Jason Aronson

[75]   Franzini, L. (2000). Humor in Behavior Therapy. *The Behavior Therapist, 23,* 23-41.

[76]   Nevo, O., Aharonson, H., & Klingman, A. (1998). Improving sense of humor. In W. Ruch (Ed.) *The Sense of Humor: Explorations of a Personality Characteristic* (pp. 385-404). Berlin, Germany: Mouton de Gruyter.

[77]   Fry, W. F. (1978). Humor: Boon and curse. Address given at the *Annual Convention of the American Orthopsychiatric Association*, San Fransisco, CA.

[78]   McGhee, P. E. (Ed.). (1979). *Humor: Its Origin and Development*. San Francisco, CA: W.H. Freeman.

[79]   Scogin, F., & Polio, H. (1980). Targeting and the humorous episode in group process. *Human Relations, 33,* 831-852.

[80]   Goldstein, J. (1976). Theoretical notes on humor. *Journal of Communication, 26(3),* 104-112.

[81]   Napier, A. & Withaker, C. (1978). *The Family Crucible*. New York: Harper and Row.

[82]   Yalom, I. (1985). *Theory and Practice of Group Psychotherapy*. New York: Basic Books.

[83]   Kahn, W. A. (1989). Toward a sense of organizational humor: Implications for organizational diagnosis and change. *Journal of Applied Behavioral Sciences, 25,* 45-63.

[84]   Pierce, R. (1994). Use and abuse of laughter in psychotherapy. In H. Strean (Ed.), *The use of Humor in Psychotherapy* (pp. 105-111). Northvale, NJ: Jason Aronson.

[85]   Salameh, W. A. (1987). Humor in Integrative short-term therapy (ISTP). In W. F. Fry Jr & W. A. Salameh, (Eds.), *Handbook of humor and Psychotherapy: Advances in the Clinical Use of Humor* (pp. 195-240). Sarasota, FL: Professional Resource Exchange.

In: Humor and Health Promotion
Editor: Paola Gremigni

ISBN: 978-1-61942-657-3
© 2012 Nova Science Publishers, Inc.

Chapter 11

CLOWNS IN HOSPITALS

Alberto Dionigi,[1,2], Roberto Flangini[2] and Paola Gremigni[3]
[1]Department of Education, University of Macerata, Italy
[2]Association "l'Aquilone di Iqbal" APS, Cesena, Italy
[3]Department of Psychology, University of Bologna, Italy

Abstract

In recent decades, humor has become to be considered as an important component of mental and physical health other than a mere socially desirable individual's trait. Clown therapy represents a peculiar way of using humor in order to promote people's well-being. Clown therapy officially started in 1986 and presently, it is easy to meet clown doctors in hospitals. Nevertheless, it is necessary to clarify their position and role, because when thinking about clowns in hospitals, ordinary people see them as just volunteers dressing in a clown's clothes whose primary purpose is to entertain hospitalized patients. As clown doctors, two of the authors of this chapter know that this activity is much more than that. To become a successful clown doctor is required a thorough and accurate training, because his mission is challenging. The real goal of this professional is to work with the patient's emotion, to reduce anxiety related to hospitalization, treatment and the disease itself. To regularize all the Clown Care Units spread across the globe, many Federations of clowns have been set up in many countries. Their goal is to determine the role and status of clown doctors, along with providing adequate training.

INTRODUCTION

Dr. Thomas Sydenham, an eminent physician who lived in the 17th century, used to say that the arrival of a brilliant clown exercises a more beneficial impact on the health of a town than the arrival of twenty asses laden with drugs [1]. This statement clearly shows how clown therapy is not an invention of our time. Clown therapy is defined as the implementation of clown techniques derived from the circus world to contexts of illness, so as to improve people's mood and state of mind [1]. Clowns have probably worked in hospitals since the time of Hippocrates, as doctors of that era thought that a good mood positively influenced the healing process. However, the presence of professional clowns working in hospitals as part of the healthcare team dates back to thirty years ago. The birth date of clown therapy dates back to 1986, when Karen Ridd in Winnipeg and Michael Christensen in New York independent to each other began the practice of clown in broad pediatric hospitals. Karen Ridd (Robo the Clown), a child life specialist, founded the first Canadian therapeutic clown program at Winnipeg Children's Hospital. Almost simultaneously, Christensen, a famous clown of the Big Apple Circus, stable in New York, founded the Big Apple Circus Clown Care. This was founded after that Christensen's brother (another clown working in the Big Apple Circus) was hospitalized for cancer in the Presbyterian Hospital, in New York. During his staying in the hospital, he was frequently visited by his fellow colleagues that came to his room dressed in their usual clown suit [2]. The medical staff noted that the arrival of clowns in the hospital had a beneficial effect on the other hospitalized patients: these strange and peculiar visitors amused patients and made them laugh. The most significant outcome of these visits was that patients felt happier and, as their mood improved they needed to take fewer drugs.

Unfortunately, Christensen's brother died, but before dying, he gave him as a gift a leather doctor's bag. After the death of his brother, Michael started to wonder what use he could make of that bag and decided to use it to act as a clown (doctor) in the hospital. Michael, whose clown's nickname was Mr. Stubbs, decided to work in pair with a female clown, known as Great Grandma. So, in 1986 the first couple of clown doctors entered the hospital wards and started the first clown therapy intervention in USA. Dr. Stubbs and all the Big Apple Circus artists created moments of pleasure to animate children's staying during their hospitalization in the pediatric wards. They then found the first Clown Care Unit (a stable support unit formed by clowns). This event was followed by other clowns in Boston, Los Angeles, San Francisco and throughout the United States. In a few months, other 17 projects in pediatric hospitals distributed throughout the country were carried out involving about 90 professional clowns and 200,000 patients.

These experiences acted as catalysts for many programs around the world, so other associations of clown therapists were set up and many clowns left the world of the circus and entered hospitals and health care settings to work as clown therapists.

For example, the first Clown Care Unit in Europe was set up in France by Caroline Simonds. Caroline was one of the first clown doctors who worked with Big Apple Circus Clown Care Unit in New York City. In 1991 she decided to move to France and to set up the association Le Rire Medecine.

Two years later, in 1993, Jan and André Poulie founded the Theodora Foundation in Switzerland, in memory of their mother, Théodora. Nowadays, over 160 Theodora Giggle Doctors work in 8 countries.

Ridd and Christensen represent two main approaches to the way clowns work in hospital: the solo therapeutic clown (Robo) and clown doctors who work in pairs (Mr. Stubbs and Great Grandma). Although there are also other models of practice for clown working in hospitals, in this chapter we refer to the activity of a specially trained professional artist, not a medical doctor, who works in hospital or health care facility as an integral component of the health care delivery system.

HUMOR AND CLOWNING

One of the most salient aspects related to clowning is humor. The purpose of clowning is to bring smiles and laughter to an audience of all ages. Contrary to popular opinion, clowns are not strictly children's entertainers, as adults may enjoy clowns too. An effective clown makes people laugh so humor is his main instrument. He should be able to accept humor as an integral part of life, improve his personal sense of humor, listen and learn how other people recognize and use humor, and be prepared to respond to other people's humor.

Sigmund Freud was so interested in humor and wit to devote an entire book to this fascinating construct. In *Jokes and Their Relation to the Unconscious* [3], Freud analyzed the relationship between laughter, humor and their role in discharging repressed instinctual energy, due to sexual and aggressive impulses. Freud thought that the release of libidinal energy (both aggressive and sexual) is the source of *tendentious jokes*, while the cognitive "joke-works" are called *non-tendentious* jokes. As an effect of the unconscious, a joke has a recurring nature and leads to the end of psychical energy release. Here, we have Freud's description of laughter: "We should say that laughter arises if a quota of psychical energy, which has earlier been used for the catharsis of particular psychical paths has become unstable, so that it can find free discharge" [3: 147].

From his view point, humor is necessary to deal with life adversity and everyday life, as people generally tend to be unhappy. Children, in fact, tend to laugh easily, but grown-ups have more difficulties in spotting the funny side of things. A research states that children usually laugh 400 times a day, whereas adults only 15 [4]. Where do the other 385 laughter go? Growing up we tend to lose our spontaneity, which remains a characteristic trait of children.

In Freud's opinion humor is a tool that allows individuals to find happiness even in adverse events and circumstances. He calls it a defense mechanism. Today we might state that humor is a coping strategy. Although Freud did not analyze the relationship between humor and good health, he believed that it is not possible to be happy without having a sense of humor and without using it.

During the last half of the 20th century, a tremendous change happened in health's research: clinicians, medical doctors, and psychologists began to study the effects of laughter both on the body and mind, from a scientific perspective. It was in this scenario that clowning had the possibility of being introduced into the hospital and became the currently well-known practice.

CLOWN THERAPY AND HEALTH

Although physicians and philosophers have been making claims about health benefits of humor and laughter for centuries, this idea has become increasingly popular only in recent decades. In 1979, Norman Cousins published an account of his recovery from ankylosing spondylitis following a self-prescribed treatment regimen based on daily laughter and vitamin C [5]. The subsequent popularization of alternative approaches to medicine gained humor, laughter and their therapeutic benefits widespread acceptance [6]. In addition, the medical world began to get more serious consideration of the healing power of humor and the positive emotions associated with it [7]. All these aspects favored the formal establishment of the clown therapy and sanctioned its official entry in hospitals, where the clowns had worked occasionally, from ancient times.

In many ways, the hospital setting is the antithesis of the home environment. Illness and death often cast a shadow of intense seriousness, interfering with the expression of the full range of emotions. As we have seen, a person laughs about 15 times a day [4]. In hospitals, however, this figure can drop to zero.

Hospitalization is considered an adverse event in life, usually causing distress that may become traumatic, especially for children [8]. Even a minor pediatric hospitalization can have negative consequences on the emotional, behavioral, cognitive, and educational development of a child [9]. Feelings of tension, uneasiness, and anxiety are some of the many symptoms that children may experience during the hospitalization period [10,11].

Parental anxiety is also most common during hospitalization due to the perception of the child's pain and their personal worries and fears [12]. In particular, if a child has to undergo surgery, parents are expected to develop high levels of anxiety. Interestingly, research has shown that children's preoperative anxiety is associated with parental anxiety [10]. Hence, some hospitals have developed, over time, various programs of support for hospitalized patients. These programs include various forms of art therapy and play therapy for children. Nowadays, it is very likely to find hospital rooms provided with DVD players that play comic movies and library shelves filled with comic books. In addition, in recent years, clown therapy has become an integral part of the hospital setting. Clowns and their humor have entertained human beings for centuries. However, there is little scientific literature that demonstrates a significant research evidence base on the effectiveness of clown humor as a therapy within children's hospitals/units.

In pediatrics, humor is increasingly present in the hospital setting, and it often employs clowns based on the assumption that humor is associated with the well-being of patients [9]. Clinical staff has noted that the main advantage of humor therapy is represented by its distracting technique, which keeps the patients' minds away from concerns related to their illness and consequent depressed mood, thus promoting a healthy expression of emotions [13].

A qualitative study of children's perceptions of hospital clown humor, using the draw and write/draw and tell techniques, showed that children appreciate the beneficial effects of a clown visit to them during their hospital stay [14]. In fact, before the clown visit, the majority of children's written comments made to annotate their drawings were negative (i.e., scared, sad, worried, nervous, etc.). Subsequent to the clown doctor visit there was a significant increase in the positive written comments with no negative verbal comments recorded.

Another qualitative study reported that children liked playing with clowns, during their hospital stay. The majority of parents agreed that the presence of clown doctors has a positive impact on sick children and their families. The majority of the pediatricians who participated in the study also agreed that the presence of clown doctors has a positive impact on sick children and their families during a hospital stay [15].

A survey to address the impact of therapeutic clowning from the perspectives of pediatric health care professionals and parents of hospitalized children reported similar findings [16]. In terms of how staff viewed the work of the therapeutic clown, 88% believed it was to engage children in play; a large number of employees (76%) believed that clowns were a part of the health care team, and 93% of staff believed that the clown program was beneficial to the hospital. For parents, 88% viewed the role of the clown as making children happy. The majority of parents (80%) enjoyed the clown visits, and believed their children did too; 94% of parents acknowledged that their child was happier following a clown visit than was before.

The literature on humor in hospital wards across different age levels shows that not only patients and medical staff benefit from humor, but interactions involving humor between hospital staff and patients foster an atmosphere in which laughter and humor self-perpetuates [14]. Other investigations report that humor has beneficial effects on stress related to terminal illnesses, on pain tolerance, and on cognitive functions such as memory and anxiety [6].

However, clear outcomes cannot be assessed from descriptive data obtained from surveys. Comprehensive studies using experimental designs and inferential statistics should be used to do an in-depth analysis of therapeutic clowning in pediatric settings.

Two pilot studies at Columbia University [17,18] focused on the effectiveness of clowns as distractive presences during cardiac catheterization and invasive procedures in a pediatric oncology day clinic. Results showed that, during cardiac catheterization, there were significant decreases in observed child suffering, in child self-reported distress and parent-rated child distress with the clowns present. As a result, physicians found that the procedure was significantly easier to implement with the clowns present than without them. In addition, positive changes in the behavior and mood of health care providers were observed when the clowns were around.

An Italian randomized controlled study investigated the effects of the presence of clowns on a child's preoperative anxiety during the induction of anesthesia and on the parent who accompanied the child [19]. The clown group was significantly less anxious than the control group, during anesthesia induction. Similar findings were cited in other studies. A recent quasi-experimental study examined the effects of medical clowns on psychological distress of allegedly sexually abused minors during pediatric anogenital examinations [20]. Results indicated that children accompanied by a medical clown during examination expressed less fear, reported reduced pain levels and had reduced quantities of invasive thoughts.

Another controlled study investigated whether clown intervention could reduce preoperative fear of children undergoing minor surgery, taking into consideration also parental anxiety [21]. Compared to the control group of children accompanied only by parents, the group of children accompanied by parents and a couple of clowns showed a decrease in preoperative worries and emotional responses both in children and parents.

Other studies, that investigated the same issue with rigorous scientific methods, reported less encouraging results than those mentioned above. In a randomized controlled study, the experimental group of pediatric patients showed an increase in self-reported and parent-reported psychological well-being immediately after a clown visit, compared to the control group, but these effects were not maintained four hours later [22]. Another recent study investigated the effect of the presence of a hospital clown on children treated with botulin toxin in an outpatient setting (botulin toxin injection is a painful procedure and a stressful experience for the child). Results indicated that not all children, the majority of whom had spastic cerebral palsy, showed beneficial effects from the presence of a clown [23]. The effect of the clown was significantly related to patient gender. Girls were found to have a significantly shorter period of crying when the clown was there. For children younger than 8 years, the impact on boys was negative.

Overall, the existing studies concerning clown performances found decreased levels of distress in the child and parents and increased cooperation of children who undergo medical procedures [9,19]. These studies show that those children who benefited from clown performances felt less concerned about hospitalization, medical procedures, illness and their negative consequences; they also reported a more positive emotional states (felt happier and calmer) than those who did not benefit from clown therapy. These results seem to support the hypothesis that humor and specifically the clown doctor's presence may reduce the suffering of hospitalized children. Nevertheless, the results are not unique and consistent across the studies, especially the most recent. In addition, not all the studies are methodologically exempt from criticism. Therefore, the promising findings of several studies concerning the positive effect of the clown therapy in the hospital wards need to be verified with scientifically rigorous research designs and measures.

Finally, an area that is promising but still understudied is that of clowning for older people and staff in residential facilities. Recent research carried out in Canada as part of the "Down Memory Lane" project suggests that elder clowns may help seniors improve communication skills, mood, and quality of life [24,25,26]. Elder clowns may also help some older people with dementia connect to their immediate surroundings, and restore a sense of autonomy to individuals who have very little control over their lives. This activity is especially helpful for residents who do not receive many visitors. In addition, the presence of elder clowns can have a positive effect on the feelings of staff members caring for older people. A demonstration of the increasing interest in this area is the fact that the prestigious medical journal *The Lancet* has recently published a paper, in the section dedicated to the art of medicine, on the work of elder clowns [27].

THE CLOWN DOCTOR'S PROFILE

Clown doctors are highly skilled professional performers who have undergone an audition process and initial training to work in the sensitive hospital setting. Once they are allowed into health care settings, clown doctors collaborate with the medical and paramedical staff, to allay the anxiety and fear that the hospitalized children and their family feel.

The difference between clown and clown doctors is significant and noteworthy. The term 'clown doctor' specifically may refer to:

- Volunteers who have carried out a specific training to improve their psychological skills and capacity of clowning within various professional contexts they may work (e.g. hospitals, communities, etc.);
- Non-professional artists who have been trained as a professional clown doctors;
- Professional artists (not volunteers) with a show-business or theatrical experience who have been specifically trained in order to adjust their artistic skills to medical and clinical settings [1].

Therefore, a clown doctor is someone who (regardless of his/her qualification) operates in the context of distress using the technique of clowning and integrating it with knowledge of psychosocial health so as to act on emotions and change them. Clown doctors should be seen as providers of support and practical support during treatment programs for hospitalized children and adults.

Play, spontaneity, lightheartedness, humor and creativity are the key ingredients in the healing process. Clown doctors serve both as catalysts for change and gauges of health along the way. Clown therapy is based on performance that fosters humor, creates a light-hearted atmosphere, and relaxes the person at both physical and mental level [28].

The purpose of clown therapy is to be ironic about medical practices, in order to alleviate certain states of anxiety that can be exceedingly distressful for children and adults who are suffering. It also aims to support children's caregivers. This practice focuses specifically on the "healthy part" of the patient in order to influence the "affected part" and speed up the recovery process [1].

Clown doctors are not physicians. In fact, they are a peculiar kind of artist and each of them develops a distinctive clown doctor *persona*. Everyone has a distinct and unique character, logo and name. For example, Dr. Giraffe wears ears, horns and a detachable tail, Dr. Chic wears a traditional dress shirt, Scottish kilt and a French beret [29]. In addition to their own clothing, each clown doctor has a personal and decorated white medical coat. This makes the white coats of the medical staff less scary and, at the same time, identifies clown doctors as part of the medical staff. Moreover, the clown doctor's medical model has the goal of parodying the medical routine in order to help children adjust to their new environment and the intimidating medical jargon and procedures.

Clown doctors often carry a variety of props in their pockets or their "doctor bags" (e.g., slide whistles made from syringes, telephones made from stethoscopes, traditional musical instruments of all kinds, etc.) [28]. Essentially, any object, medical device or toy that is found in a patient room can be transformed and used as a theatrical tool. Finally, and most importantly, all the clown doctors wear a red nose that is also called "the smallest mask in the world" [13]. This is the glue that holds all the clown doctors' characters together. The red nose or make-up mask of the clown, like a dramatic character or role, is both caring and liberating, enabling the expression of what lies buried beneath our real life roles. "Having something to hide behind is a vehicle, rather than an obstacle, to self-exposure. Illusion in theater does not lead to elusion of truth but to confrontation with truth" [30: 7].

The clown doctors usually work in pairs. One performer plays the role of the "white clown" who represents the rational voice of reason and the orderly decision maker. His partner plays the role of "August", a fun loving, emotional character who is also the problem maker [31]. Each person has his own style, set of practices, comic gags, gestures, vocabulary, and voice. Some make no use of a spoken language, whereas others use a certain kind of voice or a funny nonsense way to communicate.

Therapeutic clowns in paediatric settings use soft games and fun to provide sick children with another method for emotional expression, control and social interaction during their hospitalization. The design of therapeutic clowning is to reduce stress for patients and their families during hospitalization and treatment [28]. For this reason, doctor characters evolved from the clown's natural affinity with authority figures: in the circus, the ringmaster; in the hospital, the doctor. In addition, clown doctors often work in pairs, to encourage creative interpretation, to release the child from pressure to participate, and to provide professional and emotional support [29].

As every clown has a particular characteristic, they use something unique both in the gestures and the voice. Yet every clown doctor shares specific skills, traits and sensitivity. Thus, they need specific performing skills. The abilities to improvise and clowning are the most important. Many performers have a specialized expertise such as music, comedy, mime, magic, or puppetry. They need to be able to work as a duo and a team. In addition, essential qualities include monitoring and listening skills, along with the potential to be gentle, sensitive and caring. Clown doctors play with their hearts fully opened. It is necessary to remember that children in hospital have little control, and clown doctors give them choices, always asking for permission to enter the room or bedside space.

Clown doctors must be seen as competent professional figures, able to assist hospitalized people, working along with the medical staff to promote people's well-being. They usually perform their work wearing a colored coat, in order to perform the irony game on the real doctors, the "serious" ones. That gives the patients a less scary idea of the medical staff [31].

Moreover, it must be said that clown doctors' intervention is not mandatory or imposed. Children and adults may always evaluate and have the right to decide whether they want their company or not. This aspect is extremely valuable for children, because they acquire the power to make their own decisions in an environment where the others take all the calls for them.

If clown doctors note that a family or a member of a family does not want to be disturbed by clowns, they take a step behind, end their intervention and run away. Before leaving, they tend to attract the attention of the patient or family in a gentle, non-invasive way, making a timid greeting or smiling kindly.

Interventions of the clown doctors are based both on improvisation and on clowning techniques that they have learnt, during the course they attended. Crucial aspects of performing as clown doctors are spontaneity and sincerity, in order to carry out the original comic feature that they are thought to possess, so they are often guided by the inspiration of the moment. In taking inspiration from circumstances, they try to change the situation by transforming the emotional state into a more positive one (that is called "climax"). They must always observe the reactions, work on what is beneficial for the child, waiting for feed-back, responding accordingly, also paying attention to possible errors [2].

Children usually participate actively in the games of the clown doctors, as, for example, in the resolution of basic conflicts or in completing funny magic tricks.

Clowns usually employ music, improvised games using the standard clown's art. They engage patients and their family with improvised scenes in order to help them in coping with the disease and circumstances for which they are in hospital. The child feels that his assistance is necessary to the clown, and indeed it is necessary. This reinforces the sense of confidence and self-esteem in himself and others, reiterates its willingness to cooperate with others, and stimulates the growth process.

ABILITIES REQUIRED TO BE A CLOWN DOCTOR

Clown doctors must possess abilities, the most salient of which are a good sense of humor, be empathetic and be a bright clown. Clown doctors must be especially able to listen empathically to the emotional state of people in hospital as well as paying attention to the context in which the relationship occurs. A second key structure is represented by the clowning abilities (e.g., slapstick, jugglery, mime, and so on). As said earlier, they must possess a good sense of humor in order to generate laughter in others. In summary, the required criteria for a Clown Doctor are [31]:

- Artistic skills from the art of the clown.
- Psychological skills in order to interact with others.
- Self-care and responsibility.

During the preparation and training program for becoming a clown doctor, candidates are involved in studying and practicing in different areas. For what matter artistic disciplines, they will learn about clowning technique, pantomime, and theatrical improvisation, team working skill and the principles of common prestidigitation and juggling. In addition, candidates study subjects, such as gelotology, psychology, communication, anthropology and social science. They also learn basic notions on diseases, hospital rules, privacy rules, self-care routine (grooming, bathing, dressing, toileting, eating), and practice in different settings.

There is not a universal rule, but many federations of clown doctors determine some basic criteria. To attend the course people must possess a High School degree, have a balanced personality, excellent listening skills, abilities to work in pairs and artistic skills.

This criteria are compulsory because, in order to carry out their activities, clown doctors are expected to master specific artistic skills adapted from the clowning, such as humor, comedy, theatrical improvisation and creativity. Since they work with people of all ages, clown doctors must also possess good interpersonal skills and adequate knowledge of psychology and social science. They are also required to develop an adequate degree of autonomy and control in order to determine the most appropriate methodologies for the different areas of intervention.

It is mandatory to attend specific training to become a clown doctor. As said earlier, the training comprises two parts: a theoretical and a practice one. Both are proposed and implemented through a qualifying course of vocational training. The course clearly provides the theoretical foundations in the areas addressed below. However, the practical experience is gained by taking part to role play activities and by practicing within the clinical setting. The training can be considered as completed when the clown doctor has spent a sufficient time in the health care setting working with a tutor (an expert clown doctor). The tutor provides ongoing supervision, monitors the new clown doctor's psychological attitude and corrects possible mistakes.

Even after obtaining a clown doctor degree, it is strongly recommended that clown doctors attend refresher courses and request ongoing supervision.

Clown doctors must be able to organize their practice in accordance with the other professionals of the centre where they work [31]. If needed, they should be able to arrange their performances themselves by contacting the centre where they intend to work and according to their tools. During their performance, clown doctors are required to refer to theatre expression techniques as much as possible because they have to bear in mind that the goal is to change the emotional state of the patient and the environment they are in. Clown doctors can do so by bringing their performance to the "climax" and finishing it by making sure they leave a positive feeling behind. They must pay attention to the emotional impact and consequences of their action and to what the patient and their relational world need. They must always seek the addressed person for allowance and abide rejection.

Finally, it should be reminded that clown doctors are not a substitute for other clinical professionals (e.g. nurses, doctors and so on) but they support medical personnel in their work. Clown doctors have a function that differs from other professionals' in the hospitals (e.g., art therapists, music therapists, and volunteers in general). Clown doctors maintain their specific role and can work in teams with the other health care professionals.

CLOWN FEDERATIONS

"Red Noses" are considered as providers of services to individuals. Hence, given the breadth and importance of their functions, in recent years an increasing need to clarify their role and responsibilities, their tools, training methods has been arisen.

In several countries have been set up different Federations whose purpose is to provide a point of reference to the many Clown Care Units. The Federations integrate health and social professionalism with competence. It stems from the necessity of clarifying the clown doctor's work and standardizing the vocational training required to become one. Furthermore, Federations provide adequate training and a code of ethics. They usually bring various organizations together, which have decided to set up a Clown Care Unit. They are point of reference for institutions and individuals who want to give a support service and help people in need by means of professional and competent clown doctors. This allows a person operating with a comprehensive approach and interacting in complex settings such as hospitals. Clown doctors work closely with the medical team and identify the patient's overall situation, so as to modify and adjust their performance.

Every Federation shares together some purposes. Firstly, every institution puts the beneficiaries in the foreground. The goal is to protect patients, providing them professional assistance and an appropriate support by using non-invasive and acceptable practice that is suitable to their individual physical and psychological conditions.

Secondly, they attempt to determine the role of the clown doctor distinctly and his actions from other recreational activities, animation, entertainment and social health. Since clown doctors provide services that are directly connected to the medical sphere, their adequate training is paramount. Clown doctors need right competences that can help them behave appropriately within the health care setting. The role of these institutions is to develop clown doctors as professional therapists of mental and physical health; in this way, medical staff can rely on safe and professional services that may help to facilitate the therapeutic relationship between them and their patients.

It is especially critical that clown doctors use the tools clown normally use. These tools must be integrated with psycho-social and medical knowledge, in order to facilitate communication, thus paying a keen attention to the relational dynamics. They can be also reformulated in a paradoxical way so as to act on emotions that can be accordingly transformed from negative to positive one.

In order to become a clown doctor, each Federation determines specific mandatory education that must be attended. Every course comprises both theoretical and practical training. Clown doctors can work with people of different ages, planning their performances on the basis of a training model and a structured methodology. They always need to negotiate their objectives with the other professionals who work in the health care setting.

A Clown Docto's Experience

Here, below, we want to report a story that involved directly one of us (Roberto Flangini) [32]. It is about a child who was recovered for cancer. We believe it may help understanding what does it involve working as a clown doctor and what we can expect as a result of this practice.

The Skin of the Dinosaurs

Starting from May 2008, the Clown Care Unit that Roberto Flangini coordinates set up a regulation program about clown doctors' work, in order to study and come to guidelines. The study was conducted in an Oncohaematology hospital where one aspect of significant relevance and weight is efficient sterilizing of materials and people. The first step in which clown doctors were involved was to attend a specific training both theoretical and practical. Clown doctors initiated their education by observing the medical staff while medicating adult patients, and studying the characteristics of the setting. After that, they attended training to adjust their usual games and tools (e.g., plastic red noses, colored coats, plastic balloons used to make sculptures, and so on) to the environment. Clowns started to work in the department of Oncohaematology in April 2009, directly with children and always supervised by a trained psychologist and psychotherapist.

The story we want to say is about a six-year old boy that we call Nicholas (pseudonym) who was hospitalized in a large urban pediatric clinic, from September 2008 till October of the same year for a total of 44 days. Nicholas was hospitalized because of an acute myeloid leukemia and during his staying underwent a surgery in order to have a marrow-bone transplant. After this event, he was again hospitalized several times, but for most short periods. Nicholas' pathology was quite serious, but a valuable aspect was the close relationship between his family members: they were remarkably close to each other and able to face the traumatic event in a positive way. At the first visit with the psychologist, Nicholas appeared serious and taciturn. He did not say a word. His mother explained that her son wasn't used to give confidence to the strangers. After a while, Nicholas became angrier and started to oppose any medical treatment. The child's anger was expressed through acts of crying, screaming and blaming the mother. The psychologist decided to call the clown doctors to find a way to distract and calm the child.

Nicholas appreciated a lot the presence of the clowns, and he was able to spend more than two hours with them, forgetting his physical condition and the place where he was. After this first approach, the boy asked voluntarily to meet the clowns again, thus once a week the clowns met Nicholas, allowing him to relieve his emotional state due to his health condition.

Once discharged from the hospital, Nicholas had to return to the day hospital to check up, periodically. Each visit, the clowns were at his side. After seven months, Nicholas' conditions got worse, and the medical staff communicated that there wasn't anything left to do for him.

During his hospitalization, Nicholas had the opportunity to experience his illness in a lighter way. Clown doctors, obviously, did not cure Nicholas; rather they helped him facing adversity, changing his emotional and psychological mood and taking insight about his illness.

Nicholas wanted to have the company of the red noses during his last trip, as well as the educators.

During his recovery, Nicholas tried to make up a dinosaur (his parents were used to purchase a periodical magazine where every week there was a new piece). Unfortunately, in the last days of his life, Nicholas did not make it finish building the dinosaur, because one last piece was missing: and that was the skin.

Nicholas knew that he would have never been able to complete the toy, and he was worried, anxious and angry. Because of the situation, the clown doctors decided to make a game with Nicholas. They decided together to create a new skin by themselves using clay. The clowns, Nicholas's family and some other children were engaged, for a couple of days, in finding the clay, handling it, coloring it, and placing it on the toy. This was not only a game. It represented also a new state of psycho-oncology in the disease where the new skin (the clay one) embodied a new dimension, covering the truth to discover a new state of mind which leads to mental awareness of the self. One day, the last of Nicholas's life, he closed his eyes while embracing the completed dinosaur. At that moment, the toy became a comprehensive and meaningful representation for the family in their journey of processing the grief. For that family, the dinosaur became (and it is still today) a memory connected to an object that represented an atavistic world.

The role of the clowns here was not to cure or treat the child. The work of the red noses consisted of making the disease more acceptable and changing the emotional state of the family. Clown doctors are not actually medical doctors they are interpreters of emotions.

CONCLUSION

Clowns and hospitals are currently a normal match. However, clown doctors have a long history. Some reports say that the clowns have worked in the hospitals since the time of Hippocrates. An entire page of a French Journal in 1908 was dedicated to a drawing of a nurse who dressed as a clown while working in a pediatric hospital. In recent years, there has been a considerable interest in this activity. Everybody knows the story of Dr Patch Adams, who in the seventies put on a red clown nose and changed the way of taking care about people. It was only in 1986 that professional clown doctors began to work in hospitals, in USA and Canada. After that experience, many hospitals decided to create a clown program to support recovered patients. Clown doctors address the psychosocial needs of the child as a patient in a unique way. Clown doctors help children reduce their scary of medical procedures by making a parody of the hospital routine. Oversized medical equipment, 'red-nose' transplants, 'cat' scans, humor checks and funny bone examinations are all part of the fun. Therefore, we believe that integrating clown doctors into the medical staff of hospitals is useful and appropriate, because clowns and children are a natural combination.

Research found that the presence of clowns during the hospitalization of children is an effective intervention for managing child and parents' anxiety. Although several researches have tried tested the effectiveness of clown therapy in decreasing anxiety and anger, few of them use a controlled or evidence-based design. Therefore, there is a requirement of further studies to produce stronger evidence to the positive effects of the clown therapy.

Finally, we need to focus on an extremely critical point represented by the abilities that a clown doctor must possess to work in a hospital. We strongly encourage people intentioned in taking part to this fascinating world to attend a well-qualified and recognized course. Only in this way, the work of clowns in conjunction with other health care personnel can promote patient satisfaction and compliance.

We conclude citing an anthropological study that compared the Big Apple Circus Clown Care Unit with non-Western healers, especially shamans [32]. This study found many similarities, from a superficial resemblance represented by costumes, music, sleight of hand, and puppet/spirit helpers, to a similarity in the meanings and functions of their performances. In fact, both clown and shaman in their performances violate natural and cultural rules, help patient and family deal with illness, and use suggestion and manipulation of medical symbols in attempting to relieve their patients' distress. The anthropologist suggested that clown doctors can provide complementary therapy that may increase the efficacy of medical treatment.

REFERENCES

[1]   Dionigi, A., & Gremigni, P. (2010). *Psicologia dell'umorismo.* Roma: Carocci.
[2]   Flangini, R. (2010). La terapia del sorriso. Fondamenti teorici e implicazioni operative. In G. F. Ricci, D. Resico & L. Pino (Eds.), *Il clown professionale nei servizi alla persona* (pp. 32-40). Milano: Franco Angeli.
[3]   Freud, S. (1960 [1905]). *Jokes and their Relation to the Unconscious.* New York: Norton.
[4]   Hassett J. & Houlihan, J. (1979). Different Jokes for Different Folks. *Psychology Today, January,* pp. 64-71.
[5]   Cousins, N. (1979). *Anatomy of an Illness.* New York: Norton.
[6]   Martin, R. A. (2004). Sense of humor and physical health: Theoretical issues, recent findings, and future directions. *Humor: International Journal of Humor Research 17*(1/2), 1–19.
[7]   Martin, R. A. (2007). *The Psychology of Humor.* New York: Academic Press.
[8]   Golden L., Pagala M., & Sukhavasi S. (2006). Giving toys to children reduces their anxiety about receiving premedication for surgery. *Anesthesia & Analgesia 102,* 1070–1072.
[9]   Vagnoli, L., Bastiani, C., Turchi, F., Caprilli, S., & Messeri, A. (2007). Preoperative anxiety in pediatrics: Is clown's intervention effective to alleviate children discomfort? *Algia Hospital, 2,* 114–119.
[10]   Kain, Z. N., Mayes, L. C., & Caramico, L. A. (1996). Preoperative preparation in children: a cross-sectional study. *Journal of Clinical Anesthesia, 8,* 508–514.
[11]   Kain, Z. N., Mayes, L. C., Weisman, S. J., & Hofstadter, M. B. (2000). Social adaptability, cognitive abilities, and other predictors for children's reactions to surgery. *Journal of Clinical Anesthesia, 12,* 549–554.
[12]   Lamontagne, L. L., Hepworth, J. T., Salisbury, M. H., & Riley, L. P. (2003). Optimism, anxiety, and coping in parents of children hospitalized for spinal surgery. *Applied Nursing Research, 16,* 228–235.

[13]   Farneti A. (2004). *La maschera più piccola del mondo. Aspetti psicologici della clownerie*. Bologna: Alberto Perdisa.

[14]   Weaver, K., Prudhoe, G., Battrick, C. & Glasper, E. A. (2007). Sick children's perceptions of clown doctor humour. *Journal of Children's and Young People's Nursing, 1*,(8): 359-365.

[15]   Battrick, C., Glasper, E. A., Prudhoe, G., & Weaver, K. (2007). Clown humour: the perceptions of doctors, nurses, parents and children. *Journal of Children's and Young People's Nursing, 1*(4), 174-179.

[16]   Koller, D. & Gryski, C. (2008). The Life Threatened Child and the Life Enhancing Clown: Towards a Model of Therapeutic Clowning. *eCAM, 5*(1), 17–25.

[17]   Slater J., Gorfinkle K., Bagiella E., Tager F., & Labinsky E. (1998). *Child Behavioral Distress During Invasive Oncologic Procedures and Cardiac Catheterization with the Big Apple Circus Clown Care Unit*. Columbia University, NY: Rosenthal Center for Complementary and Alternative Medicine.

[18]   Smerling, A. J., Skolnick, E, Bagiella, E., Rose, C., Labinsky, E., &, Tager F. (1999). Perioperative clown therapy for pediatric patients. *Anesthesia & Analgesia, 88,* 243–56.

[19]   Vagnoli, L., Caprilli, S., Robiglio, A., & Messeri, A. (2005). Clown doctors as a treatment for preoperative anxiety in children: A randomized, prospective study. *Pediatrics, 116,* 563–567.

[20]   Tener, D., Lang, N., Ofir, S., & Lev-Wiesel, R. (2011). The Use of Medical Clowns as a Psychological Distress Buffer during Anogenital Examination of Sexually Abused Children. *Journal of Loss and Trauma.* DOI: 10.1080/15325024.2011.578025

[21]   Costa Fernandes, S., & Arriaga, P. (2010). The effects of clown intervention on worries and emotional responses in children undergoing surgery. *Journal of Health Psychology, 15*(3), 405-415.

[22]   Pinquart, M., Skolaude, D., Zaplinski, & K., Maier, R. F. (2011). Do Clown Visits Improve Psychological and Sense of Physical Well-being of Hospitalized Pediatric Patients? A Randomized-controlled Trial. *Klinische Padiatrie, 223*(2), 74-78.

[23]   Hansen, L. K., Kibaek, M., Martinussen, T., Kragh, L., & Hejl, M. (2011). Effect of a clown's presence at botulinum toxin injections in children: a randomized, prospective study. *Journal of Pain Research, 4,* 297–300.

[24]   Warren B. (2008). Healing laughter: the role and benefits of clown doctors working in hospitals and healthcare. In B. Warren (Ed). *Using the Creative Arts in Healthcare and Therapy* (pp. 213–228). London and New York: Routledge.

[25]   Warren B. (2009). Spreading sunshine down memory lane: how clowns working in healthcare help promote recovery and rekindle memories. In N. T. Baum, (Ed.), *Come to your Senses: Creating Supportive Environments to Nurture the Sensory Capital Within* (pp. 37–44). Toronto: MukiBaum,

[26]   Spitzer P. (2011). The Laughter Boss. In L. Hilary, & T. Adams (Eds.),. *Creative Approaches in Dementia Care* (pp. 32–53). Hampshire and New York: Palgrave Macmillan,

[27]   Warren B. & Spitz P. (2011). Laughing to longevity—the work of elder clowns. *The Lancet, 378(13)*, 562-563.

[28] Carp, C. E. (1998). Clown therapy: the creation of a clown character as a treatment intervention. Two archetypes of human sexuality. *The Arts in Psychotherapy, 25(4),* 245–255.

[29] Simonds, C. & Warren, B. (2001). *Le Rire Medecin: Le Journal de Dr. Girafe*. Paris, FR: Albin Michel.

[30] Emunah, R. (1994). *Acting for Real: Drama Therapy Process, Technique, and Performance*. New York: Brunner/Mazel.

[31] Flangini, R. (2010). Strumenti operativi del clown: una panoramica di insieme. In G. F. Ricci, D. Resico & L. Pino (Eds.), *Il clown professionale nei servizi alla persona* (pp. 126-137). Milano: Franco Angeli.

[32] Flangini, R. (2009). *La relazione d'aiuto nel sostegno in psico-oncologia pediatrica: la funzione del care giver nell'elaborazione della malattia e del lutto* (Unpublished Dissertation). Rome, Italy: Università Cattolica del Sacro Cuore.

In: Humor and Health Promotion
Editor: Paola Gremigni

ISBN: 978-1-61942-657-3
© 2012 Nova Science Publishers, Inc.

Chapter 12

GELOTOPHOBIA: THE FEAR OF BEING LAUGHED AT

Tracey Platt[1] and Giovannantonio Forabosco[2]
[1]University of Zurich, Switzerland
[2]Psychotherapist, Italy

ABSTRACT

Being ridiculed and laughed at by others typically leads to shame that is emotionally painful and aversive. While some wipe this off more easily or even share the laughter, for others an anticipatory fear of being laughed at exists, which may go along with a generalized conviction of ones own ridiculousness. The aim of this chapter is to explore gelotophobia; i.e., the fear of being laughed at. It has long been common to distinguish between laughing with and laughing at, but while research investigated the positive use of laughter and humor in social interactions, the effects of laughing at or ridiculing were neglected. The chapter describes those with a fear of being laughed at and the development of the concept of gelotophobia from clinical observations to a worldwide-identified individual difference disposition towards laughter and ridicule, how it is measured and how it affects people who experience it. Special attention will be given to the humor of gelotophobes. The chapter will also show how the fear of being laughed at stands apart from its close relation social phobia, how it has co-morbidity with other diagnosed psychological problems and how it relates to dental issues. Gehotophobia, as a form of humorlessness goes along with reduced well-being, which is apparent in lower life satisfaction and a lack the gratification that comes from immersing themselves in challenging activities; i.e., the lack flow experiences. Furthermore, the results on how fearing laughter negatively affects the establishment of adult, pair-bonded relationships, as opposed to other dispositions towards laughter, will be presented. Finally, ideas on positively interacting with gelotophobes, considering these will be individuals who more often require social care will be considered.

INTRODUCTION

This chapter will address the fear of being laughed at – gelotophobia [1]. In order to understand this phenomenon it is first essential to understand the role of laughter. More specifically, how laughing at and laughing with creates an ambiguity, which is difficult for someone with a fear of being laughed at to differentiate. If they do or can understand this difference it is possible that the fear is so overwhelming the result is the same [2]. Gelotophobes assume all the laughter is directed at them in a negative, malicious, way. They seem to perceive all good-natured humor as negative derision. As laughter is such an integral part of human interaction, this fear permeates many social aspects, making it crucial for well-being and a healthy life. Since the first observations of gelotophobia, an instrument to measure it has allowed for it to be reliably assessed outside of a clinical setting. Both the scale and the concept of the fear of being laughed at have been validated across 73 countries with different patterns emerging across different cultures for the different intensities of gelotophobia, which will be discussed as well in the chapter. Once there was the possibility to assess gelotophobia, it was also possible to show how to discriminate gelotophobia from its close relation social phobia. This is necessary due to the many similarities shared between the two phobias. The development of gelotophobia and how it prevails over a lifetime will also be discussed along with other cognitive and dynamic aspects focusing on how it relates (or not) to humor, smiling and wit. Within the community the population of psychiatric patients is a particularly vulnerable group. Understanding the problems and difficulties they face is critical for their mental health. As the fear of being laughed at was expected to be more problematic in this subpopulation, the relations for different diagnosed categories and gelotophobia were investigated.

As this study confirmed higher fear of being laughed at in this group than a normal control group and among those who had years in the care system, which makes the findings discussed of particular importance to those who work with people with these issues. A further exploratory study within the field of dentistry investigated smoking habits, halitosis and gelotophobia. Although no correlations were found between smoking habits and gelotophobia, there was a correlation between self perceived halitosis and gelotophobia. Thought provoking explanations for this are discussed in detail. Finally, the consequences of gelotophobia and how it effects a person's subjective well-being is considered and how it impairs the affective components such as joy. Also the negative impact of the fear of being laughed at on the development and maintenance of good relationships are highlighted. How looking more closely at a population where was expected that the people predominantly should be in or have been in long-term adult relationships, allowed to show the difficulties faced by those that do not see the positive nature of laughing along with others. This also allowed for the introduction of two further dispositions towards laughter, namely, gelotophilia (the joy of being laughed at) and katagelasticism (the joy of laughing at others) [3].

The two additional constructs offer a broader perspective to how people deal with being laughed at and ridiculed. Derived from reports given by participants, in a study by Ruch and Proyer [3], the new variables suggested alternative responses to that solely of the gelotophobic response. When asked to give an example of the worst event that they could think of, in relation to being laughed at, most individuals gave embarrassing situations or times they behaved inappropriately. Yet some people replied that there could not think of a "worst" example, as being laughed at was a positive thing. Others emerged whom particularly derived pleasure from laughing at the mishaps of others; these were the katagelasticistic group.

LAUGHER: LAUGH WITH AND BEING LAUGHED AT

Traditionally, humor research distinguished between *laughing with* and *laughing at* others. This can be exemplified by the words that we use in everyday language. Schmidt-Hidding [4] collected all English words relating to the comic and grouped them according to frequency and meaning. He identified four key words in the field, namely "humour", fun, mock/ridicule and wit, which he located at the corners a rhombus with satellite words surrounding them (nb. The English spelling of humo(u)r has been used where it has been literally quoted). Two of them, "humour" and "mock/ridicule" formed the end poles of a bi-polar dimension, and these words represent the antagonism between laughing with and laughing at well. Clustered around the key term humor are terms like, "quaint", "pleasantry", "whimsical", "teasing," "bantering", "playfulness," and "nonsense." Some of these have relations to the fun and wit but they all share a benevolent nature, and all of these would be used when people are laughing with someone. Oh the other pole of the dimension clustering around the key word "mock/ridicule" there are terms like "cynic", "sarcasm", "deride", "rally", "taunt", "twit", "sneer," and "scoff". Thus a variety of words are used in everyday language, which are associated with laughing at. Laughing at typically involves a target, while laughing with does not exclude but includes the target person.

It should be noted that humor has not always been used to refer to a benevolent quality of laughter. Schmidt-Hidding [4,5: 8]describes historic shifts of the meaning of the term humor. From this it is clear that both humor and wit were used interchangeably until the rise of humanism made a clear distinction between events that reflect *laughing with* and *laughing at*. Before, during the 17th century a "humour" referred to someone of "odd" character that elicited the laughter of others. Later, a more tolerant and benevolent form of "good humour" was used, that did not relate to laughing at but laughing along with the imperfections of the world. Also, more recently, humor as a character strengths emphasizes the benevolent forms of humor and it is postulated that humor contributes to the good life. Indeed, laughing with people has been found to go along with rather pleasant forms of social interactions. Bachorowski and Owren [6] were able to show that in dating situations, women who laughed out loud with the male, made him more interested in meeting her again. Even of this evidence can be argued as only benefiting the woman, it does highlight the integral part that laughing with others plays for relationship development. More direct evidence for both sexes can be found in a workplace setting, where group laughter interventions have shown to enhance morale, resilience and the belief that one has personally efficacy [7]. Laughter in small groups has also been shown to reduce stress . Thus *laughing with* others has definite social and health benefits. This function of laughter is a signal that rewards the witty humorist. It signals to the witty person that you are not only paying attention but also that you actually understand the context of the humor and that you are responding to it positively. Weisfeld [8] elucidated this positive reinforcement cycle. He described how the gratitude of the audience, which in turn, elicits pride, rewards the reciprocator.

Laughing at is different. It is rather probable that laughing at others was among the earliest forms of laughter. Locating laughing at from the perspective of early man, MacHovec [9] theorized that the first humans amused themselves mimicking their opponents and by mocking their differences, weaknesses or deformities. This idea supports that of Gruner [10] who postulated that laughter originated as an aggressive display of victory over a challenger, thus the winner *laughs at* the loser. Monro [11] stated that emotional states such as triumph (and anxiety) are accompanied by smiling and laughter and this would fit too in the triumph over another. Even in modern life, where fighting is not quite such a usual or socially accepted behavior, we can still see through investigating jokes that they are used to laughing at a target deemed "people joke not about good things or virtuous people but about failure and wickedness and about matters they might well find disturbing outside the context of the joke" [12, 13]. Theoretically, this form of humor behavior falls into that of the disparagement theory or put down humor [14]. Although some argue that it is playful aggression, the disparagement and the subgroup of that, namely, superiority theory states that humor stimuli (the causes of the laughter) are generated where one protagonist aggressively disparages against another person.

Nobody likes to be the butt of a joke, the object of derisive laughter or ridicule. However, even though there are many arguments for the beneficial effects of laugher in social interactions, some people do not see this side of laughter to the point they fear it assuming it is a negative putdown. This fear is known as gelotophobia--the fear of being laughed at [1].

RESEARCH ON GELOTOPHOBIA

When we think that another person has breeched some social norm, is acting dishonorably, is worthless, vile or simply doing something that would be considered beneath us, we typically would feel contempt or scorn. Laughing at or ridiculing the wrongdoer is one of the ways we can show our disapproval, thereby inducing shame and guilt in the person exposed by this derision. Shame, rather than guilt and embarrassment is the self-conscious emotion which has been claimed to be experienced following events where people are made to feel others have exposed their inferiority [15]. Also, shame is a significantly painful experience, more so than guilt [16], and it is therefore understandable that generally people try to avoid the derision of others. Laughter has been seen as a means to correct deviant behavior and to foster conformity, through its ability to evoke emotionally painful shame. However, there are individual differences in the propensity to shame, and for some being laughed at will be very painful and they will try to avoid derision. Others will be less affected and still others, for example those with a disposition to joy and positive emotions might even share the laughter, at least when at lower levels of ridicule [3]. For those with a low threshold for shame (and a high threshold for joy) observing a smile or hearing laughter irrespective of the context, will more likely induce the feeling of shame, fear and anxiety rather than responding with joy and reciprocate the laughter.

Such people, presenting for clinical treatment lead to a pathological fear of being laughed at being identified and named *gelotophobia*, from the Greek *gelos* meaning laughter and phobos for fear [17]. These individuals were described as having shame anxiety, i.e., those that fear the pain of shame induced by ridicule and laughter [17,18,19]. A graphical model of the proposed putative causes and consequences of gelotophobia was produced by Ruch [20] that systematized the clinical observations of Titze (see Fig. 1).

Causes

Consequences

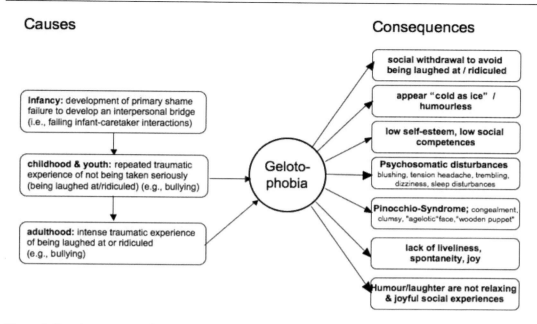

Figure 1. Putative causes and consequences of gelotophobia as proposed by Titze (Ruch, 2004) Redrawn with permission of the author.

In Figure 1 Titze`s postulate is that gelotophobia originates from one of three types of events over a lifespan from infancy to adulthood. During infancy there can be a failure to develop an interpersonal bridge to the caregiver. In childhood and adolescence gelotophobia can develop from repeated, traumatic experiences of being ridiculed or not being taken seriously. In adulthood it was proposed that gelotophobia may be caused by intense traumatic experiences of being ridiculed, which differs from the repeated element of the childhood hypothesis [1,18,19]. The model also states there are several consequences of gelotophobia, for example, social withdrawal, low social competences, lack of liveliness, spontaneity and joy, a cold as ice appearance, and a lack of pleasurable effect due to the social aspects of humor and laughter. The model developed from experience with clients (see also the vignette in 2009) and is subject of empirical investigation since assessment tools were developed. The initial clinical assessment was based on observations during the interaction with the client involving several elements. One important criterion for the assessment of gelotophobia is "… the patients' pronounced sensitivity with regard to any kind of humorous remarks. ... In this context, they mostly will react ''agelotically,'' i.e., their face will grow stiff and their possible polite smiling will freeze." [19: 37].

TOOLS FOR THE STANDARDIZED ASSESSMENT OF GELOTOPHOBIA

There are different approaches for the standardized assessment of the fear of being laughed at. The current standard is the GELOPH<15> [21], a self-report questionnaire containing 15 items to be answered in a 4-point format (1 = strongly disagree; 4 = strongly agree). The GELOPH<15> was based on the GELOPH<46>, which was a pilot form containing a list of 46 items. It was occasionally referred to as the long form of the

GELOPH<15> which is not correct as it was more a list of items used to verify the concept of gelotophobia [1] but due to its unclear dimensionality the computation of a total score was not foreseen.

There is also the Picture-GELOPH, a semi-projective test, which was used in a study by Ruch, Altfreder and Proyer [22]. This experimental version consists of 20 drawings depicting social situations that involve two or three persons, each of which may or not be saying something. One person, the target, has a speech or thought balloon above his or her head where the test-taker write down what the target person in each situation is presumably thinking or most likely saying. The content of those writings either reflects a fear of being laughed at (sample answer ''why are they laughing at me?''), an enjoyment of the situation (e.g., cheerful statements) or is neutral (expressing neither fear nor enjoyment of the situation). Scores from 1 to 5 are assigned to each of the 20 answers. The total score correlates .64 with the GELOPH, and it also correlates -.64 with liking positively motivated laughter [22].

Finally, a *Structured Gelotophobia Interview* has been developed that is currently being examined for its validity [23]. It contains a list of 20 questions relating to a variety of issues regarding the onset of the fear of being laughed at, typical ways of dealing with it, thoughts, emotions and actions while being laughed at, as well as socio-demographic variables. It provides supplemental information to the GELOPH in as much as it includes more facets of the model (see Figure 1); for example, how people deal with the fear and how intense their responses to ridicule are. No definite evidence of the amount of overlap with the GELOPH<15> scores has been provided so far; however, Platt et al. [23] present several case studies, that shows that high scorers in the questionnaire show a rich variety of gelotophobic symptoms.

The GELOPH<15> was developed in several stages on the basis of the 46 items. This original list of 46 items covered the gelotophobic symptomatology broadly [1], including the domains of a paranoid sensitivity towards mockery of others, fear of the humor of others, critical self-consciousness of their own bodies, critical self-consciousness of their own verbal and non-verbal communicative functions, social withdrawal, general response to the smiling and laughter of others, discouragement and envy when comparing with the humor competence of others, but also traumatizing experiences with laughter in the past. In the initial study a principal components analysis of the 46 items yielded a strong gelotophobia factor and two minor factors. The final questionnaire (i.e., the GELOPH<15>) contains only items loading highly on the first factor and additionally the items needed to discriminate well between a group of gelotophobes and several comparison groups [21].

The scale turned out to be clearly unidimensional in a sample of adults and it typically had a high internal consistency [24,25]. However, in samples of individuals with high fear of being laughed at some sub-factors might emerge. Indeed, in a sample of high scorers (i.e., those who had at least a *slight* fear of being laughed at) a three-factor solution emerged in which components of coping with derision (by control, withdrawal, or internalizing), paranoid sensitivity to anticipated ridicule, and disproportionate negative responses to being laughed at could be distinguished.

USING THE GELOPH TO IDENTIFY GELOTOPHOBES AND LEVELS OF THE FEAR OF BEING LAUGHED AT

While the above-mentioned assessment tools converge to an appreciable extent, the question arises whether the GELOPH indeed measures the pathological fear of being laughed at as originally described among patients. Ruch and Proyer [1,21] studied samples of clinically diagnosed gelotophobes, shame-based as well as non shame-based neurotics, and normal controls that were compared on the basis of their answers to the 46 items of the pilot form of the GELOPH. It was not only demonstrated that the fear of being laughed at existed as a homogeneous dimension, the group of patients with diagnosed gelotophobia came out on top of the dimension (followed by shame based neurotics, which were in turn higher that both normal controls and the non-shame based neurotics which did not differ from each other). Most importantly, the GELOPH<15> identified 92.93 % of the clinically diagnosed gelotophobes correctly, i.e., as having at least a slight fear of being laughed at. As this result was found in the sample that was also used to derive the items, an independent replication is needed. Nevertheless, the instrument is sensitive to detect the fear of being laughed at.

Moreover, the GELOPH gives a quantitative assessment of the intensity of that fear. People are assumed to vary between having absolutely no fear of being laughed at, through a borderline area, to slight, marked or pronounced and extreme fear. If there is no fear then participants either strongly or moderately disagree to all statements (yielding scores between 1.0 and 2.0). The borderline area reaches from moderately disagreeing to moderately agreeing to less than half of the statements; i.e., between a total score of 2.0 and 2.5. The cut-off-score for slight gelotophobia was set at 2.5 as this was where a) the distributions of the clinically tested gelotophobes and normal people overlapped, b) individuals agree to half of the items (i.e., every second symptom applies) and c) where two standard deviations added to the mean is. The standard deviation in various countries was roughly .50 and this was chosen to be the unit for segmenting the levels of fear.

The segment between 2.5 and 3.0 defines slight fear; this refers to people who have moderately agreed to at least half of the statements (and moderately disagreed to less than half of the items). The range of 3.0 to 3.5 defines marked or pronounced fear, where people moderately agree to statements and also strongly agree with up to half of them. Finally, we speak of extreme fear when the mean score is between 3.5 and 4.0; i.e., when people strongly agree to between at least half and all of the statements on the GELOPH<15> [21]. These categories should be seen as descriptive cut-off points; and it should be remembered that they are formed using the observed mean scores and not the true scores.

It is exactly the distribution of people who fall into each class of gelotophobia that differs between healthy individuals and clinical populations. It was already mentioned above that gelotophobes score highest in the GELOPH, but also shame-based patients (37.95%) and patients with Aspergers syndrome (45 %) [26] yielded a high percentage of individuals with at least a slight fear. Not all clinical groups yield high scores; among patients with no shame symptoms gelotophobia is rather infrequent (6.80%). No study of a broad variety of clinical groups with established diagnosis (ICD or DSM) and information on co-morbidity has been conducted so far. The results of the clinical groups available so far are discussed later in this chapter.

To examine whether the fear of being laughed at is universal, can be measured in all countries via the GELOPH and to study whether the percentages of gelotophobia differ between countries a large cross-cultural study involving 93 samples from 73 countries was conducted [25]. This large study utilized 43 different language translations and sampled over 22,000 people. Most importantly, the fear was found in every single country. Also across all samples the reliability of the 15-item GELOPH questionnaire was high (mean alpha of .85). Interestingly, of multiple samples derived from one country, the scores tended to be (with a few exceptions) highly similar.

Although gelotophobia was found on every populated continent and in every country tested, there were also differences in the percentage of gelotophobes, and the distribution of slight, marked and extremes differed as well. Table 1 summarizes the results from all studies published so far. In these studies at least 200 males and females (most often students) did fill in the gelotophobia questionnaire. The results are based on 10 language versions and cover mostly European countries, but also samples from the Middle East, Asian, and the Americas.

Table 1 shows that the overall percentage of gelotophobia in the different countries ranges from the lowest, Denmark with 1.61 percent to England and Romania with 13 percent (i.e., 8 times more often). Clearly, at least these low and high gelotophobic countries do differ significantly from each other in terms of the prevalence rate. These country differences are also reflected in the mean GELOPH total score (Denmark: $M = 1.43$, $SD = .38$; England: $M = 1.80$, $SD = .59$; Romania: $M = 1.92$, $SD = .50$); i.e., the difference in the mean level is approximately one standard deviation, which is a strong effect size.

It is also evident that extreme fear of being laughed at is very rare, and slight fear is most frequent in such samples. The distribution across countries for the different cut off point ranged from slight Denmark with 1.21 percent to 10 percent in England and Romania. Marked gelotophobia ranged Denmark 0.40 percent to Germany with 4.02 percent. Of the sixteen countries presented only nine had a population with extreme gelotophobia with Canada, China, Czech Republic, Denmark, Italy, Romania, and Russia yielded no score at all. The extreme scores ranged from Poland with 0.20 percent to England with 1 percent. While the latter differences might be due to chance, the percentage of slight gelotophobia (and the total percentage of gelotophobes) varies markedly across countries.

SOCIAL PHOBIA AND GELOTOPHOBIA

There is no argument that elements of gelotophobia closely resemble aspects of social phobia. Indeed, one can argue that they are just one and the same, that gelotophobia is just "social phobia repackaged" [40]. Therefore it is important to understand what exactly is social phobia and what components these anxieties share and where they differ.

Although the first mention of a psychiatric term social phobia (*phobie des situations sociales*), was made in the early 1900s and psychologists used the term "social neurosis" to describe extremely shy patients in the 1930s [41], what is known today as social phobia was first defined by Issac [42] as the second, of four, of the most common phobias caused by external stimuli observed in adult clinical patients. Isaac Marks [42] claims that although most people live with a normal level of fear, they can go about their daily lives. However, when their fears become too intense the stimuli would be avoided and these are the people who seek help for their phobia problems. However, social phobia was not included into the Diagnostic and Statistical Manual of Mental Disorders until the third edition in 1980.

Table 1. Percentage (%) of gelotophobes for individual countries, as derived from published studies

Authors	Reference	Country	M	SD	Total	Slight	Marked	Extreme
Samsom et al. (2010)	[27]	Canada	1.65	0.50	8.57	7.35	1.22	0.00
Proyer et al. (in press)	[28]	China	1.84	0.44	7.31	6.54	0.77	0.00
Carretero-Dios et al. (2010)	[24]	Colombia	1.79	0.48	8.53	6.64	1.42	0.47
Hrebickova et al. (2009)	[29]	Czech Republic	1.77	0.46	6.28	5.23	1.05	0.00
Führ et al. (2009)	[30]	Denmark	1.43	0.38	1.61	1.21	0.40	0.00
Platt et al. (2009)	[31]	England	1.80	0.59	13.0	10.00	2.00	1.00
Ruch & Proyer (2008)	[1]	Germany	1.75	0.57	11.65	6.83	4.02	0.80
Sarid et al. (2011)	[32]	Israel	1.53	0.49	5.90	4.09	1.36	0.45
Forabosco et al. (2009)	[33]	Italy	1.71	0.50	7.12	4.75	2.37	0.00
Kazarian et al. (2009)	[34]	Lebanon	1.86	0.46	7.08	6.06	0.51	0.51
Chlopicki et al. (2010)	[35]	Poland	1.66	0.47	7.30	5.72	1.38	0.20
Ruch, Proyer, & Popa (2008)	[36]	Romania	1.92	0.50	13.0	10.00	3.00	0.00
Stefanenko et al. (2011)	[37]	Russia	1.75	0.45	7.41	6.48	0.93	0.00
Hrebickova et al. (2009)	[29]	Slovakia	1.65	0.47	6.14	4.55	1.36	0.23
Carretero-Dios et al. (2010)	[38]	Spain	1.84	0.49	8.53	6.64	1.42	0.47
Samson et al. (2011)	[39]	Switzerland	1.69	0.45	5.38	3.95	1.21	0.22

The DSM-III lists a standardized classification, which allows levels of social phobia (or social anxiety disorder as it is called in the DSM-III) to be measured against a list of defining and diagnostic criteria. From this growing body of literature has been developed the criteria for social anxiety disorder. The DSM requirement for being diagnosed with social phobia says that a person has to have a marked and persistent fear of one or more social or performance situations in which the person is exposed to unfamiliar people or to possible scrutiny by others. The individual fears that he or she will act in a way (or show anxiety symptoms) that will be humiliating or embarrassing. Exposure to the feared social situation almost invariably provokes anxiety, which may take the form of a situationally bound or situationally predisposed panic attack. The person recognizes that the fear is excessive or unreasonable. The feared social or performance situations are avoided or else are endured with intense anxiety or distress. The avoidance, anxious anticipation, or distress in the feared social or performance situation(s) interferes significantly with the person's normal routine, occupational (academic) functioning, or social activities or relationships, or there is marked distress about having the phobia. The fear or avoidance is not due to the direct physiological effects of a substance (e.g., a drug of abuse, a medication) or a general medical condition and is not better accounted for by another mental disorder. If a general medical condition or another mental disorder is present, the fear in the first criteria is unrelated to it [43] (DSM IV, 1994). From this list it is very clear how some of these behaviors are met for those of gelotophobia. Yet the fear of being laughed at, so far, is not considered as a criterion for social phobia.

That being said, the fear of being laughed at was first mentioned in the context of social fears over one hundred years ago a French psychiatrist, Paul Hartenberg. He defined in his book *Les timides et la timidité* [44] how timid people had unwarranted fear and shame and embarrassment, which they felt in the presence of other people and which affected their psychosocial competencies. This was combined with physiological symptoms (e.g. trembling, blushing, speech disturbance and disturbance in visceral and secretory functions), as well as psychological symptoms (e.g. derangements in the processes of attention, reflection, volition and memory). Most importantly, Hartenberg [44] suggested that one of the characteristics of the timid was that they have a *fear of ridicule*; which he relates this to their fearfulness of self-disclosure and in expressing their opinions. However, unlike the early observations that seemed to include the fear of ridicule, the latter ones did not. So, one could be excused for assuming that gelotophobia is just the forgotten or "lost" facet of social phobia.

There does exist, however, evidence that although the two phobias do indeed share similarities, they retaining some distinct facets. Edwards, Martin and Dozois [45] investigated the relation between gelotophobia, memories of being teased during childhood and adolescence and different measures of social anxiety and specific fears. They found that gelotophobia was associated with higher levels of remembered teasing about their social behavior and about academic excellence but not about family background, appearance or performance. They also confirmed that gelotophobia was strongly related to three measures of social anxiety but not to specific fears that related to such topics as death, illness, injury, animals and situations. Yet even when controlling for social anxiety there remained a strong relation between gelotophobia and a history of remembered having being teased in childhood and adolescence. They concluded that gelotophobia was related to but distinct from social phobia and that it was the specific element, namely the laughter of other during being teased and ridiculed that was significant.

Furthermore, in a study that looked directly at the relationship between measures of social phobia and gelotophobia, [38] was confirmed that Social Anxiety and Distress (SAD) and Fear of Negative Evaluation (FNE, both by Watson & Friend, [46]) scales overlapped with the fear of being laughed at but were able to show that it was not identical to it. While the SAD and FNE correlated highly with the GELOPH <15> not all high scorers in the scales expressed a fear of being laughed at. Investigating the findings further, confirmatory factor analysis revealed that a measure model where one general factor of social anxiety was specified, or another one where two different factors were defined (gelotophobia vs. social anxiety assessed by SAD and FNE) showed a very poor fit to the data. Thus the authors concluded that the fear of being laughed was not fully accounted for by the measures of social phobia. Hence this warrants the existence of gelotophobia as a concept overlapping but distinctive of social phobia.

COGNITIVE AND DYNAMIC ASPECTS IN GELOTOPHOBIA

By the nature of the construct, gelotophobia should be most strongly predictive of an individual's stance towards humor and laughter. However, humor and laughter are different from each other, as is smiling. Furthermore, one has the ability to produce a smile, a laugh or humor as well as being able to respond to other people's smiles, laughter and humor; for this reason the production and perception should be differentiated. Also, there are different types of smiles and laughter [47], and also humor is seen as a multidimensional construct [48] (Ruch, 2008).

According to Titze [19](also see Figure 1) the general state of gelotophobes is "agelotic", i.e., they are not able to appreciate the benefits of laughter. Titze postulated that the origin of this state might derive from the fact that the patients frequently experienced their early reference person(s) as lacking a smiling face. Therefore, the children experience themselves as being unconnected to others and do not interpret laughter as a positive element of shared identity. Gelotophobes experience their peers as hostile strangers who treat them in a cold, sarcastic, and disparaging way, and the weapon these strangers use is derisive laughter. Gelotophobic patients feel uneasy and fear being humiliated by those who face them with laughter and smiling. For them, a smiling face might hide a mind with evil intentions. Of course, there is alternative interpretation to the dynamics outlined above. For example, a genetic interpretation might be that parents low in the capacity to experience joy and humor most likely will produce off-spring that are low in joy and humor, even if these kids were adopted and not raised by the parents.

Several studies investigated the relationships between humor, laughter and fear of being laughed at [49]. An early study investigated participant's reactions to a variety of laughter samples that were auditory presented [22]. They found, for example, that gelotophobes and non-gelotophobes do not differ in their reaction to negatively motivated laughter (i.e., derision, *schadenfreude*) but those without a fear of being laughed at appreciate positively motivated laughter (i.e., hearty, joyful) more than gelotophobes do. Furthermore, more complex social situations involving laughter did affect gelotophobes and non-gelotophobes differently. Those without a fear of being laughed at react to playful teasing scenarios primarily with joy and to the laughter in ridicule situations with sadness, anger and shame. For those that fear laughter all laughter is bad laughter: they respond to laughter situations of both qualities (ridicule and teasing) as if it was ridicule [50]. In a further pioneering study Ruch, Beermann, and Proyer [51] investigated humor of gelotophobes and rightfully asked the question whether feeling ridiculous equals being humorless. Studying a large set of humor scales they found that gelotophobia was both positively and negatively related to humor but also orthogonal to certain forms. Since then several new studies were conducted that produced results in line with the pioneering studies but also adding new facets and perspectives. These findings are summarized in Table 2.

Table 2 summarizes the findings relating to humor, laughter, and wit as derived from different published and unpublished studies. Essentially, the results converge and give a meaningful pattern. As expected, the gelotophobes have a different stance towards laughter, e.g., they do not recognize laughter generated by positive motivation as such. They attribute more negative motivations to laughter by others, and hearing laughter does not improve their mood to a more positive one. They also don't laugh at themselves genuinely when presented distorted photographs of them taken secretively before the experiment. Regarding their habitual mood and frame of mind, gelotophobes are serious rather than playful, and grumpy and sad rather than cheerful. They do not like comedians, and in terms of traditional comic styles they are more characterized by satire, sarcasm and cynicism than by fun and nonsense. They characterize their humor style as inept, socially cold, and mean-spirited, and they report less frequently the use of humor as a means for coping style. They indulge less often in self-enhancing and affiliative humor styles.

However, overall one cannot conclude that feeling ridiculous equals being humorless, as several components of humor were uncorrelated or only slightly negatively correlated (e.g., finding jokes and cartoons funny) to the fear of being laughed at. Furthermore, the results might depend on the nature of the instruments used. For example, while gelotophobes see themselves as "inept" and lacking humor competencies, they do not differ from those without a fear of being laughed at when writing funny captions to cartoons. Platt, Ruch and Proyer [49] argued that the gelotophobes' low level of cheerfulness and the lack of a playful frame of mind might impair the development of humor skills and enhance the likelihood that humorous messages will be processed in a serious frame of mind and thereby elicit negative emotions.

As described in the earlier part of this chapter, sharing a good laugh with others is positive and makes you feel good. One of the seven points made by George Vaillant in his book on adult development, Aging Well [53], for predicting healthy aging was to have an adaptive coping style and part of that was having a good sense of humor and being able to laugh with others. In a study that postulated the possibility of a late onset of gelotophobia due to being laughed at for age related vulnerabilities, Platt, Ruch and Proyer [49] found that for remembered instances of being gelotophobic there was trend of steady decrease from ages twenty to fifty years old. If, however, you still had gelotophobia by that age, it would remain consistent. This remembering back over a lifetime also allowed to see if gelotophobia came and went over a lifespan, yet this pattern was not observed. Gelotophobia came and went or came and stayed, there was no coming, going and coming again.

A further study conducted with the elderly participant (> 60-years) group asked if the different dispositions towards laugher really does help coping with age related vulnerabilities. Platt and Ruch [53] measured the three dispositions towards laughter (gelotophobia, gelotophilia and katagelasticism) as well as fourteen known age related vulnerabilities (e.g. illness, isolation, relationships, lack of control, sensory impairment). They asked participants over 60 if they had experienced but never worry about one of the vulnerabilities or never experienced and also did not worry about it or, if they had experienced one of the fourteen vulnerabilities and worry about it or worry about it even though they never experienced it.

Gelotophobia correlated positively with worrying about the vulnerabilities irrespective of whether the person had experienced it or not. It also negatively correlated with the number of vulnerabilities where people are not worrying (whether or not they experienced them). Also, the total number of vulnerabilities they worry about increased with the fear of being laughed at, but the total number of problems experienced was uncorrelated with gelotophobia. So having gelotophobia does not mean they experience more problems but it does seem to go along with worrying about more of them, even if they had not experienced them. Gelotophilia (i.e., the joy of being laughed at) only correlated with the number of problems experienced but not worried about. Gelotophiles did report more problems that were not worrisome. So it seems this disposition towards laugher did not prevent the problems either but even if they had experienced them the vulnerability was overcome and not something to worry about. Katagelasticism (i.e., the joy of laughing at others) did not correspond with anything so laughing at others as one gets older does not go along with worrying or not or experiencing a vulnerability or not. The authors suggested that empathy might play a role. Once one knows how it feels to experience problems, people are less likely to laugh about others who did.

THE FEAR OF BEING LAUGHED AT AMONG PSYCHIATRIC PATIENTS

Focusing on a specific sub-population, that of people with a psychiatric diagnosis, some thought provoking questions arise. First of all, is the phenomenon of gelotophobia expected to be more present and severe than in non-psychiatric subjects? And, if this is the case, are there any significant differences among the various diagnostic categories? What are the psychopathological elements, which are supposed to be more closely associated with gelotophobia?

There is however one preliminary question to be addressed on the matter. Is there any particular reason why a psychiatric patient should more likely score higher on a gelotophobia index? Such a belief may even be considered part of a stereotype according to which mentally ill people should be full time affected by all sort of psychological problems. Clinical experience and knowledge show that, even in the most severe cases, there may be areas of personality, which are symptoms free, functioning, and capable of positive performances; and that there may be periods of time of significant recovery also in the disturbed areas. From this perspective, no general statement should be made as to a binding association between a psychiatric diagnosis as such and gelotophobia. On the other hand, gelotophobia involves many aspects that are relevant and crucial in a healthy personality, and are symptoms related, or generating, in an individual with a pathological condition. Cognitivity, the capability of a functional thinking ability, the way others, and oneself, are perceived and evaluated, affective experiences, feelings and emotions, the relational, social dimensions, all tend to some extent to be negatively affected in a gelotophobic condition. And as some, and often many, of these elements are critically present, either as a central or as a concomitant feature of the psychopathological conditions, it is reasonable to expect some problematic manifestation also as regards the "fear of being laughed at".

Table 2. Humor, smiling, laughter, and wit as correlates of gelotophobia[1]

Positive correlates/high scores go along with	Negative correlates/low scores go along with
Bad mood (STCI-T)	Affiliative humor (HSQ)
Boorish humor style (HBQD) (students only)	Benign humor style (HBQD)
	Competent humor style (HBQD)
Cynical comic style (SchmHd)	Coping humor (CHS)
Factor grumpy (vs. cheerful) (HUWO)	Earthy humor style (adults only)
Factor serious (vs. playful) (HUWO)	High positive and lowered negative affect
Finding aggressive humor aversive	after hearing laughter
Finding distorted photographs of oneself in	Factor cheerful (vs. grumpy) (HUWO)
an experiment aversive and showing more	Factor playful (vs. serious) (HUWO)
facial markers of negative emotions	Finding distorted photographs of oneself in
Finding sexual humor aversive (3WD)	an experiment funny and showing more
Give more answers expressing mockery	Duchenne displays (smiles and laughter)
and fear of being laughed in a semi-	Fun as comic style (SchmHd)
projective cartoon evaluation task	Funniness of incongruity-resolution humor
Ironic comic style (SchmHd)	(3WD)
Inept humor style (HBQD)	Funniness of nonsense humor (3WD)
Laughter depicts "embarrassed" person	Laughing at yourself (SHS)
Mean-spirited humor style (HBQD)	Laughter depicts "happy" person
Negative laughter perceived as "not	Liking comedians
dominant"	Negative laughter perceived as "dominant"
No change in mood (positive, negative)	Nonsensical comic style (SchmHd)
after hearing laughter	Playfulness and positive mood (SHS)
Positive laughter perceived as "neutral"	Positive laughter perceived as "pleasant"
Repressed humor style (HBQD) (adults	Reflective humor style (HBQD) (students
only)	only)
Sarcastic comic style (SchmHd)	Self-enhancing humor (HSQ)
Satirical comic style (SchmHd)	Sense of humor (SHS)
Self-defeating humor style (HSQ)	Socially warm humor style (HBQD)
Seriousness (STCI-T) (adults only)	Trait cheerfulness (STCI-T)
Seriousness and negative mood (SHS)	
Socially cold humor style (HBQD)	

Uncorrelated with/high and low scores may go along with	
Aggressive humor (HSQ)	Fluency of punch line production (CPPT)
Finding incongruity-resolution humor	Funniness of sexual humor (3WD)
aversive (3WD)	Originality of produced punch line (CPPT)
Finding nonsense humor aversive (3WD)	

Note. 3 WD = 3 Witz-Dimensionen humor test, CHS = Coping Humor Scale, CPPT = Cartoon Punch line Production Test, HBQD = Humorous Behavior Q-Sort Deck, HSQ = Humor Styles Questionnaire, HUWO = Humor Words, SchmHd = comic styles according to Schmidt-Hidding; STCI-T = State-Trait-Cheerfulness Inventory. For size of correlations and further description of these studies and the measures used, see the original articles.

[1] Updated from Platt, Ruch, & Proyer (2010).

In order to test which hypothesis had more empirical support, a preliminary study was conducted in an Italian research project. A group of psychiatric patients (N = 34; 17 males; 17 females) and a group of controls (N = 36; 16 males; 20 females) were examined. The investigating tool was an Italian version of the GELOPH<46>. Answers are given on a four point Likert-scale from 1 (= strongly disagree) to 4 (= strongly agree). The psychiatric group had a significantly higher mean score (2.27; SD = .67) on the gelotophobia scale than controls (M = 1.45; SD = .34). In this exploratory study no differences among diagnostic categories emerged (the number of cases was too limited to have enough subjects in each category for statistical analysis).

A more extended and articulated study was subsequently conducted [33], which included a total of 194 Ss, 100 patients (53 male, 43 female, 4 missing; age ranging from 22 to 64) and 94 controls (35 male, 58 female, 1 missing; from 20 to 77 years). As an investigating tool the Italian version [54] of the GELOPH<15> was employed. A participant was defined as a "psychiatric patient" if he/she attended a psychiatric service at the time of the study, and had a record in the individual clinical file reporting a diagnosis established by a psychiatrist of a public institution (Dipartimento di Salute Mentale, Mental Health Department), according to the criteria of the Diagnostic Statistic Manual for Mental Disorders (DSM IV, American Psychiatric Association 1994). The GELOPH<15> was self-compiled, except for a few cases in which the interviewer administered it, due to difficulties of the patient (no substantial differences were anyway detected in relation to the administering modality).

The main result was that the patients group had a mean score on GELOPH<15> significantly higher than the normal control group (Patient: M = 2.25, SD = .58; Normal controls: M = 1.79, SD = .46; t = 6.0; p<.001). The mean score for the patients (2.25) was not far from 2.5, the threshold beyond which the individual enters the critical gelotophobic area. All the various diagnoses had been grouped into 5 broad categories keeping a criterion of internal homogeneity: 1. personality disorders; 2. schizophrenia disorders; 3. mood disorders; 4. anxiety disorders; 5. eating disorders. A comparison of the mean scores on the GELOPH<15> showed that there were differences associated with the diagnostic group. A one-way ANOVA resulted having a highly significant effect, $F(5, 188) = 11.965, p<.0001$. In particular, from lower to higher mean scores, Normal Controls scored 1.80 (SD = .46), Anxiety Disorders 2.01 (SD = .44), Mood Disorders 2.08 (SD = .59), Eating Disorders 2.24 (SD = .37), Personality Disorders 2.52 (SD = .56), and Schizophrenic Disorders 2.53 (SD = .57). It is worth noting that the mean score for the controls is very close to that found in a study with a wider sample of Italian subjects[33] (Forabosco et al., 2009; see Table 1). This can therefore be considered so far a standard value of reference for the Italian population. Interestingly, and not surprisingly, the sub-group of patients with paranoid schizophrenia (n = 7) had by far the highest score (M = 2.88). This is consistent with the typical persecutory world in which the patient affected by this form of disorder tangentially lives. This is a world where being laughed at may be rather easily (mis-) perceived as an act of aggression. Age and gender did not influence the scores, except that male individuals with schizophrenic disorder scored higher.

These results, in general, seem to associate a higher level of gelotophobia to what may be assumed as a higher degree of severity as regards the diagnosis. A first intuitive interpretation of this observation is that in, say, an individual with a schizophrenic disorder more psychological dimensions, also relevant in order to be more or less sensitive to being laughed at (be it real or imagined), are compromised in the pathological condition, in comparison with, for instance, an individual with a mood disorder. That may be not the only explanation is suggested by an additional finding. The years of care for each patient were also reported and compared with the means scores on GELOPH<15>. Years of attendance (less than a year, one to five years, more than five years), was assumed as an independent variable and the gelotophobia scores as a dependent variable. Years in care had a significant effect on degree of gelotophobia ($\underline{F}(2, 93) = 8.293$, $p < .001$): the longer the attendance the higher the score on GELOPH<15>. Still this may be due to the fact that the time spent in psychiatric care can be considered an indirect indicator of severity of the condition. But in addition, the longer the time in a "psychiatric patient" position the higher the probability of difficulties connected to a negative social perception, and even to the stigma which targets people with mental problems: a position in which being laughed at hardly is a benign experience. Other aspects are worth being taken into account. For instance, Ivanova [55] reports that patients with schizophrenia and affective disorders, when reading a joke, tend to identify with the mocked character, and this in turn might have an effect on gelotophobia.

A limit of the study conducted in Italy was that patients highly deteriorated or in an acute phase were not included. Therefore no generalizations are possible for this kind of subjects, who are not many in number, but a very important part of psychiatric care and research. Another aspect, which was not examined, was medication: how do psychotropic medicines influence a gelotophobic attitude and reaction? These are some of the most interesting lines for future investigation.

One possible, and striking, comparison in terms of research is with an investigation carried out in Russia [37,55,56]. Samples of 34 psychiatric patients and of 40 controls were examined using a Russian version of the GELOPH<15>. The results had an impressive similarity with the outcome of the Italian study: the control group $M = 1.61$ ($SD = .40$); the patients group $M = 2.22$ ($SD = .60$). What this similarity in results, in countries so different under many relevant aspects, appears to suggest is that there seem to be some underlining factors connecting gelotophobia and psychopathological conditions which are not influenced, at least not in a decisive way, by differences in social and cultural variables. This too is in need of being more deeply explored, also considering that the same Russian study found the relevance of a socio-cultural factor: people from a small town had higher gelotophobia scores than people from Moscow. The proposed explanation was that in a greater town people benefit from a higher degree of anonymity, which might be used as a shield protecting from the fear of being laughed at.

"THE DENTISTRY ENVIRONMENT"

The presence of gelotophobia may be, and has been, detected, in a revealing way, also in some other settings, different and even distant from the psychiatric ones, but still broadly connected with health care. An investigation was conducted in a specific dental care environment, namely that of "dental hygiene" which was presented [57]. Three phenomena were taken into consideration to examine whether and how they interact, halitosis, smoking habit, and gelotophobia. The two first are of obvious interest in the dental field, having to do with the oro-dental apparatus in many ways. Halitosis may be or signal a problem as a sign/symptom of some malfunction, and it is a relational issue, often connected with negative emotions, such as embarrassment. Smoking habit is considered to be responsible of many severe diseases, and has very controversial social implications.

One straight connection between smoking and halitosis is that the smoker's breath is chemically affected by the habit. No previous research work was available which could suggest how specifically gelotophobia relates to these phenomena. Therefore, it was an open exploratory hypothesis that was advanced. A total of 64 subjects (29 males; 35 females) were examined in the waiting room of a dental service. Three questionnaires were administered: the GELOPH<15>, a Smoking Habit Questionnaire, and the Halitosis Questionnaire [58]. Results showed that self perceived halitosis and smoking habit (number of cigarettes per day) were correlated ($r = .47$; $p<.05$); no correlation was found between smoking habit and gelotophobia; self perceived halitosis and gelotophobia presented a low but significant correlation ($r = .243$; $p <.05$). Smokers seem likely to be aware of (or believe they have) breathing problems, at least partly caused by the habit. As for the association between gelotophobia and halitosis, one possible, and theoretically stimulating, explanation is that a connecting element may be provided by the experience of shame, which is a crucial component both in gelotophobia [1] and in the way people typically feel about halitosis particularly when is publicly detected and mentioned [58]. The same does not seem to apply to the smoking habit. In general, other feelings appear to be involved, such as that of a sense of guilt for the damage the habit may cause to oneself and to others (for similarities and differences between shame and guilt [15] . A provocative question in this frame of (dental) hygiene may be advanced: shame and fear of being laughed at are emotions, which is safe and health to avoid and prevent. Yet would, or would not, in the particular and notable case of smokers, a dose of shame and even more of ridicule be a valid deterrent against a risky behavior?

GELOTOPHOBIA AND SUBJECTIVE WELL-BEING

The fear of being laughed at, as a form of humorlessness, can be seen as a factor severely impairing subjective well-being. Subjective well-being has affective and cognitive components. The former relates to both the presence of positive affect and the absence of negative affect. The latter relates to the evaluation that ones life is satisfactory—either as a whole (general life satisfaction) or in certain areas of life, such as satisfaction with work or relationship (domain satisfaction).

Figure 1 and the research quoted above show that the affective component is impaired, as high gelotophobia goes along with a lack of liveliness, spontaneity, joy, cheerfulness and humor (i.e., low positive affect) and the presence of psychosomatic complaints, shame, fear etc. (i.e., presence of positive affect). This is also replicated in the fact that gelotophobes are introverted (low positive affect) and emotionally unstable (high negative affect). Proyer, Ruch, and Chen [28] studied the relationship between fear of being laughed at and satisfaction with life in Austria, China and Switzerland using the Satisfaction with life scale. [59] They find that gelotophobia correlated negatively (between -.29 and -.40) in the three countries. That is, fearing being laughed at is a predictor of low satisfaction with life. They also investigated which of the three traditional orientations to happiness (i.e., life of pleasure, life of engagement, and life of meaning; see Seligman [60] are impaired. It turned out that in all three countries those fearing ridicule especially are low in life of engagement (coefficients between -.16 and -.31), suggesting that gelotophobes seem to lack the gratification that comes from immersing themselves in challenging activities; i.e., the lack flow experiences.

Well-being and making life worth living is the aim of the Positive Psychology [61]. To flourish in life Seligman argues requires a person to thrive in five components. Those are positive emotion, engagement and interest, relationships, meaning and purpose, and achievement (abbreviated to PERMA). While gelotophobes are markedly lower in positive emotion and engagement, nothing much can be said about achievement so far. However, there is indirect evidence for one of the other main facets of PERMA that helps an individual to flourish, namely to be in a *good relationship*. No questionnaire study was conducted so far on the quality of relationships of gelotophobes, but it is of interest to look at relationship status; i.e., life data.

GELOTOPHOBIA, WELL-BEING AND RELATIONSHIP STATUS

Prior studies of gelotophobia [1,33,49] all noted, as an aside to their respective studies, participants who were not in a relationship tended to score higher in gelotophobia. However, as relationships were not the main focus of those studies, the relationship status was not carefully defined and remained a basic demographic question that correlated negatively with gelotophobia. Another aspect these particular studies had in common was that they used younger participants. This in itself is no problem but it really would not be telling if many of them reported being single, as being single would, more than likely, be the norm. This left the open question: Are gelotophobes, who really want a relationship, and are still actively looking for a partner, remaining single due to the fear of being laughed at?

In order to fully answer this question there was a logical need for using a much older participant sample. This allowed to investigating where gelotophobia accounted for problems in relationships, at an age where an established relationship is usual and expected. To ensure that it was indeed gelotophobia as the disposition that affected relationship status two other dispositions towards laughter and ridicule were included that allowed to see if a good relationship is impaired only by gelotophobia, namely gelotophilia and katagelasticism.

The study consisted of people 60 years old and older (N = 148). In the study nine items regarding relationship status were asked. The items were chosen to reflect on the living arrangements as well as the marital status. The items and the distribution across all participants (irrespective of disposition) are shown in Table 3.

Table 3 shows that of all the nine dimensions of relationship status, 54% were married. The second largest group of people was those who were single and not looking for a partner. However, 5.8% of the sample of over 60 year olds were not in a long-term relationship and were still actively looking for a partner.

The relationship status was then correlated with the mean levels of gelotophobia, gelotophilia and katagelasticism. Being in a relationship (either living alone, with someone, being married) went along with higher scores in gelotophilia and lower scores in gelotophobia compared to not being in a relationship. It turned out that the highest scores were the singles that were not in a long-term relationship, but actively looking (*M* = 2.62) or not actively looking (M = 2.15). Singles that were in a long-term relationship were actually lowest (M = 1.88), and comparable to those in a relationship be they living with someone (M = 1.98) or married (M = 1.93). Widowed (M = 2.02) and divorced (M = 1.91) were in between. Thus, relationship status did matter in the fear of being laughed at. A different pattern emerged for gelotophilia. Here the highest scores were found for divorced (M = 2.79) and the lowest for separated but still married (M = 2.00). Katagelasticism did not show any significant effect. The highest groups were the widowed (M = 1,95) and the married (M = 1.96); the latter with men (M = 2.13) exceeding the women (M = 1.72). The highest level of katagelasticistic answers came from the people living with someone - In a relationship with them (M = 1.70) and the lowest from the singles actively looking for a long-term relationship (M = 1.12).

Table 3. Percentage of participant response to relationship status

Status	Percentage
Not in a long-term relationship but actively looking	5.8%
Not in a long-term relationship but not actively looking	14.2%
In a long-term relationship	5.8%
Living with someone but not in a relationship with them	0.0%
Living with someone and in a relationship with them	2.8%
Married	54%
Separated but still married	3.5%
Divorced	9.9%
Widowed	4.3%

Note: N = 148.

Overall, this suggests that being in a relationship was a potent predictor of which strategy a person adopts towards being laughed at. If a person was in a relationship, irrespective of actually living with the significant other, they tended to give gelotophilic answers, meaning they were able to laugh at their selves and enjoyed it when others laughed at them. By measuring the more detailed relationship status (for example being single and actively looking for a partner and being single and not looking for a partner), this study was able to elucidate the differences within this status and find precisely what the role the laughter dispositions played in maintaining a relationship. Actively seeking a partner shows that the person is discontent with their single status. This implies it is not a situation they would choose but something prevents them establishing a serious relationship, even though they desire it.

The joy of having others laugh at you does have a more social context. Indeed, without the audience's engagement and appreciation of the gelotophiles offering of embarrassing situations to be laughed at, the revelation would not be necessary or could even foolhardy. Thus, gelotophilia must require a certain social skill, which one could develop being in a close relationship. This would also answer why those in a relationship are lower in gelotophobia. The relationship with someone else might moderate the fear of being laughed at, as laughter styles can be explored in the relative safety of a close relationship.

An explanation as to why those who were single predominantly had the highest scores of gelotophobia could be due to laughter having a social aspect. Sharing laughter is bonding "People who laugh together stay together" is a well-used aphorism. Having a good sense of humor is a prerequisite in most dating advertisements and gelotophobes seem to lack it (see Table 2). So it seems inevitable that having a fear of laughter will disadvantage the sufferer in social situations and also in attracting a mate and sustaining a relationship. This was clearly shown from the results. Those with the highest scores in gelotophobia were not in a relationship but were actively looking. Meaning their single status was not what they wanted and the thought of having a partner was something they desired.

CONCLUSION

The aim of this chapter was to explore gelotophobia; i.e., the fear of being laughed at. It was evident from the first case-studies, which were used to elucidate the concept that gelotophobes had difficulty perceiving the difference between laughing with and laughing at. It went on to show how prevalent the fear of being laughed at is on a global scale, as well as showing how this overall score can be broken down further into a continuum ranging from none to extreme fear of being laughed at. Through extensive cross-cultural studies the construct of gelotophobia moved from a pathological fear to an individual difference in the general population. Gelotophobia was found in every country tested and this should be highly relevant considering the difficulties in making and maintaining social interactions and relationships.

Although gelotophobia shares many aspects with social phobia, investigations into this have shown that there are unique differences, which should be considered. Not all social phobes have gelotophobic tendencies and for those who do have a hyper-sensitivity towards being laughed at and are undergoing treatment for social phobia, may find that the help they are receiving, needs to have a more specific focus dealing with the very aspect that sets it apart from social phobia. Therefore understanding gelotophobia is crucial for clinicians and applied counselors who offer support for people with social phobia, social anxiety and general anxiety disorder.

The chapter also showed that gelotophobia goes along with still looking for a life partner, even at an age where one would expect them to be strongly pair-bonded and in a stable adult relationship. There is evidence that not being in a thriving relationship is detrimental to overall well-being and so it could be argued that in older age it will be these very people who lack social support that require interventions of a social nature, perhaps from healthcare or nursing homes. People working in these fields should also be made aware of the implications of trying to be playful with such older people as doing so will cause even more stress for them. These people will not be able to judge the playfulness or the attempts to be cheerful, as these will be seen as ridicule and not something positive. Retaining a serious demeanor will allow the gelotophobes in care to feel like they are taken seriously, which is important for them, especially as these people will be more affected by old age vulnerabilities and worry about them, even if they have not been directly affected by them. A similar argument can be made for psychiatric patients (especially the paranoid schizophrenics) where there is often seen a higher co-morbidity with gelotophobia.

As well as the care aspects of psychiatric patients with gelotophobia that have been alluded to, the studies conducted so far also highlighted some highly pertinent further research questions. As generally gelotophobia research is still in the early stages, more in-depth studies in areas known to have a higher prevalence of gelotophobia have a lot of potential not only in corroborating what has already been found but could also take the field into new directions.

Looking at the fear of being laughed at from the perspective of dentistry raised a valid question, namely, what would be the positive aspects of laughing at someone? Especially if doing so could correct a negative and anti-social habit such as smoking. Could the pay off of inducing shame and stimulating gelotophobia really is of therapeutic value?

ACKNOWLEDGMENTS

This study has been facilitated by a research grant from the Swiss National Science Foundation (SNSF; 100014_126967-1).

REFERENCES

[1] Ruch, W., & Proyer, R. T. (2008). The fear of being laughed at: Individual and group differences in gelotophobia. *Humor: International Journal of Humor Research, 21*, 47-67.

[2] Proyer, R. T., & Ruch, W. (2010). Dispositions towards ridicule and being laughed at: Current research on gelotophobia, gelotophilia and katagelasticism. *Psychological Test and Assessment Modeling, 52*, 49-59.

[3] Ruch, W., & Proyer, R. T. (2009). Extending the study of gelotophobia: On gelotophiles and katagelasticists. *Humor: International Journal of Humor Research, 22 (1/2)*, 183-212.

[4] Schmidt-Hidding, W. (1963). *Humor und Witz [Humour and Wit]*. München: Huebner.

[5] Ruch, W. (2007) (Ed.). *The Sense of Humor: Explorations of a Personality Characteristic*. Berlin: Mouton de Gruyter.

[6] Bachorowski, J., & Owren, M. J. (2001). Not all laughs are alike: Voiced but not unvoiced laughter readily elicits positive affect. *Psychological Science, 12*, 252-257.

[7] Beckman, H., Regier, N., & Young, J. (2007). Effect of workplace laughter groups on personal efficacy. *Journal of Primary Intervention, 28*, 167-182.

[8] Weisfeld, G. E. (1980). Human social motivation. In D. R. Omark, F. F. Strayer, & D. G. Freedman (Eds.), *Dominance Relations: An Ethological View of Human Conflict and Social Interaction* (pp. 273-286). New York: Garland STMP Press.

[9] MacHovec, F. J. (1988). *Humor: Theory, History, Applications*. Springfield, IL: Charles C. Thomas Publisher.

[10] Gruner, C. (1978). *Understanding Laughter: The Workings of Wit and Humor*. Chicago: Nelson-Hall.

[11] Monro, D. H. (1951). *Argument of laughter*. Melbourne: Melbourne University Press.

[12] Brottman, M. (2004). *Funny Peculiar: Gershon Legman and the Psychopathology of Humor*. Hilldale, NJ: Analytic Press Inc.

[13] Davies, C. (2011). *Jokes and Targets*. Bloomington, IN: Indiana University Press.

[14] Zillman, D., & Stocking, S. H. (1976). Putdown humor. *Journal of Communication, 26,* 154-163.

[15] Tangney, J. P., Miller, R. S., Flicker, L., & Barlow, D.H. (1996). Are shame, guilt and embarrassment distinct emotions? *Journal of Personality and Social Psychology, 70,* 1256-1269.

[16] Tangney, J. P. (1993). Shame and guilt. In C. G. Costello (Ed.). *Symptoms of Depression* (pp. 161-180). New York: Guilford Press.

[17] Titze, M. (1996). The Pinocchio complex: Overcoming the fear of laughter. *Humor & Health Journal, 5,* 1–11.

[18] Titze, M. (1997). Das Komische als schamauslösende Bedingung [The funny as an elicitor of shame]. In R. Kühn, M. Raub, & M. Titze (Eds.), *Scham – ein menschliches Gefühl* [Shame – A human emotion] (pp. 169–178). Opladen, Germany: Westdeutscher Verlag.

[19] Titze, M. (2009). Gelotophobia: The fear of being laughed at. *Humor: International Journal of Humor Research, 22* (1/2), 27-48.

[20] Ruch, W. (2004). *Gelotophobia: A useful new concept? IPSR Spring 2004 Colloquium Series,* Department of Psychology, University of California at Berkeley, Berkeley, USA, 10th March 2004

[21] Ruch, W., & Proyer, R. T. (2008b). Who is gelotophobic? Assessment criteria for the fear of being laughed at. *Swiss Journal of Psychology, 67,* 19-27.

[22] Ruch, W., Altfreder, O., & Proyer, R. T. (2009). How do gelotophobes interpret laughter in ambiguous situations? An experimental validation of the concept. *Humor: International Journal of Humor Research, 22 (1/2),* 62-89.

[23] Platt, T., Ruch, W., Hofmann, J., & Proyer, R. T. (2011). Extreme fear of being laughed at: Components of gelotophobia. Manuscript submitted for publication.

[24] Carretero-Dios, H., Proyer, R. T., Ruch, W., & Rubio, V. J. (2010). The Spanish version of the GELOPH<15>: Properties of a questionnaire for the assessment of the fear of being laughed at. *International Journal of Clinical and Health Psychology, 10,* 345-357.

[25] Proyer, R. T., Ruch, W., Ali, N. S., Al-Olimat, H. S., Andualem Adal, T., Aziz Ansari, S. et al. (2009). Breaking ground in cross-cultural research on the fear of being laughed at (gelotophobia): A multi-national study involving 73 countries. *Humor: International Journal of Humor Research, 22* (1/2), 253-279.

[26] Samson, A. C., Huber, O., Ruch, W. (2011). Teasing, ridiculing and the relation to the fear of being laughed at in individuals with Asperger's syndrome. *Journal of Autism and Developmental Disorders, 41,* 475–483.

[27] Samson, A. C., Thibault, P., Proyer, R. T., & Ruch, W. (2010). The subjective assessment of the fear of being laughed at (gelotophobia): Adaptation of the French version of the GELOPH<15>. *European Review of Applied Psychology/Revue Européenne de Psychologie Appliquée, 60,* 247-253.

[28] Proyer, R. T., Ruch, W., & Chen. G.-H. (in press). Positive psychology and the fear of being laughed at: Gelotophobia and its relations to orientations to happiness and life satisfaction in Austria, China, and Switzerland. *Humor: International Journal of Humor Research.*

[29]   Hrebickova, M., Fickova, E., Klementova, M., Ruch, W., & Proyer, R. T. (2009). Strach ze zesmesneni: Ceská a slovská verze dotazníku pro zjistovani gelotofobie [The fear of being laughed at: Czech and Slovak version of a questionnaire for gelotophobia]. *Ceskoslovenska Psychologie, 53*, 468-479.

[30]   Führ, M., Proyer, R. T., & Ruch, W. (2009). Assessing the fear of being laughed at (gelotophobia): First evaluation of the Danish GELOPH<15>. *Nordic Psychology, 61*, 62-73.

[31]   Platt, T., Ruch, W., & Proyer, R. T. (2009). Gelotophobia and bullying: The assessment of the fear of being laughed at and its application among bully victims. *Psychology Science Quarterly, 51*, 135-147.

[32]   Sarid, O., Ruch, W., & Proyer, R. T. (2011). Gelotophobia in Israel: On the assessment of the fear of being laughed at. *Israel Journal of Psychiatry and Related Sciences, 48*, 12-18.

[33]   Forabosco, G., Ruch, W., & Nucera, P. (2009). The fear of being laughed at among psychiatric patients. *Humor: International Journal of Humor Research, 22*, 233- 252.

[34]   Kazarian, S. S., Ruch, W., & Proyer, R. T. (2009). Gelotophobia in the Lebanon: The Arabic version of a questionnaire for the subjective assessment of the fear of being laughed at. *Arab Journal of Psychiatry, 20*, 42-56.

[35]   Chlopicki, W., Radomska, A., Proyer, R. T., & Ruch, W. (2010). The assessment of the fear of being laughed at in Poland. Translation and first evaluation of the Polish GELOPH <15>. *Polish Psychological Bulletin, 41*, 172-181.

[36]   Ruch, W., Proyer, R. T., & Popa, D. E. (2008). The fear of being laughed at (gelotophobia) and personality. *Anuarul Institutului de Istorie "G. Baritiu" din Cluj-Napoca, Series Humanistica", VI*, 53-68.

[37]   Stefanenko, E. A., Ivanova, E. M., Enikolopov, S. N., Proyer, R. T., & Ruch, W. (2011). Diagnosing the fear of being laughed at diagnostics: Russian adaptation of the gelotophobia questionnaire (in Russian). *Psihologicheskij Jurnal, 32*, 94-108.

[38]   Carretero-Dios, H., Agudelo Vélez, A. D., Ruch, W., Platt, T., & Proyer, R. T. (2010). Fear of being laughed at and social anxiety: A preliminary psychometric study. *Psychological Test and Assessment Modeling, 52*, 108-124.

[39]   Samson, A. C., Proyer, R. T., Ceschi, G., Pedrini, P. P., & Ruch, W. (2011). The fear of being laughed at in Switzerland: Regional differences and the role of positive psychology. *Swiss Journal of Psychology, 70*, 53-62.

[40]   Findlay, B. M. (2011). Gelotophobia: Is it just social anxiety repackaged? *Paper presented at the International Society of Humor Studies (ISHS) Congress*, 2011, July 5-9, Boston, MA.

[41]   Schilder, P. (1938). Social neurosis. *Psychoanalytic Review, 25*, 1-19.

[42]   Marks, I. M. (1970). The classification of phobic disorders. *The British Journal of Psychiatry, 116*, 377-386

[43]   American Psychiatric Association. (1994). *Diagnostic and Statistical Manual of Mental Disorders, 4th ed*. Washington, DC: American Psychiatric Association.

[44]   Hartenberg, P. (1901). *Les timides et la timidité [The socially anxious and social anxiety]*. Paris: Félix Alcan.

[45]   Edwards, K., Martin, R. A., & Dozois, D. J. A. (2010). The fear of being laughed at, social anxiety and memories of being teased during childhood. *Psychological Test and Assessment Modeling, 52*, 94-107.

[46]   Watson, D., & Friend, R. (1969). Measurement of social-evaluative anxiety. *Journal of Consulting and Clinical Psychology, 33*, 448-457.

[47]   Ruch, W., & Ekman, P. (2001). The expressive pattern of laughter. In A. W. Kaszniak (Ed.). *Emotion, Qualia, and Consciousness* (pp. 426-433). Tokyo: Word Scientific Publisher.

[48]   Ruch, W. (2008). The psychology of humor. In V. Raskin (Ed.), *A Primer of Humor* (pp. 17-100). Berlin: Mouton de Gruyter.

[49]   Platt, T., Ruch, W., & Proyer, R. T. (2010). A lifetime of the fear of being laughed at: An aged perspective. *Zeitschrift für Gerontologie und Geriatrie, 43*, 36-41.

[50]   Platt, T. (2008). Emotional responses to ridicule and teasing: Should gelotophobes react differently? *Humor: International Journal of Humor Research, 21(2)*, 105-128.

[51]   Ruch, W., Beermann, U., & Proyer, R. T. (2009). Investigating the humor of gelotophobes: Does feeling ridiculous equal being humorless? *Humor: International Journal of Humor Research, 22 (1/2)*, 111-143.

[52]   Vaillant, G. (2002). *Aging Well. Surprising Guideposts to a Happier Life from the Landmark Harvard Study of Adult Development*. Boston, MA: Little, Brown and Company.

[53]   Platt, T., & Ruch, W. (2010). Gelotophobia and age: Do dispositions towards ridicule and being laughed at predict coping with age-related vulnerabilities? *Psychological Test and Assessment Modeling, 52*, 231-244.

[54]   Forabosco, G., Dore, M., Ruch, W., & Proyer, R. T. (2009). Psicopatologia della paura di essere deriso. Un'indagine sulla gelotofobia in Italia. *Giornale di Psicologia, 3*, 183-190.

[55]   Ivanova, A. (2005). Psychological mechanisms of sense of humor disorders in patients with schizophrenia and cyclothymia. A qualitative analysis. *Paper presented at the 17th annual conference of the International Society for Humor Studies*. 2005, June 13-17, Youngstown, OH, USA.

[56]   Ivanova, A., Stefanenko, E., Enikopolov, S., Proyer, R. T., & Ruch, W. (in press). The fear of being laughed at in healthy people and psychiatry patients. Assessing gelotophobia in Russia. *Bridging Eastern and Western Psychiatry*.

[57]   Forabosco, G., Forabosco, A., Cavalli, L., & Galeoni, C. (2010). Le implicazioni psicologiche dell'alitosi. *Paper presented at the Conference Alitosi 2010. Informazioni e competenze cliniche*. 2010, December 11, Modena, Italy.

[58]   Nardi, G. M., Forabosco, A., Forabosco, G., Musciotto, A., Campisi, G., & Grandi, T. (2009). Halitosis: a stomatological and psychological issue. *Minerva Stomatologica, 58*, 435-44.

[59]   Diener, E. D, Emmons,R.A., Larsen,R.J. & Griffin, S. (1985). The Satisfaction With Life Scale. *Journal of Personality Assessment, 49, 71-75*

[60]   Seligman, M.E.P. (2002). *Authentic happiness: Using the New Positive Psychology to Realize your Potential for Lasting Fullfilment*. Free Press: New York

[61]   Seligman, M. E. P. (2011). *Flourish: A New Understanding of Happiness, Well-Being - and How to Achieve Them*. Free Press: New York.

In: Humor and Health Promotion
Editor: Paola Gremigni

ISBN: 978-1-61942-657-3
© 2012 Nova Science Publishers, Inc.

Chapter 13

HUMOR MEASUREMENT

Giulia Casu and Paola Gremigni

Department of Psychology, University of Bologna, Italy

Abstract

Some of the most recent trait-oriented, self-report instruments for measuring humor are briefly described. Assessment tools can be classified according to their primary measurement objective: Sense of humor, humor creation and/or humor appreciation, humor coping, and humor styles.

Most instruments measure a global sense of humor that is the extent to which individuals tend to laugh, smile, create and express humor in their lives.

Some instruments treat humor as a uniform construct, whereas others assess different components of humor. Few humor measurement tools address the potentially harmful uses of humor, and different humor styles are measured by two instruments only.

Researchers can choose a variety of tools to measure self-reported humor with acceptable psychometric properties. Instrument choice should be guided by consideration of the aim of the study and the operationalization adopted for humor.

INTRODUCTION

Using humor has positive effects on different areas of everyday life, such as education, work and marriage. Thus, many scholars have been trying to develop appropriate measures of humor, and different types of tools are now available in the literature. Such tools include informal surveys, joke telling techniques or diary methods, joke/cartoon tests, and trait- and state-oriented self-reports [1]. Other instruments do not measure sense of humor directly, but use humor to assess various aspects of individuals' personality. Others measure different phenomena (e.g., coping strategies) but include also subscales assessing humor.

Natural observations and semi-structured interview have also been used. Similar qualitative approaches are unquestionably useful, yet they cannot address individuals' interpretations of humorous stories and jokes nor one's perceived amount of humor use and humor production ability, as well as the perceived effects of such humorous productions on others.

Currently, questionnaires are preferred by researchers, with most questionnaires being addressed to adult individuals.

We will focus here on some of the most recent trait-oriented self-report instruments that are available for assessing humor in adults. Four different categories have been identified, according to the first measurement objective: sense of humor, humor creativity and/or humor production, humor coping, and humor styles.

SENSE OF HUMOR

Situational Humor Response Questionnaire (SHRQ)

The Situational Humor Response Questionnaire (SHRQ) [2] measures the frequency with which individuals smile, laugh and respond with cheerfulness in a variety of life situations. It is composed of 21 items describing both pleasant (7 items) and unpleasant situations (11 items).

The first 18 items include descriptions of ordinary life situations. Respondents indicate the extent to which they typically would laugh in such situations, using a 5-point Guttman-type scale, ranging from 1 (I would not have been particularly amused) to 5 (I would have laughed heartily). The last three items are self-descriptive and evaluate the overall extent to which individuals are amused and laugh in a variety of situations. Examples of items:

> "You were watching a movie or TV program with some friends and you found one scene particularly funny, but no one else appeared to find it humorous."
> "You were wakened from a deep sleep in the middle of the night by the ringing of the telephone, and it was an old friend who was just passing through town and had decided to call and say hello."

Reliability was acceptable. Internal consistency coefficients (Cronbach's alpha) ranged from .70 to .85, and test-retest reliability over a 4-week interval was .70.

Construct validity was supported by correlations between SHRQ scores and frequency and duration of spontaneous laughter during unstructured interviews, rated humor of monologues produced by participants, peer ratings of participants' amount of mirth and inclination to use humor as a coping strategy, and a measure of positive mood [3-4].

SHRQ scores were not significantly related to scores on the Marlowe-Crowne Social Desirability Scale [5], suggesting that the SHRQ is not subject to social desirability biases. Nevertheless, Ruch and Deckers [6] found some significant correlations between SHRQ total scores and the *Lie* scale of the Eysenck Personality Questionnaire-revised (EPQ-R) [7], suggesting that funniness reactions are not socially desirable in certain situations.

Evidence of SHRQ validity also emerged in subsequent studies. SHRQ scores were positively related to frequency of laughter over a three-day period [8] and extraversion [6,9], and negatively associated with neuroticism [6]. Positive associations were also found between psychoticism and items of the SHRQ describing risk, non-conformity, and embarrassing events in which the respondent or another person is involved [6]. Other studies that used the

SHRQ found significant positive correlations between SHRQ scores and the *Metamessage sensitivity* subscale of the Sense of Humor Questionnaire (SHQ-MS) [10] (r from .32 .39, p < .01) [3, 11], *Personal liking of humor* subscale of the SHQ (SHQ-LH) (r = .25, p < .001) [11], *Emotional expressiveness* subscale of the SHQ (SHQ-EE) (r = .40, p < .001) [11], Coping Humor Scale (CHS) [3] (r from .39 to .44, p < .05) [3,11,12] *Humor creation* subscale of the Multidimensional Sense of Humor Scale (MSHS-HC) [13] (r = .42, p < .001), *Humor appreciation* subscale of the MSHS (MSHS-HA) (r = .22, p < .05), Humor Initiation Scale (HIS) [14] (r = .53, p < .001) [15], *Humor creation* subscale of Ziv's Sense of Humor Questionnaire (SHQZ-HC) [16] (r from.49 to .53, p < .001), *Humor appreciation* subscale of the SHQZ (SHQZ-HA) (r from .48 to .50, p < .001) [11,15], *Affiliative* humor style subscale of the Humor Styles Questionnaire (HSQ-AF) [17] (r = .27, p < .001), and the *Self-enhancing* humor style subscale of the HSQ (HSQ-SE) (r = .43, p < .001) [17]. On the other hand, the SHRQ was negatively associated with social avoidance, distress [18], and depression [9].

In their factor analytic study, Thorson and Powell [19] suggest that the SHRQ is a tool for assessing individuals' propensity to smile and laugh *per se,* rather than a measure of sense of humor. Consistently with such hypothesis, SHRQ scores were found to be unrelated with humor ratings of jokes and cartoons [20]. One weakness of the SHRQ is that the situations described in the first 18 items refer too specifically to college students' experiences and look somewhat anachronistic.

Sense of Humor Questionnaire (SHQ)

The SHQ [10] is a 21-item instrument for measuring the cognitive, social, and affective dimensions of humor thorough three subscales. Each item is rated on a 4-point Likert scale ranging from 1 (very difficult/not at all) to 4 (very easily/yes indeed).

Metamessage sensitivity scale (SHQ-MS; 7 items) assesses the cognitive dimension of humor, which is described as the ability to identify humorous stimuli. Example items:
"Do you easily recognize a mark of humorous content?"
"I can usually find something comical, witty, or humorous in most situations."

Personal liking of humor scale (SHQ-LH; 7 items) represents the social dimension that reflects an appreciation of humorous individuals and situations. Example items:
"Persons who are always out to be funny are really irresponsible types not to be relied upon."
"It is my impression that those who try to be funny really do it to hide their lack of self-confidence."

Emotional expressiveness scale (SHQ-EE; 7 items) assesses the affective dimension, which measures one's comfort in expressing emotions, including humor. Example items:
"If I find a situation very comical, I find it very hard to keep a straight face even when nobody else seems to think it's funny."
"I appreciate people who tolerate all kinds of emotional expression."

Reliability was not entirely satisfactory. Internal consistency coefficients (Cronbach's alpha) were .60, .75, and below .20 for *Metamessage sensitivity, Liking of humor*, and *Emotional expressiveness*, respectively. Test-retest reliability ranged between .58 and .78 over a 4-week interval. Moreover, no significant correlations were found between the SHQ and the Marlowe-Crowne Social Desirability Scale [5], suggesting that the SHQ is not subject to social desirability biases [21].

In subsequent studies, the SHQ-MS reported significant correlations with the MSHS-HC ($r = .39$, $p < .05$) [12], SHRQ ($r = .32$, $p < .01$) [3], and the CHS ($r = .38$ to .51, $p < .05$) [3,12], whereas SHQ-LH was significantly related to the CHS ($r = .33$, $p < .01$) [3]. In addition, the *Metamessage sensitivity* scale was found to be the best predictor of the emotional consequences of a stressor, when considering various senses of humor measures, and it was related to more positive affect and reduced anxiety both before and after exposure to a stressful situation [12]. In a study by Deaner and McConatha [9], negative correlations were found between the total SHQ and depression scores. In another study [11], all the three SHQ scales showed significant correlations with both the SHQZ-HA ($r = .27$, .33, and .41 for SHQ-MS, SHQ-LH, and SHQ-EE, respectively; $p < .001$) and the SHQZ-HC ($r = .39$, .24, and .39 for SHQ-MS, SHQ-LH, and SHQ-EE, respectively; $p < .001$).

A factor analysis conducted by Thorson and Powell [19] yielded a 6-factor solution: *Negative attitudes towards humorous people* (7 items); *Getting the joke* (3 items); *Affable outlook* (2 items); *Inappropriate humor* (3 items); *Humorous people* (4 items); and *Social worth of humor* (3 items). The SHQ has been largely criticized, as it has consistently showed unacceptable reliability levels, with Cronbach's alpha values of .51 [19].

Due to its inacceptable internal consistency, the *Emotional expression* scale was not included in a shorter version of the SHQ (SHQ-6) [22], which was developed for inclusion in epidemiological surveys. The SHQ-6 measures individuals' ability to perceive and enjoy humor and humorous people in their lives. This brief instrument is composed by three *Metamessage sensitivity* and three *Liking of humor* items, and uses a 4-point Likert scale ranging from 1 (very difficult/not at all) to 4 (very easily/yes indeed).

An overall sense of humor score is computed, since factor analysis revealed a single-factor structure. Cronbach's alpha coefficient was .85, suggesting good internal consistency. Validity was supported by significant correlations with the HSQ-AF ($r = .54$, $p < .001$) and the HSQ-SE ($r = .45$, $p < .001$), whereas no significant correlations emerged between the SHQ-6 and the *Aggressive* and *Self-defeating* scales of the HSQ. The HSQ-6 can be used with individuals aged 15 years and older.

Sense of Humor Scale (SHS)

The Sense of Humor Scale (SHS) [23] is usually employed within the McGhee's humor development program [24]. Originally, the SHS was composed by eight 5-item subscales measuring different humor-related behaviors: *Enjoyment of humor, Seriousness and negative mood, Playfulness and positive mood, Laughter, Verbal humor, Finding humor in everyday life, Laughing at yourself, Humor under stress*. Respondents rate each item on a 7-point Likert scale, ranging from 1 (strongly disagree) to 7 (strongly agree).

An investigation of the psychometric properties of English and German versions of SHS was realized by Ruch and Carrell [25].

Reliability coefficients for the total SHS were high, with Cronbach's alpha values of .92 (US sample: N = 263) and .90 (German sample: N = 151). Internal consistency coefficients for the six SHS subscales ranged from .56 (*Laughter*; German sample) to .80 (*Laughing at yourself*; US sample) [25]. Factor analyses with oblique rotation were conducted separately for the two samples. A general factor of humor skills (composed of the original *Enjoyment of humor*, *Laughter*, *Verbal humor*, *Finding humor in everyday life*, *Laughing at yourself*, and *Humor under stress* subscales) and a playful vs. serious factor (composed of the original *Seriousness and negative mood*, and *Playfulness and positive mood* dimensions) emerged [25].

Construct validity was supported by positive correlations between the SHS subscales and trait cheerfulness: correlations with trait cheerfulness ranged from .52 (*Laughter*) to .80 (overall SHS), and from .47 (*Humor under stress*) to .83 (overall SHS) in the US and German samples, respectively [25]. In both samples, *Playfulness and positive mood* was the SHS component most highly correlated with trait cheerfulness (rs = .65 and .75 in the US and German sample, respectively; $p < .001$). In a recent study [26], the SHS showed significant positive correlations with the *socially warm* (r = .57, $p < .001$), *competent* (r = .23, $p < .05$), and *earthy* (r = .21, $p < .05$) dimensions of the Humorous Behavior Q-Sort Deck (HBQD) [27,28].

Psychometric analyses led McGhee [23] to divide the SHS into three parts, corresponding to three separate scores:

Playful vs. serious attitude (8 items). Example items:
    "I have a lot of fun in my life."
    "I prefer friends who are generally pretty serious."
Positive vs. negative mood (8 items). Example items:
    "I have a lot of joy in my life."
    "I am often depressed."
Sense of humor (24 items). *Sense of humor* is composed of the following 4-item scales:
Enjoyment of humor. Example items:
    "When I go to the movies, my preference is generally to see a good comedy."
    "It is important for me to have a lot of humor in my life."
Laughter. Example items:
    "I have a heartier, more robust laugh than most people."
    "I feel comfortable laughing, even when others aren't."
Verbal humor. Example items:
    "I often tell funny stories."
    "I often create my own spontaneous puns."
Finding humor in everyday life. Example items:
    "I often find humor in things that happen at work."
    "I often share with others the funny incidents I observe, or that happen to me."
Laughing at yourself. Example items:
    "I have no troubles poking fun on my physical imperfections."
    "I find it easy to laugh when I am the butt of the joke."
Humor under stress. Example items:
    "My sense of humor rarely abandons me under stress."
    "I often use my sense of humor to control the effect of stress on my mood."

A final Humor Quotient is computed for this part, by giving the *Laughing at yourself* and *Humor under stress* scales higher weights. Total sense of humor rating turned out to be positively related to trait cheerfulness (r .18, p < .01) and extraversion (r = .15, p < .05) [29].

State-Trait Cheerfulness Inventory – Trait Part (STCI-T)

The State-Trait Cheerfulness Inventory (STCI) [30] measures the dimensions of cheerfulness, seriousness, and unpleasant mood as both states (STCI-S) and traits (STCI-T). Although the STCI is not properly a measure of sense of humor, it addresses emotion-related traits that are considered to be parts of the temperamental basis of humor [31]. For the Trait part (STCI-T), three different forms are available: a long form composed by 106 items (STCI-T<106>); a standard form consisting of 60 items (STCI-T<60>), and a short form with 30 items (STCI-T<30>). Items in all three forms are rated on a 4-point Likert scale, ranging from 1 (strongly disagree) to 4 (strongly agree). Internal consistency coefficients were found to be high, with Cronbach's alpha values ranging from .86 to .96 for the STCI-T<106> and from .80 to .94 for the STC-T<60> [30]. The survey was also found to be temporally stable, with test-retest reliability coefficients ranging from .77 to .86 for the STCI-T<106> (N = 103; 4-week interval) and from .73 to .86 for the STCI-T<60> (N = 68, 3-week interval) [30]. Validity was assessed through correlations between the self-report and the peer-evaluation forms, which were found to be adequate [30].

The STCI-T<106> [30] is composed of three subscales:

Trait Cheerfulness (STCI-T CH; 38 items) reflects cheerfulness as a temperamental trait that facilitated the expression of humor. Example items:
"I am a cheerful person."
"Laughing has a contagious effect on me."
Trait Seriousness (STCI-T SE; 37 items) assesses the tendency to prefer humorlessness activities and expressions. Example items:
"In my life, I like to have everything correct."
"In everything I do, I always consider every possible effect and compare all pros and cons carefully."
Trait Bad mood (STCI-T BM; 31 items) describes the prevalence of a sad and ill-humored mood. Example items:
"Compared to others, I really can be grumpy and grouchy."
"I often feel so gloomy that nothing can make me laugh."

The STCI-T<60> measures the same dimensions as the STCI-T<106>, but using three 20-item subscales (STCI T CH, STCI-T SE, and STCI-T BM).

A recent study that used the STCI-T<60> [26] found that the STCI-T CH was positively associated with the socially warm (r = .56 to .70, p < .001) and the earthy humor styles (r = .26, p < .001), the HSQ-AF (r = .69, p < .001), HSQ-SE (r = .58, p < .001), and HSQ-SD (r = .16, p < .05). On the other hand, the STCI-T SE was negatively correlated with the socially warm (r = -.35 to -.45, p < .001) and earthy humor styles (r = -.15 to -.24, p < .05), the HSQ-AF (r = -.45, p < .001), HSQ-SE (r = -.24, p < .01), and HSQ-AG (r = -.34, p < .001). Finally, the STCI-T BM was negatively related to the socially warm (r = -.35 to -.56, p < .001) and competent (r = -.22 to -.24, p < .01), earthy (r = -.16, p < .05), and benign (r = -.21, p < .01) humor styles, the HSQ-AF (r = -.50, p < .001), and HSQ-SE (r = -.36, p < .001). For a more detailed description of the STCI, see Ruch and Hofmann's Chapter in this book.

HUMOR CREATIVITY AND HUMOR APPRECIATION

Ziv's Sense of Humor Questionnaire (SHQZ)

The Sense of Humor questionnaire [16] is composed of two 7-item scales for the measurement of two components of humor: humor appreciation and humor creation. Items are rated using a 7-point Likert scale ranging from 1 (very rarely) to 7 (very often), and a total sense of humor score is computed from adding the two subscale scores together.

Humor creativity scale (SHQZ-HC) measures the ability to perceive unconventional relationships between people, objects and ideas and talent for entertaining others. Example item:
    "When I want to achieve some purpose, I use humor."
Humor appreciation (SHQZ-HA) assesses the ability to appreciate messages containing humor creativity. Example item:
    "I find many situations laughable."

Validation sample was composed of three hundred and forty four high school students. Internal consistency was acceptable, with Cronbach's alpha values of .66, .73, and .81 for *Humor creativity, Humor appreciation* and total sense of humor, respectively [11]. Concurrent validity was demonstrated for the SHQZ, with significant correlations between each of its subscales and the *Humor creation* and *Humor appreciation* scales of the MSHS (rs = .49 and .38 for SHQZ-HA, respectively; rs = .71 and .33 for SHQZ-HC, respectively; p < .001), the HIS (rs = .56 and .67 for SHQZ-HA and SHQZ-HC, respectively; p < .001), and the SHRQ (rs = .50 and .53 for SHQZ-HA and SHQZ-HC, respectively; p < .001) [15], the CHS (rs = .48 and .49 for SHQZ-HA and SHQZ-HC, respectively; p < .001), and all three subscales (*Metamessage sensitivity, Liking of humor, Emotional expression*) of the SHQ (rs = .27, .33, and .41 for SHQZ-HA, respectively; rs = .39, .24, and .39 for SHQZ-HC, respectively; p < .001) [11].

Multidimensional Sense of Humor Scale (MSHS)

The Multidimensional Sense of Humor Scale [13] is one of the most used multidimensional measures of sense of humor, being available in several languages. It is a 24-item self-report scale designed to assess both humor creation and humor appreciation. Respondents rate each item on a 5-point scale ranging from 0 (strongly disagree) to 4 (strongly agree).

Data obtained from three independent samples were subjected to principal components analyses with Varimax rotation, leading to retention of 24 items divided into four subscales.

Humor creativity and use of humor for social purposes (MSHS-HC; 11 items). Example items:
> "I'm confident that I can make other people laugh."
> "I can ease a tense situation by saying something funny."

Coping with humor (MSHS-CH; 7 items). Example items:
> "Coping by using humor is an elegant way of adapting."
> "Uses of humor help to put me at ease."

Humor appreciation (MSHS-HA; 2 items). Items:
> "I appreciate those who generate humor."
> "I like a good joke."

Attitudes toward humor (MSHS-AH; 4 negatively phrased items). Example items:
> "People who tell jokes are a pain in the neck."
> "I'm uncomfortable when everyone is cracking jokes."

Internal consistency reliability of the total scale was excellent, with a Cronbach's alpha coefficient of .92. A more recent study that used the MSHS [32] reported Cronbach's alpha values ranging from .57 (*Humor appreciation* and *Attitudes toward humor*) to .93 (*Humor creation*).

The MSHS was positively associated with optimism ($r = -.40$ with the Levy scale [33], $p < .001$) and self-esteem ($r = -.57$ with the Negative Self-esteem Scale [34], $p < .05$), and negatively associated with depression ($r = -.18$, $p < .05$) [35,36]. *Humor creativity* was positively related with exhibition and dominance (exhibition: $r = .28$ in males and .32 in females; dominance: $r = .24$ in males and .16 in females; $p < .001$). *Coping with humor* and *Attitudes toward humor* were negatively related to death anxiety (MSHS-CH: $r = -.23$ in males and -.19 in females, $p < .001$; MSHS-AH: $r = -.12$ in females, $p < .001$) [36].

The MSHS has been used in numerous studies, showing associations with multiple variables. For example, overall sense of humor was positively related with warmth, gregariousness, assertiveness, excitement seeking, positive emotions, and intrinsic religiosity [36]. Nevertheless, one study found that only the *Humor creativity* and *Coping humor* scales showed significant correlations with other humor scales [12]. Specifically, *Humor creativity* was related with the *Metamessage sensitivity* scale of the SHQ ($r = .39$, $p < .05$), whereas both MSHS-HC and MSHS-CH showed positive correlations with the CHS (rs = .47 and .46, respectively; $p < .05$). In another study [17], the MSHS was the only one of six instruments to be significantly associated with all four subscales of the HSQ. In addition, a recent study showed that all the four dimensions of the MSHS were positively correlated with the *Affiliative* (rs from .43 to .72, $p < .01$) and *Self-enhancing* (rs between .27 and .58, $p < .01$) subscales of the HSQ, whereas the MSHS-HC and the MSHS-CH subscales were also associated with the *Aggressive* humor subscale of the HSQ (rs = .32 and .21, respectively; $p < .01$) [32].

Humor Orientation Scale (HO)

The Humor Orientation Scale (HO) [37] assesses individuals' enactment of humorous messages in interpersonal situations. It is a 17-item scale that uses a 5-point Likert scale ranging from 1 (strongly disagree) to 5 (strongly agree). Examples of items are as follows:

"I regularly tell jokes and funny stories when I am with my group."
"Of all the people I know, I'm one of the funniest."

A confirmatory factor analysis was conducted on data from 275 university students, showing a good fit for both one-factor and two-factor (frequency and effectiveness of humor use) models. The one factor solution was supported by item-total correlations (equal or above .5), and Cronbach's alpha value ($\alpha = .90$).

Higher Humor Orientation scores were found to be associated with a higher number of situations in which respondents stated that they "would use" humor and a reduced number of situations in which they "would not use" humor. The HO scores were also correlated with the humor complexity index, which was calculated as the total number of categories of humor used, over six different possible categories of entertaining behaviors (e.g., nonverbal, other-orientation, expressiveness).

Finally, significant, positive correlations emerged between HO scores and the amount of specificity and planning in written accounts in which participants described those behaviors they would show in a hypothetical situation aimed at "wittily communicating to get a new person to like them". In other words, individuals predisposed to use humor tended to produce funniness without substantial planning, and included more descriptions and dialogue details in their accounts than others.

Internal consistency reliability turned out to be high, with a Cronbach's alpha value of .89 [29,37], and test-retest reliability over an 8-week interval was .70 (N = 37) [37].

In subsequent studies, the HO was found to be positively related to the STCI-T CH (r = .63, p < .0001) and extraversion (r = .63, p < .001), and negatively associated with neuroticism (r = -.37, p < .0001), psychoticism (r = -.30, p < .0001), STCI-T SE (r = -.14, p < .05), and STCI-T BM (r = -.50, p < .0001) [29]. Moreover, HO scores significantly correlated with scores on the RHAI (r = .51, p < .0001) [29].

One weakness is that the HO scale does not measure the use of humor to communicate, but rather it addresses the inclination to engage in jokes and humorous story telling [29]. As a matter of fact, one item only refers specifically to the communicative uses of humor ("I use humor to communicate in a variety of situations").

Richmond Humor Assessment Instrument (RHAI)

The Richmond Humor Assessment Instrument (RHAI) [38] measures individuals' propensity to use humor as a verbal and nonverbal communicative tool. It is composed of 16 items with a 5-point response format ranging from 1 (strongly disagree) to 5 (strongly agree). Example items:

"Being humorous is a natural communication orientation for me."

"Even funny ideas and stories seem dull when I tell them." (reverse item).

The internal consistency of the RHAI was found to be high, with a Cronbach's alpha value of .89 [29]. Construct validity was supported by positive correlations with extraversion ($r = .42$, $p < .0001$) and the STCI-T CH ($r = .39$, $p < .0001$), whereas negative correlations were found between the RHAI and both neuroticism ($r = -.16$, $p < .05$) and the STCI-BM ($r = -.27$, $p < .0001$) [29]. Moreover, RHAI scores were significantly associated with HO scores ($r = .51$, $p < .001$) [29].

Principal component analysis was realized on the data obtained from 448 university students, who received a modified version of the RHAI, with items adjusted to fit the classroom setting (e.g., "Being humorous is a natural communication orientation for my teacher", "Even funny ideas and stories seem dull when my teacher tells them"). One single factor emerged, with a Cronbach's alpha value of .95 [29].

HUMOR COPING

Coping Humor Scale (CHS)

The Coping Humor Scale (CHS) [3] is a well-established, valid and reliable measure of how humor is deliberately used as a coping strategy. Its 7 items are rated on a 4-point scale, ranging from 1 (strongly disagree) to 4 (strongly agree). Example items:

"I usually look for something comical to say when I am in tense situations."
"I have often felt that if I am in a situation where I have to either cry or laugh, it's better to laugh."

Internal consistency coefficient (Cronbach's alpha) in the validation study was .61 ($N = 56$), and corrected item-total correlations ranged from .11 to .54.

Construct validity is confirmed by positive correlations between the CHS and both the SHQ-MS ($r = .51$, $p < .001$) and the SHQ-LH ($r = .33$, $p < .01$). Moreover, it was found that participants with higher scores on the CHS reported lower mood disturbance in spite of increased negative life events. A further evidence of validity was provided by correlations with peer ratings of use of humor in stressful situations, and rated funniness of monologues produced by participants while watching a stressful film. Nevertheless, CHS scores did not correlate with the use of humor in non-stressful situations.

No significant correlations were found between the CHS and the Marlowe-Crowne Social Desirability Scale [5]. This indicates that the CHS is not affected by social desirability.

In subsequent studies using the CHS, a Cronbach's alpha coefficient of .75 emerged [39], and test-retest reliability coefficient was found to be .80 over a 12-week period [40].

Construct validity of the CHS is supported by positive correlations with extraversion ($r = .43$, $p < .01$) [36], the HSQ-AF ($r = .33$, $p < .001$), HSQ-SE ($r = .55$, $p < .001$), and HSQ-AG ($r = .21$, $p < .01$) [17].

A confirmatory factor analysis conducted by Nezlek and Derks [41] revealed that all but one CHS items met the criteria to be valid measures of the underlying construct.

This 6-item version of the CHS showed acceptable internal consistency (Cronbach's alpha = .75). It was also positively associated with the amount of social interaction, enjoyment and confidence in social interaction, showing satisfactory validity.

The CHS has been largely used to evaluate the stress-moderating effects of humor, showing satisfactory predictive validity [4]. An empirical study examining the relationships between humor and burnout among female nursing education faculty (N = 192) showed that use of humor as a coping strategy was negatively associated with depersonalization and positively related to accomplishment [39]. In addition, it was found that a higher score on the CHS was negatively related to loneliness, depression and stress, and positively associated with self-esteem and quality of life [40,42,43].

Relational Humor Inventory (RHI)

The Relational Humor Inventory (RHI) [44] was developed for measuring the use of humor in the marriage relationship. Respondents are asked to report their own and their partner's use of humor within the marital couple, by rating 16 items on a 7-point Likert scale ranging from 1 (not at all accurate) to 7 (very accurate). Principal component analysis conducted on data from 136 participants yielded three subscales:

Instrumental humor (8 items), which reflects the extent to which marital partners use humor to avoid tension or reduce negative feelings. Example items:
"I use humor to get out of a fight with my partner."
"When my partner feels sad or upset, I try to make him/her see the funny side of the story."
Positive humor (5 items), which describes positive aspects of humor, such as humor appreciation and closeness. Example items:
"Joking with my partner makes me feel closer to him/her."
"I believe that my partner appreciates my humorous remarks."
Negative humor (3 items), which addresses the use of humor to express hostility or manipulate the partner. Example items:
"Occasionally, I tend to make jokes at my partner's expense."
"Sometimes I use humor to put my partner down."

Internal consistency reliability was acceptable, with Cronbach's alpha coefficients ranging from .72 (*Couple humor*) to .84 (*Instrumental humor*).

Construct validity was supported by correlations with other humor and relationship measures. For example, the *Partner positive humor* subscale was significantly related to marriage intimacy (rs = .48 and .49 for husbands and wives, respectively; p < .001) and satisfaction (rs = .55 and .43 for husbands and wives, respectively; p < .001), whereas the *Partner negative humor* subscale was associated with avoidant interaction between partners (husbands: r = .39, p < .05; wives: r = .55, p < .001). Moreover, for both wives and husbands, *Positive humor* subscales (husbands: r = .33, p < .05; wives: r = .53, p < .001) and *Instrumental humor* (husbands: r = .45, p < .001; wives: r = .38, p < .05) were related to the SHQZ-HC.

Authors suggest using the RHI in family psychotherapy settings, and propose to consider positive humor as relationship strength, negative humor as a failure of constructive communication, and instrumental humor as a couple's ability to deal with sensitive issues.

Questionnaire of Occupational Humorous Coping (QOHC)

The Questionnaire of Occupational Humorous Coping (QOHC) [45] is a self-report tool designed to assess humorous coping strategies for dealing with work-related demands, and can be used in a broad range of work settings.

The development process was based on Gross's model of emotion regulation [46], which distinguishes between antecedent-focused and response-focused emotion-regulating coping. It is composed of 23 behavioral descriptions of coping strategies and uses a 5-point Likert-type scale ranging from 1 (never) to 5 (very often).

Factor analysis was conducted on data from 2094 healthy Dutch employees, and four factors emerged, describing four different forms of humorous coping.

Antecedent-focused coping (QOHC-AF; 9 items) describes the attempt to reappraise a situation by using humorous behaviors. Example items:
"When technical problems interfere with my work, I concentrate on the funniness of the situation."
"A humorous perspective on things helps me to deal with pressure due to demands at work."
Response-focused coping (QOHC-RF; 4 items) refers to the ability to use humorous behavior in order to relieve, avoid or reduce pre-existing stress or negative feelings. Example items:
"When I encounter problems at work, I try to laugh away my worries."
"In uncomfortable situations I try to suppress my feelings by being witty."
Instrumental, aggressive/manipulative coping (QOHC-IAG; 7 items). Example items:
"When a colleague gets on my nerves, I use humor to get back at him or her."
"If I need a colleague to do something extra for me, I use humor to make him or her do it."
Instrumental, affiliative coping (QOHC-IAF; 3 items). Example items:
"Humor helps me to take a verbal confrontation with a colleague less seriously."
"When a colleague's behavior bothers me, I let him or her know by making an appropriate joke."

Internal consistency reliability was satisfactory, with Cronbach's alpha coefficients ranging from .73 (QOHC-IAF) to .82 (QOHC-AF); test-retest reliability for the total QOHC was assessed on a small sample (N = 20) after a 4- to 5-month interval, and seems to be promising (r = .71).

Criterion-related validity was assessed through analysis of correlations with other humor measures. All four QOHC subscales showed significant correlations with the MSHS and HSQ subscales: correlations with MSHS-HA ranged between .11 (QOCH-RF) and .16 (QOHC-

IAG), with MSHS-HC from .39 (QOCH-RF) to .47 (QOHC-IAG), and with MSHS-CH from .43 (QOCH-IAF) to .54 (QOCH-RF) ($p \le .001$).

Correlations with the HSQ-SE ranged from .30 (QOCH-IAG) to .58 (QOCH-AF) ($p < .001$), with HSQ-SD from .24 (QOCH-AF) to .45 (QOCH-IAG) ($p \le .001$), with HSQ-AF from .21 (QOCH-AF) to .30 (QOCH-IAF) ($p \le .05$), and with HSQ-AG from .24 (QOCH-AF) to .40 (QOCH-IAG) ($p \le .05$). The only no significant association was between the QOCH-RF and the HSQ-AF.

The QOCH-RF and QOCH-IAG subscales were also associated with the CHS, with correlations of .50 and .48, respectively ($p \le .001$).

Predictive validity of QOHC subscales for job-related satisfaction and affect was generally low (rs from .04 to .09, $p \le .05$). Nevertheless, positive correlations between antecedent-focused humorous coping and positive job-related affect and job well-being were slightly higher ($r = .16$, $p \le .001$), as were those between instrumental humorous coping (aggressive/manipulative type) and negative job-related affect ($r = .11$, $p \le .001$).

HUMOR STYLES

Humor Styles Questionnaire (HSQ)

The Humor Style Questionnaire (HSQ) [17] is a reliable, temporally stable and valid measure which can be used to assess humor styles in individuals from adolescence to old age. It was developed to assess four hypothesized styles of humor use and was validated on different samples, with a total sample size of 1195. The HSQ is made-up of 32 items rated on a 7-point Likert scale, ranging from 1 (totally disagree) to 7 (totally agree). The 8-item scales emerged from principal component and confirmatory factor analyses measure two relatively benign two potentially harmful uses of humor. The *Self-enhancing* and *Affiliative* scales evaluate the uses of humor to enhance the self and improve one's relationships with others, respectively, whereas the *Aggressive* and *Self-defeating* scales measure the uses of humor to enhance the self at the expense of others, and to improve one's relationships at the expense of self, respectively. Internal consistency coefficients (Cronbach's alpha) ranged from .77 (*Aggressive*) to .81 (*Self-enhancing*), and high test-retest reliability coefficients were obtained over a 1-week interval (N = 179). Peer ratings of humor styles significantly agreed with participants' self-reports on the four HSQ scales, indicating good convergent validity.

Self-enhancing humor scale (HSQ-SE) refers to the tendency to maintain a humorous outlook on life and use humor as a strategy for emotion regulation and coping, even while in solitude. It was positively correlated with optimism ($r = .32$, $p < .01$), satisfaction with social supports ($r = .30$, $p < .001$), and desirable masculinity (agency) ($r = .27$, $p < .001$), and negatively associated with undesirable femininity (unmitigated communion) ($r = -.36$, $p < .001$) and neuroticism ($r = -.37$, $p < .001$). Example items:

> "My humorous outlook on life keeps me from getting overly upset or depressed about things."
> "I don't need to be with other people to feel amused – I can usually find things to laugh about even when I'm by myself."

266   Giulia Casu and Paola Gremigni

Affiliative humor scale (SHQ-AF) describes the tendency to laugh with others and amuse others. It was positively related to social intimacy (r =, p < .001) and desirable femininity (communion) (r = .29, p < .001), and negatively related to seriousness (r = -.31, p < .001). Example items:

"I don't have to work very hard at making other people laugh – I seem to be a naturally humorous person."

"I laugh and joke a lot with my closest friends."

Aggressive humor scale (SHQ-AG) refers to the tendency to use humor to criticize or manipulate others, without considering its effects on others. Example items:

"When telling jokes or saying funny things, I am usually not very concerned about how other people are taking it."

"Sometimes I think of something that is so funny that I can't stop myself from saying it, even if it is not appropriate for the situation."

Self-defeating humor scale (SHQ-SD) includes items reflecting the tendency to use humor in an overly self-disparaging and ingratiating manner, or as a defense to hide potential negative feelings. It was positively related to depression (r = .24, p < .001), anxiety (r = .26, p < .001), bad mood (r = .28, p < .01) and psychiatric symptoms (r = .31, p < .001), and negatively related to self-esteem (r = -.36, p < .001), psychological well-being (r =,-.24, p < .05), social intimacy (r = -.15, p < .05) and satisfaction with social supports (r = -.21, p < .001). This scale was the only one to be affected by social desirability, as it significantly correlated with the Marlowe-Crowne Social Desirability Scale [5]. Example items:

"I let people laugh at me or make fun at my expense more than I should."

"When I am with friends or family, I often seem to be the one that other people make fun of or joke about."

The *Self-enhancing* and *Affiliative* humor scales are both positively related to cheerfulness (r = .55 and .65, respectively; p < .001), self-esteem (r = .28 and .21, respectively; p < .001), and psychological well-being (r = .46 and .26, respectively; p < .05), and negatively associated with depression (r = -.33 and -.22, respectively; p < .001), anxiety (r = -.40 and -.27, respectively; p < .001), and unpleasant mood (r = -.37 and -.33, respectively; p < .001). In addition, individuals with either a self-enhancing or an affiliative humor style show higher extraversion (r = .28 and .47, respectively; p < .001) and openness to experience (r = .27 and .23, respectively; p < .01). The SHQ-SE and SHQ-AF scales measure constructs that are similar to those assessed by other humor measures, as they correlated in the predicted way with the SHRQ, CHS, SHQ-6, MSHS, STCI-T, and the Humor coping scale of the Coping Orientations to Problems Experienced Scale (Brief-COPE) [47].

The *Aggressive* and *Self-defeating* humor scales are both positively related to aggression (rs = .41 and .28, respectively; p < .001), hostility (rs = .29 and .38, respectively; p < .001), undesirable masculinity (rs = .46 and .21, respectively; p < .01), and negatively associated with desirable femininity (rs = -.32 and -.21, respectively; p < .01). Individuals with either an aggressive or self-defeating humor style show higher neuroticism (rs = .21 and .35, respectively; p < .05) and lower agreeableness (rs = -.59 and -.23; p < .01) and conscientiousness (rs = -.37 and -.34, respectively; p < .001). Both scales describe potentially deleterious types of humor, which are no tapped by other humor scales, as they correlate with the MSHS only.

Humorous Behavior Q-Sort Deck (HBQD)

The Humorous Behavior Q-Sort Deck [27,28] was designed to provide a comprehensive portrait of individuals' humorous style, and can be used in quantifying how similar are pairs of individuals (such as marriage partners) with regard to humor styles. The tool consists of 100 non-redundant statements (e.g., "Has difficulty controlling the urge to laugh in solemn situations"), each describing a positive or negative aspect of humor-related behavior in everyday life contexts.

Respondents are asked to sort the Q sort cards into piles from 1 to 9, according to the extent to which each statement is considered characteristic of themselves or a target person with a high sense of humor. Subsequently, cards have to be sorted so that the distribution of statemenst is 5, 8, 12, 16, 18, 16, 12, 8, 5, in order to ensure the use of the full range of values.

Principal component analysis of self-descriptions from 456 college students identified five bipolar styles of humorous conduct: *socially warm vs. cold*, *reflective vs. boorish*, *competent vs. inept*, *earthy vs. repressed*, and *benign vs. mean-spirited* humor [27,28].

Socially warm humor describes the tendency to use humor in order to promote social interaction and good will. Example items:
   "Maintains group morale through humor."
   "Uses good-natured jests to put others at ease."
Socially cold humor expresses the avoidance of cheerful behaviors. Example items:
   "Smiles grudgingly."
   "Is a ready audience but infrequent contributor of humorous anecdotes."
Reflective humor reflects the ability to discern the spontaneous humor in the doings of oneself and others. Example items:
   "Takes pleasure in bemused reflections on self and others."
   "Appreciates the humorous potential of persons and situations."
Boorish humor describes an insensitive and competitive use of humor. Example items:
   "Is competitively humorous, attempts to top others."
   "Imitates the humorous style of professional comedians."
Competent humor describes the ability to create humorous anecdotes effectively. Example items:
   "Manifests humor in the form of clever retorts to others' remarks."
   "Enhances humorous impact with a deft sense of timing."
Inept humor is characterized by limited ability to deal with humor. Example items:
   "Reacts in an exaggerated way to mildly humorous comments."
   "Spoils jokes by laughing before finishing them."
Earthy humor defines the fun in joking about taboo topics. Example items:
   "Has a reputation for indulging in coarse or vulgar humor"
   "Tells bawdy stories with gusto, regardless of audience."
Repressed humor reveals an inhibition in producing and receiving this type of jokes. Example items:
   "Is the sort of person whose sense of humor changes when feeling less inhibited."
   "Does not respond to a range of humor due to moralistic constraints."

Benign humor expresses the pleasure in intellectually tough and inoffensive humor-related activities. Example items:

"Enjoys witticism which are intellectually challenging."

"Enjoys limericks and nonsense rhymes."

Mean-spirited humor describes the use of humor to attack and disparage others. Example items:

"Occasionally makes humorous remarks betraying a streak of cruelty."

"Needles others, intending it to be just kidding."

Correlations among the card sorts of participants, asked to describe a hypothetical funny person, revealed a high agreement with respect to how a high sense of humor is expressed [48]. Moreover, social desirability ratings revealed that behaviors expressing the socially warm and competent humor styles were socially desired [28].

Internal consistency coefficients ranged from .67 (*benign vs. mean-spirited* humorous behavior) to .83 (*socially warm vs. cold* humorous behavior) [27,28].

Overall, a sense of humor was positively associated with the socially warm and competent humorous styles, whereas it was unrelated to reflective, earthy, and benign humorous behaviors. Significant correlations emerged between the socially warm and boorish humor styles and extraversion, whereas the remaining three humor styles were unrelated to it [28]. Socially warm, competent, and benign humor styles were significantly associated with agreeableness, whereas an inept humor style was associated with neuroticism [48]. The five-factor structure of the HBQD did not emerge from a subsequent factor analysis conducted on the data from 60 HBQD statements rated on a 7-point Likert scale (from 1 = extremely uncharacteristic of me to 7 = extremely characteristic of me) (HBD-R) [49]. Nevertheless, using the HBQD in a self-report format seems questionable, since it was developed for being administered by a trained observer.

CONCLUSION

The construct of humor, as we have seen, has been conceptualized in a variety of ways by scholars.

Most questionnaires were designed to measure a global sense of humor (i.e., CHS, HO, MSHS, RHAI, SHQ, SHQZ, SHRQ, SHS, and STCI-T).

Some questionnaires (i.e., CHS, HO, RHAI SHRQ, STCI-T) measure humor as a uniform dimension, whereas other instruments (i.e., HBQD, MSHS, QOHC, RHI, SHQ, SHS, and SHQZ) assess different components of humor.

Some instruments address overall sense of humor as the extent to which individuals are used to laugh, smile, create and express humor in their lives. The SHRQ measures the tendency to maintain a humorous outlook on a wide range of life events, even those embarrassing or unpleasant. On the other hand, the SHQ (through its cognitive dimension, SHQ-MS) and the *Finding humor in everyday life* subscale of the 24-item SHS seem to be more specific, as they assess the ability to recognize humorous stimuli.

Within a sense of humor, some scholars distinguish between humor creation and humor appreciation.

Humor creation is usually regarded as the ability to create comic effects, and it can be assessed using the MSHS (MSHS-HC subscale), the SHQZ (SHQZ-HC subscale), the HO, and the RHAI. HO and RHAI can be slightly differentiated from MSHS and SHQZ, as they deal with humor creation from a more general approach, by focusing on the enactment of humorous communicative messages. Nevertheless, compared to the RHAI, the HO primarily focuses on verbal humor (described as joke and storytelling). Similarly, the *competent vs. inept* humor dimension of the HBQD, and the *Verbal humor* subscale of the 24-item SHS measure the tendency to create humor and tell funny stories.

Humor appreciation, as the ability to appreciate messages containing humor creativity, can be measured by using the MSHS (MSHS-HA subscale), the SHQZ (SHQZ-HA subscale), and the *reflective vs. boorish* dimension of the HBQD. Otherwise, appreciation of humorous people and situations is assessed by the SHQ (SHQ-LH subscale), whereas the personal value usually placed on humor is addressed by the *Enjoyment of humor* subscale of the 24-item SHS.

A sense of humor has been also conceptualized as a personality characteristic or an attitude: the STCI-T measures humor temperament, differentiating it from other traits, whereas humor appreciation is considered an attitude in the SHQ and MSHS.

The moderating effect of humor on stress and the usefulness of humor in promoting effective coping and quality of life emerged in various studies [4,50,51]. The tendency to use humor as a coping strategy is assessed by some measures: the CHS, the MSHS (through its MSHS-CH subscale), the 24-item SHS (through its *Humor under stress* subscale), the RHI (through its *Instrumental* subscale), and the QOHC. Such instruments (or subscales) measure the extent to which humor is used to deal with stressful life situations. Differently from other instruments, the RHI assesses the use of humor coping to avoid marital tensions, or reduce negative feelings within marriage relationships. Similarly, the QOCH measures humor use to deal with work-related demands.

Different humor styles have received relatively little attention in the questionnaire literature; thus, they are assessed by the HBQD and HSQD only.

Most humor measures focus exclusively on positive aspects of humor. For example, the CHS addresses humor uniquely as a productive and effective coping mechanism. Similarly, the MSHS (MSHS-HC subscale) and SHQ (SHQ-LH subscale) assess the positive, facilitative effects of sense of humor on social interactions. Nevertheless, distinguishing between deleterious and benign uses of humor is essential. Potentially damaging uses of humor are assessed by few scales, such as the RHI (*Negative humor* subscale), the QOCH (*Instrumental, aggressive/manipulative type* subscale), the HSQ (*Aggressive* and *Self-defeating* humor styles), and the *reflective vs. boorish* and *benign vs. mean-spirited* humor dimensions of the HSQD.

Finally, the ability to laugh at oneself is also considered an essential component of sense of humor. Nevertheless, it is assessed by the 24-item SHS only, through its *Laugh at yourself* scale. This use of humor is also addressed by the HSQ, yet is included as an expression of the self-defeating humor style.

In conclusion, researchers can choose from a variety of tools with acceptable psychometric properties to measure self-reported humor. Instrument choice should be guided by several considerations, including the goal of the study and the operationalization adopted for humor.

The present chapter is not exhaustive, as many other self-report instruments for measuring humor are currently available. We made a selection based on the availability of the validation study in the literature. Researchers also often use ad hoc tools, without reporting the psychometric properties clearly.

For detailed descriptions of questionnaire construction, item generation and characteristics of samples used in the validation process of the questionnaires described in this chapter, readers should refer to the validation studies (see references).

REFERENCES

[1]   Ruch, W. (1998). Appendix: Humor measurement tools. In W. Ruch (Ed.). *The Sense of Humor: Explorations of a Personality Characteristic* (pp. 405–412). Berlin: Mouton de Gruyter.

[2]   Martin, R. A., & Lefcourt, H. M. (1984). The Situational Humour Response Questionnaire: Quantitative measure of sense of humor. *Journal of Personality and Social Psychology, 47*, 145-155.

[3]   Martin, R., & Lefcourt, H. (1983). Sense of humor as a moderator of the relation between stressors and mood. *Journal of Personality and Social Psychology*, *45*, 1313–1324.

[4]   Martin, R. A. (1996). The Situational Humor Response Questionnaire (SHRQ) and Coping Humor Scale (CHS): A decade of research findings. *Humor: International Journal of Humor Research*, *9*, 251–272.

[5]   Crowne, D. P., & Marlowe, D. (1960). A new scale of social desirability independent of psychopathology. *Journal of Consulting Psychology*, *24*, 349–354.

[6]   Ruch, W., & Deckers, L. (1993). Do extraverts "like to laugh": An analysis of the Situational Humor Response Questionnaire (SHRQ). *European Journal of Personality*, *7*, 211-220.

[7]   Eysenck, S. B.., Eysenck, H. J., & Barrett, P. (1985). A revised version of the psychoticism scale. *Personality and Individual Differences*, *6*, 21-29.

[8]   Martin, R. A., & Kuiper, N. A.(1999). Daily occurrence of laughter: Relationships with age, gender, and Type A personality. *Humor: International Journal of Humor Research, 12*, 355–384.

[9]   Deaner, S. L., & McConatha, J. T. (1993). The relation of humor to depression and personality. *Psychological Reports, 72, 755*-763.

[10]   Svebak, S. (1974). Three attitude dimensions of sense of humor as predictors of laughter. *Scandinavian Journal of Psychology, 15*, 185-190.

[11]   Ruch, W. (1994). Temperament, Eysenck's PEN system, and humor-related traits. *Humor: International Journal of Humor Research*, *7*, 209-244.

[12]   Cann, A., Holt, K., & Calhoun, L. G. (1999). The roles of humor and sense of humor in responses to stressors. *Humor: International Journal of Humor Research, 12*, 177-193.

[13]   Thorson, J. A., & Powell, F. C. (1993). Development and validation of a multidimensional sense of humor scale. *Journal of Clinical Psychology, 48*, 13–23.

[14]   Bell, N. J., McGhee, P. E., & Duffey, N. S. (1986). Interpersonal competence, social assertiveness, and the development of humor. *British Journal of Developmental Psychology*, 4, 51-55.

[15]   Köhler, G., & Ruch, W. (1996). Sources of variance in current sense of humor inventories: How much substance, how much method variance? *Humor: International Journal of Humor Research*, 9, 363–397.

[16]   Ziv, A. (1981) The self-concept of adolescent humorists. *Journal of Adolescence*, 4, 187-197.

[17]   Martin, R. A., Puhlik-Doris, P., Larsen, G., Gray, J., & Weir, K. (2003). Individual differences in uses of humor and their relation to psychological well-being: Development of the Humor Styles Questionnaire. *Journal of Research in Personality*, 37, 48-75.

[18]   Kuiper, N. A., & Martin, R. A. (1998). Is sense of humor a positive personality characteristic? In W. Ruch (Ed.). *The Sense of Humor: Explorations of a Personality Characteristic* (pp. 159-178). Berlin: Mouton de Gruyter.

[19]   Thorson, J. A., & Powell, F. C. (1991). Measurement of sense of humor. *Psychological Reports, 69,* 691-702.

[20]   Deckers, L., & Ruch, W. (1992). The Situational Humor response Questionnaire as a test of "sense of humor": A validity study in the field of humor appreciation. *Personality and Individual Differences*, 13, 1149-1152.

[21]   Lefcourt, H. M., & Martin, R. A. (1986). *Humor and Life Stress: Antidote to Adversity*. New York: Springer.

[22]   Svebak, S. (1996). The development of the Sense of Humor Questionnaire: From SHQ to SHQ-6. *Humor: International Journal of Humor Research*, 9, 341-361.

[23]   McGhee, P. E. (1996). *The laughter remedy. Health, Healing and the Amuse System: Humor as Survival Training*. Dubuque, IA: Kendall/Hunt.

[24]   McGhee, P. E. (2010). *Humor as Survival Training for a Stresses-out World: The 7 Humor Habits Program*. Bloomington, IN: Authorhouse.

[25]   Ruch, W., & Carrell, A. (1998). Trait cheerfulness and the sense of humor. *Personality and Individual Differences*, 24, 551-558.

[26]   Ruch, W., Proyer, R. T., Esser, C., & Mitrache, O. (2011). Cheerfulness and everyday humorous conduct. In Romanian Academy, *Yearbook of the 'George Baritiu' Institute of History in Cluj-Napoca* (Ed.), Series Humanistica (Vol. IX, pp. 67-87).

[27]   Craik, K. H., Lampert, M. D., & Nelson, A. J. (1993). *Research Manual for the Humorous Behavior Q-sort Deck*. Berkeley, CA: University of California, Institute of Personality and Social Research.

[28]   Craik, K. H., Lampert, M. D., & Nelson, A. J. (1996). Sense of humor and styles of everyday humorous conduct. *Humor: International Journal of Humor Research*, 9, 273–302.

[29]   Wrench, J. S., & McCroskey, J. C. (2001). A temperamental understanding of humor communication and exhilaratability. *Communication Quarterly, 49,* 170-183.

[30]   Ruch, W., Köhler, G., & van Thriel, C. (1996). Assessing the "humorous temperament": Construction of the facet and standard trait forms of the State-Trait-Cheerfulness-Inventory — STCI. *Humor: International Journal of Humor Research*, 9, 303-339.

[31] Ruch, W., & Kohler, G. (1998). A temperament approach to humor. In W. Ruch (Ed.). *The Sense of Humor: Explorations of a Personality Characteristic* (pp. 203–230). Berlin: Mouton de Gruyter.

[32] Cann, A., & Etzel, K. C. (2008). Remembering and anticipating stressors: Positive personality mediates the relationship with sense of humor. *Humor: International Journal of Humor Research, 21*, 157-178.

[33] Levy, D. A. (1985). Optimism and pessimism: Relationships to circadian rhythms. *Psychological Reports, 57,* 1123-1126.

[34] Franken, R. E., Gibson, K. J., & Rowland, G. L. (1992). Sensation seeking and the tendency to view the world as threatening. *Personality and Individual Differences, 13,* 31-38.

[35] Thorson, J. A., & Powell, F. C. (1994). Depression and sense of humor. *Psychological Reports, 75,* 1473-1474.

[36] Thorson, J. A., & Powell, E. C. (1997). Psychological health and sense of humor. *Journal of Clinical Psychology, 53,* 605-619.

[37] Booth-Butterfield, S., & Booth-Butterfield, M. (1991). Individual differences in the communication of humorous messages. *The Southern Communication Journal, 56,* 205-218.

[38] Richmond, V. P., Wrench, J. S., & Gorham, J. (2001). *Communication, Affect, and Learning in the Classroom.* Acton, MA: Tapestry Press.

[39] Talbot, L. A., & Lumden, D. B. (2000). On the association between humor and burnout. *Humor: International Journal of Humor Research, 13*, 419-428.

[40] Overholser, J. (1992). Sense of humor when coping with life stress. *Personality and Individual Differences, 13*, 799–804.

[41] Nezlek, J. B., & Derks, P. (2001). Use of humor as a coping mechanism, psychological adjustment, and social interaction. *Humor: International Journal of Humor Research, 14*, 395–413.

[42] Kuiper, N. A., Martin, R. A., & Dance, K. (1992). Sense of humor and enhanced quality of life. *Personality and Individual Differences, 13*, 1273–1283.

[43] Kuiper, N. A., & Martin, R. A. (1993). Humor and self-concept. *Humor: International Journal of Humor Research, 6*, 251–270.

[44] De Koning, E., & Weiss, R. L. (2002). The relational Humor Inventory: Functions of humor in close relationships. *The American Journal of Family Therapy, 30*, 1-18.

[45] Doosje, S., De Goede, M. P. M., Van Doornen, L. P. J., & Goldstein, J. H. (2010). Measurement of occupational humorous coping. *Humor: International Journal of Humor Research, 23*, 273–305.

[46] Gross, J. J. (2001). Emotion regulation in adulthood: Timing is everything. *Current Directions in Psychological Science, 10*, 214–219.

[47] Carver, C. (1997). You want to measure coping but your protocol's too long: Consider the Brief COPE. *International Journal of Behavioral Medicine, 4*, 92-100.

[48] Craik, K., & Ware, A. (1998). Humor and personality in everyday life. In W. Ruch (Ed.). *The Sense of Humor: Explorations of a Personality Characteristic* (pp. 63-94). Berlin: Mouton de Gruyter.

[49] Kirsh, G. A., & Kuiper, N. A. (2003). Positive and negative aspects of humor: Associations with the constructs of individualism and relatedness. *Humor: International Journal of Humor Research, 16*, 33–62.

[50] Kuiper, N. A., & Olinger, L. J. (1998). Humor and mental health. In H. S. Freedman (Ed.). *Encyclopedia of Mental Health*, vol. 2 (pp. 445-457). San Diego: Academic Press.

[51] Martin, R. A. (2001). Humor, laughter, and physical health: Methodological issues and research findings. *Psychological Bulletin, 127*, 504–519.

INDEX

one dimension, 84
openness to experience, 266
opioids, 156
opportunities, 202
optimism, 9, 104, 105, 112, 151, 156, 160, 161, 164,
    165, 175, 178, 192, 200, 260, 265
organ, 174
organism, 116
organize, 221
organs, 17
originality, 143
outpatient, 217
overlap, 34, 35, 37, 38, 63, 96, 98, 192, 234
oxygen, 93, 154

P

pain, 22, 48, 98, 99, 100, 101, 111, 149, 150, 151,
    153, 155, 156, 157, 158, 160, 164, 166, 168, 175,
    184, 194, 216, 217, 232, 260
pain management, 158
pain perception, 99, 156, 168
pain tolerance, 99, 100, 111, 152, 156, 157, 158,
    168, 217
panic attack, 238
parallel, 5
paranoid schizophrenia, 243
parenthood, 140
parents, 4, 9, 91, 138, 142, 146, 157, 216, 217, 224,
    225, 226, 239
participants, 32, 37, 89, 90, 93, 94, 95, 100, 103,
    104, 110, 125, 155, 156, 162, 163, 178, 179, 201,
    204, 230, 235, 240, 246, 254, 261, 262, 263, 265,
    268
pathogenesis, 181
pathology, 2, 3, 198, 223
pathways, 106
peer group, 180
peer relationship, 180, 187
peptides, 157
perceived health, 149
performers, 218, 219
peripheral blood, 162
permission, 220, 233
perseverance, 9
personal development, 176
personal efficacy, 186, 249
personal qualities, 180
personal relations, 180
personal relationship, 180
personality, 1, 2, 4, 6, 7, 9, 10, 12, 13, 41, 42, 79, 80,
    83, 84, 89, 95, 104, 111, 112, 150, 156, 160, 161,
    164, 165, 169, 171, 173, 175, 178, 179, 181, 183,

    184, 185, 186, 187, 188, 191, 193, 195, 208, 221,
    241, 243, 251, 253, 269, 270, 271, 272
personality characteristics, 175, 178
personality differences, 1
personality disorder, 195, 243
personality traits, 6, 80, 95, 156, 161, 164, 171, 178,
    181
pessimism, 87, 272
phenomenology, 45
Philadelphia, 43, 56, 74, 210
phobia, 199, 201, 236, 237, 238, 239, 248
phobic anxiety, 181
phonology, 33
photographs, 94, 95, 165, 171, 240, 242
physical activity, 151, 153, 163
physical aggression, 24, 112
physical health, 4, 9, 14, 149, 150, 151, 152, 153,
    155, 158, 159, 164, 165, 166, 168, 169, 173, 174,
    175, 176, 181, 184, 185, 186, 191, 208, 213, 222,
    225, 273
physical well-being, 167, 188
physicians, 215, 217, 219
Physiological, 47, 83, 108, 167
physiological arousal, 10
physiology, 40, 107, 130, 192
pilot study, 168, 181, 187
pitch, 47
placebo, 93, 157
Plato, 15, 16, 22, 206
plausibility, 15
playing, 37, 59, 70, 71, 73, 114, 115, 118, 121, 142,
    216
pleasure, 8, 17, 18, 19, 20, 22, 23, 27, 39, 49, 51, 54,
    98, 101, 102, 106, 114, 116, 120, 143, 180, 214,
    230, 245, 267, 268
Poland, 107, 236, 237, 251
polar, 231
police, 72, 164, 200
politeness, 124
population, 165, 168, 171, 230, 236, 241, 243, 248
positive attitudes, 192
positive correlation, 85, 137, 161, 178, 180, 255,
    257, 260, 261, 262, 265
positive emotions, 5, 9, 94, 95, 166, 174, 175, 178,
    182, 189, 216, 232, 260
positive mental health, 175, 178
positive mood, 11, 80, 95, 97, 101, 102, 103, 174,
    176, 181, 242, 254, 256, 257
positive reinforcement, 231
positive relationship, 88, 101, 143, 145
potato, 139
potential benefits, 173, 175, 183, 208
predictive validity, 263